Women Healers
of the World

Other Books by the Author

The Essential Herbal for Natural Health:
How to Transform Easy-to-Find Herbs into Healing Remedies for the Whole Family

The Authentic Herbal Healer:
The Complete Guide to Herbal Formulary & Plant-Inspired Medicine for Every Body System

How to Use Herbs for Natural Health Audio CD Series

Women Healers of the World

The Traditions, History, and Geography of Herbal Medicine

Holly Bellebuono

Holly Bellebuono

Foreword by Rosemary Gladstar

Watercolor Art by Tracy Thorpe

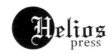

Helios press

Helios Press books may be purchased in bulk at special discounts for sales promotion, corporate gifts, fund-raising, or educational purposes. Special editions can also be created to specifications. For details, contact the Special Sales Department, Helios Press, 307 West 36th Street, 11th Floor, New York, NY 10018 or info@skyhorsepublishing.com.

Helios® and Helios Press® are registered trademarks of Skyhorse Publishing, Inc.®, a Delaware corporation.

www.skyhorsepublishing.com

10 9 8 7 6 5 4 3 2 1

Library of Congress Cataloging-in-Publication Data is available on file.

Cover design by Brian Peterson
Cover photographs provided by Holly Bellebuono, Harry Beach, Ian White, and Lillian Chang
Map and timeline designed by Nicholas Grant

Print ISBN: 978-1-62914-589-1
Ebook ISBN: 978-1-63220-194-2

Printed in China

Dedication

This book is lovingly dedicated to my mom, Carla S. Horton, RN, who set the bar high as a nurse for forty-four years and continues to be a source of strength, generosity, and creativity

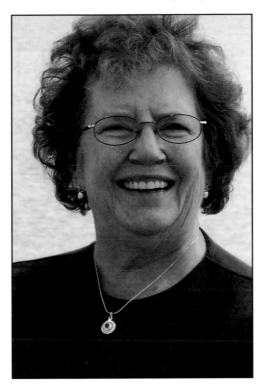

... and to the following women who participated in the creation of this book but passed away before its completion; I am honored to introduce these women who shared their transcendent passion and inspiring talent with us all. Because of their perseverance and work, we have an incredible world heritage of healing.

Because of the people in this book, we have herbalism.

For
Raylene Ha'alelea Kawaiae'a
Mary Beith
Cascade Anderson Geller
Mama Kia Ingenlath
Juliette de Bairacli Levy

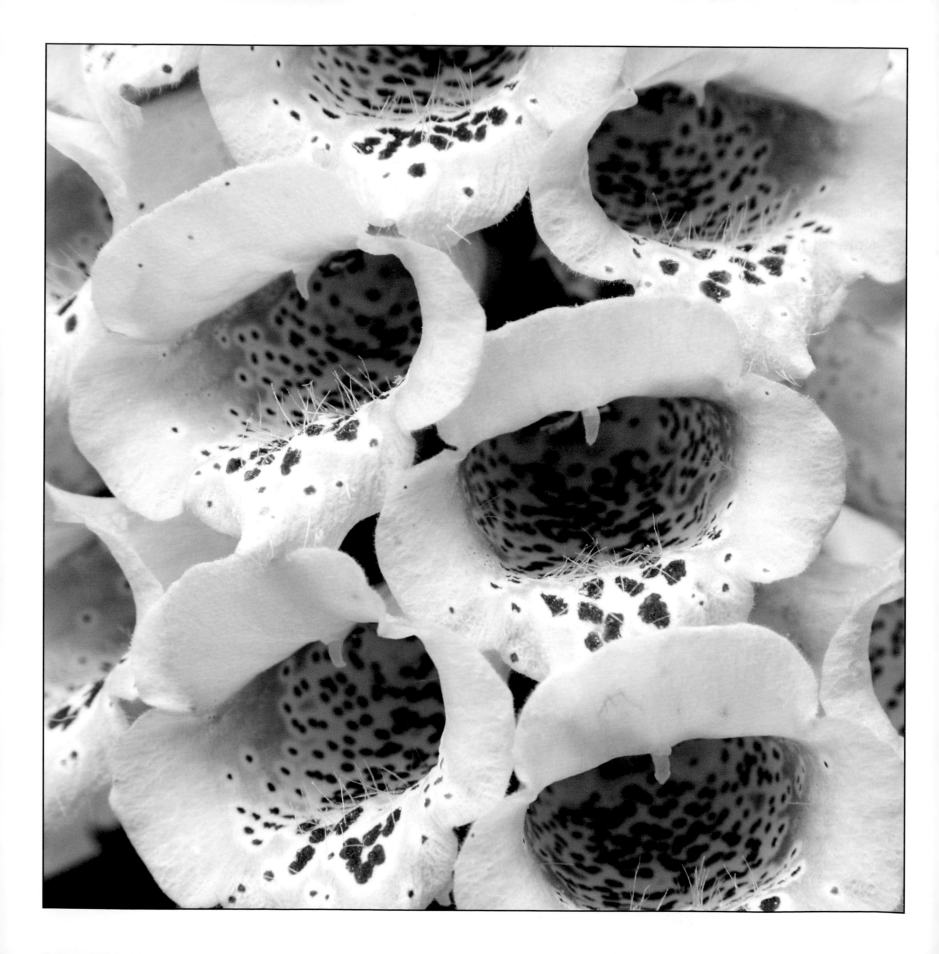

Table of Contents

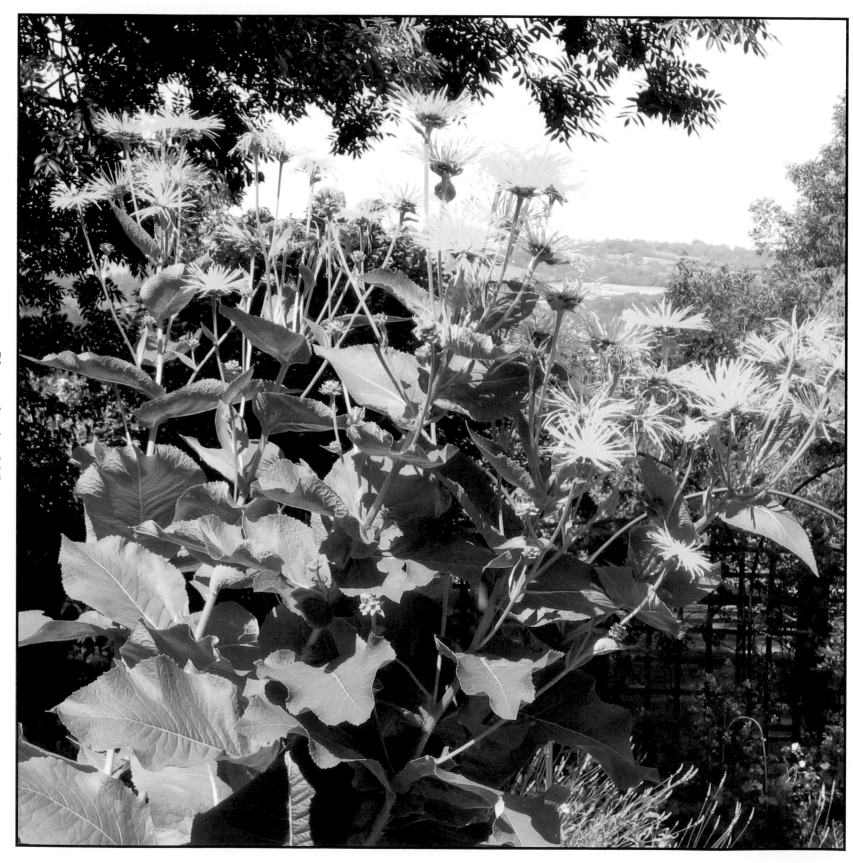

x

Foreword

"While herbalism can lend itself to encyclopedic lists of herbs and their actions, it's also rich in heritage and the stories of people. Herbalism can be the launching pad from which great people create themselves."
—Holly Bellebuono, from *The Authentic Healer*

When Holly first shared her vision with me to create a documentary on our herbal heritage by interviewing and recording the stories of women healers from around the world, I was intrigued and supportive from the start. The project sounded exciting and grand—to travel the world, interviewing, recording, and photographing the remarkable stories of women herbalists and to create a slide documentation to preserve these stories for future generations. If anyone could do this project well—and with flair—Holly could! And, of course, she did; she not only created a memorable slide presentation that has been highlighted at numerous gatherings throughout the country, but also created this beautiful and brilliant book that documents and preserves the lively stories of women healers and the rich feminine her-story of herbalism (or, her-balism).

And what a treasure this book is! Visually stunning, *Women Healers of the World* is filled with colorful photographs of herbs and the lovely, wild-hearted women who favored them; it also contains beautiful paintings, renditions of influential women healers who lived long before the advent of tape recorders or cameras. But more than just another lovely "coffee table book" to be displayed for its appealing layout, this book invites us to delve deeply into the mystery and power of herbal healing and its importance in our global history, both past and present. Holly thoughtfully includes enriching insights about the countries and geography in which each healer lives, interesting and unusual facts about the plants, herbal healing, and global herbalism.

There is much to learn here.

But at the core of this book, its essence and heartbeat, are the remarkable stories of women healers. As diverse as the pioneering spirits of Tulsi La Brun and Inez White from outback Australia to

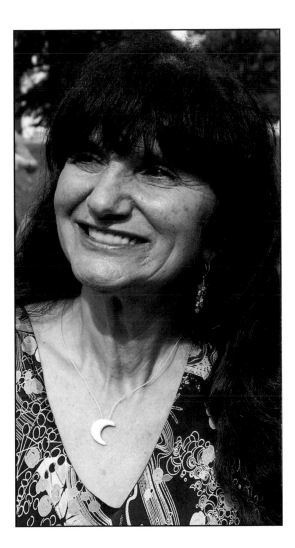

Zoubida Charrouf, the celebrated expert on Argan oil and champion of women's rights in Morocco, to the wise, gentle Polynesian elder, Auntie Velma DelaPena, who carries on the traditions of the ancient Kahunas on the island of Hawai'i, each story is inspiring, each woman empowering; the herbs weave the stories together as Holly navigates us on a journey around the world, through time, to the present.

As different and unique as each woman's story is, the central themes are similar; each woman's desire to serve humanity, to heal, their love of plants, their sense of purpose. But Holly captures something else unique, but similar, that's core to each of the storytellers and brings it to light: *the value of mentoring* and *confidence in healing*. These two principles are, I feel, the essential messages Holly brings forth through these women healers and their stories.

"*We need to take seriously our long-term influence on the children in our lives and understand that we have the power to change the future*" and "*The captain—the herbalist, the wise woman—charts the course, tests the waters, stands at the helm with confidence.*" Like adages to be remembered, she plants these thoughts firmly as though they are seeds in our hearts to be nourished, and then moves on to the next chapter . . . her next project, a new vision, navigating onward.

Holly was the perfect visionary for creating such a profoundly moving work. A dedicated and impassioned herbalist, she is well known in the herbal community for her generous teaching style, informative books, and her popular online course. For more than eighteen years, Holly has practiced her herbal craft in the small village of Martha's Vineyard, but her teachings are wide spread. A well-known presenter at herb events across the country, Holly's slide presentation, *Our Healing Heritage: Celebrating World Medicine and Women Healers* has been featured at several conferences and events. Back home in her apothecary garden on Martha's Vineyard, Holly grows, gathers, and makes herbal medicine for her community—and beyond. Like many of the woman healers she interviews, Holly was mentored by several older herbalists and is now passing her knowledge and love of plants to her own children and the children of her community. In fact, Holly *is* one of the wise women healers she writes about in this book . . . one of those who knows the *value of mentoring* and has attained *confidence in healing*. One day, someone else, perhaps one of those young herbalists she's been mentoring, will be writing Holly's personal herbal story, preserving it so that the long continuum of our herbal traditions and the stories that give them spark and bring them alive will continue on for future generations of plant lovers, healers, and green enthusiasts.

In Joy,

Rosemary Gladstar
Herbalist & Author
Sage Mountain, Vermont

"*The most beautiful experience of my life, the most enriching, is the love that the plants have taught me. To love one's neighbor is to care for them, to attend to their suffering and restore their joy of living.*"
— Bernadette Rébiénot, Gabon, Africa

A Note from the Author

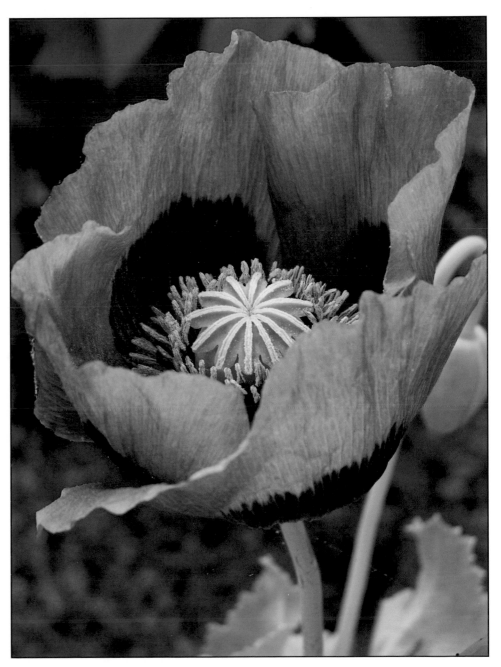

Instead of a dull encyclopedia, within these pages you'll find the stories of lively and passionate women from the far corners of our world who make plant medicine their life's purpose. They've given our generation a great gift, continuing a long and crucial heritage of botanical healing that relieves suffering and inspires ever-greater understanding.

The book's four primary parts (Plant, Body, Spirit, and Land Traditions) zero in on the subtle differences between the various methods of botanical medicine as they are practiced today, though the women listed in each category can (and often do) represent other methods. These categories are rather fluid, as the healers demonstrate their ability and interest to use other methods than simply the category into which I've placed them. For example, Dr. Zoubida Charrouf is profiled in "pharmacology," but she could easily be studied under "conservation," since she is a leader in the preservation of her country's native argan tree. Susun Weed is profiled in "spirit," but she is a strong ambassador for western herbalism, and Doña Enriqueta Contreras is a midwife but is also a self-professed shaman. Healing is, by its very nature, a multi-disciplinary approach to the body, mind, and spirit, and this book, in addition to celebrating individual healing arts, confirms the wisdom of working cross-culturally, honoring a rich array of heritages, and practicing what—in every sense of the word—is integrated medicine.

At the end of the book, you'll find a list of organizations, non-profits, and resources with which some of these women are associated. Thank you for supporting their ongoing work.

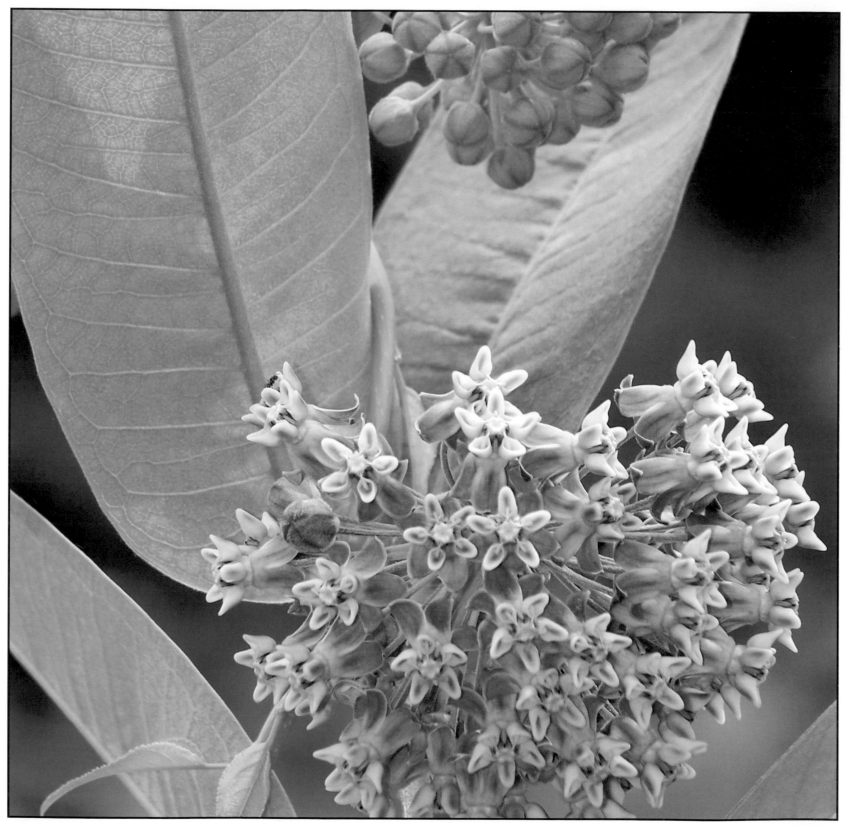

Milkweed

Introduction

For seven years, I've had the privilege of immersing myself in the world of international women who are deeply involved with healing herbs. As an herbalist (and someone bitten by the travel bug), interviewing international women for this book was an incredibly exciting time for me. Once I began calling and writing to these women, requesting interviews and sharing my ideas for the project, things happened quicker that I could have imagined: first, I interviewed several amazing herbalists in America: Rosemary, Tieraona, Susun, and Kate. Word spread about my project, and people offered the names of remarkable women I'd never heard of: Mama Kia, Doña Enriqueta, Zoubida Charrouf. Healers in Peru and England, then Australia, New Zealand, Tibet, China, Polynesia . . . When I realized how deeply these women influence the way we heal today and how they continue their culture's traditions, I knew they were important *Women Healers of the World*.

You may recognize some of these women, and others may be new to you. These are the proverbial Wise Women you've heard stories about, the legendary history makers as well as the obscure women with no names. But these women do have names—and faces and hands and hearts, and their hard work and diligence is the momentum behind our entire heritage of integrative or "alternative" medicine from which countries around the world continue to draw care and sustenance on a daily basis. This is a vast healing heritage, encompassing many global traditions, and these women—and the women who came before them—influence a wide range of effective, lucrative, and popular healing arts, from acupuncture to yoga and everything in between.

One of the most frequent questions I've received about this project is: "Is there one thing all these women have in common?" People are interested in the similarities of humanity, in the little things that make us better people and that help us understand one another. It's a way we can learn about the greater world and also reach a higher understanding of ourselves. What do we like? How do we act? Do others react the way I do? Do they deal with stress or happiness the same way I do? Is herbalism the same around the world? Is love?

Of course, the women in this book have many similarities: they are all remarkable, hard-working, kindhearted women who pursue their life's passion with drive and a sense of purpose. They are working to help other people. And they all work with plants as healers, gardeners, researchers, or conservationists; their work with plants is somehow central to their life's work. For me, this is key, as I wanted to explore and document how herbalism can become a part of women's lives in countries the world over.

But there were two intriguing similarities that all these women shared:

The Value of Mentoring

The first is that nearly all these women had been influenced—even mentored—in the healing arts or in working with plants as children by their older relatives. Many of the women I interviewed were taught healing directly from their own mothers and grandmothers. Imagine, these women—such as Rosemary Gladstar, Ada-Belinda DancingLion, Bernadette Rébiénot—began a lifelong journey of healing and connection because their mothers and grandmothers inspired and taught them. The family connection is strong, it seems, in the heritage of herbal healing. HRH Princess Basma bint Ali learned and was encouraged to pursue botany by her father; Dr. Lillian Chang received the knowledge from many generations in her family—sixty-four, to be exact; Cascade Anderson Geller continued the herbal wisdom learned from her grandmother; and Dr. Phuntsog Wangmo studied with her aunt and older brother the ancient Tibetan medical practices that she now fervently shares with the world.

Each of us has a rich opportunity to share our knowledge and life history with the young ones near us. We have the chance to profoundly influence a child's life simply by being with her and opening doors of opportunity that set a spark in her mind.

We need to take seriously our long-term influence on the children in our lives and understand that we have the power to change the future. The women healers in this book are changing the world as a result of the encouragement and support they received from their (often maternal) mentors. The sciences of environmentalism, ethnobotany, ecology, and modern medicine would do well to nurture this profound (and often overlooked) influence.

Confidence in Healing

The second similarity that struck me as I put together these interviews was something I had not considered and was surprised to see. I had always been under the impression that healing—true healing—was a kind, sweet, compassionate, gentle thing—a nourishing thing, something that was done slowly and over time and with great care.

And it certainly is that. Many of the women I spoke with are soft-spoken, immensely compassionate people who are true healers and are accomplishing a nourishment of the world's soul that is long overdue and immeasurably needed. These are the solace-givers, the tea makers, the dream-weavers. We need them, and I thank them.

But I also came across healers who worked from the opposite direction: instead of talking softly, they speak loudly, fiercely even—from the heart but with a powerful punch. People such as Susun Weed, Doña Enriqueta Contreras, and other shamans I met on my journey but were not included in this book, such as Levon Ohai, pitch their voices into the tumult and demand results. They do not back down from political pressures that have burdened healers for millennia; they do not flinch when faced with the mystery of death or the fear of failure. They teach that under no circumstances can you be a true healer if you do not have one very important thing: confidence in yourself.

Of course, I said to them, everyone in the "healing profession" is more or less confident. Doctors and nurses are schooled to be confident.

But no, these people taught me. What does it mean to truly believe in yourself as a healer, beyond the shadow of a doubt? Traditional Hawai'ian kahuna and shaman Levon Ohai told me that the healing arts require a measure of confidence above and beyond other arts. "Are you sure of your mixtures?" he asked. "Will this mixture you gave me heal me? Yes, I say, it will. It's knowledge with Spirit (*Akua*). Make no mistakes. The objective," he clarified, "is to save a life. Not to build a bridge or a house. We are not carpenters or engineers. We are healers. *We save lives*. It takes an extra effort to know how to save a life from disease. You have to be sure. How sure are you?" He pinned me with a penetrating stare. "Sure enough to put your life on it?"

Zapotecan elder Doña Enriqueta Contreras agreed, saying this is an indigenous philosophy, this practice of surety, confidence, and inner faith. Of not guessing but working until you are completely certain before you enter medical practice. "Before you even enter the camp, before you even walk in, you must have a huge discussion with yourself," she told me. "You must evaluate yourself, and where your light is. You must have a light inside of you, and ask yourself: is it secure, are you confident in yourself as a healer? If you're not, and you give a recommendation and say, '*Maybe* it will help,' are you translating confidence or doubt?"

Healers are Navigators

This strength of character is shared by all the women in this book, whose voices can murmur and then bellow in a single sentence, who can instill in others that effervescent quality of understanding without which none of us would pursue the next creative act. Most of all, all the great herbalists—ancient and contemporary—seem to teach us how to *navigate* our courses through life. The captain of a ship does not navigate by guessing or by assuming someone else will take the wheel when the waters get rough. The captain—the herbalist, the wise woman—charts the course, tests the waters, and stands at the helm with confidence.

If we are willing to learn these lessons, we can become the leaders and healers that will nurture our traditions and safeguard them for our children and future generations. It was only because this knowledge was nurtured and protected by our ancestors such as Hatshepsut, Mary Prophetissa, Trotula of Salerno, and Marie-Henriette LeJeune-Ross that these traditions still exist. And it will be thanks to today's wise women such as Auntie Velma DelaPena,

Anne McIntyre, Isla Burgess, Jody Noé, Mary Beith, Dr. Chang Yi Hsiang, Dr. Tieraona Low Dog, and all the other women in this book that our grandchildren will have this same access to knowledge when they are ready to take the wheel and guide their ships to safe harbor.

In these pages, we will traverse the myriad landscape of world healing traditions, exploring the immense variety of customs and colors with which botanical medicine tinctures our world. We'll delight in global geography, etymology and world culture. But above all, we will celebrate these extraordinary women herbalists—and it is my hope that within these pages you will find heroes as well as friends.

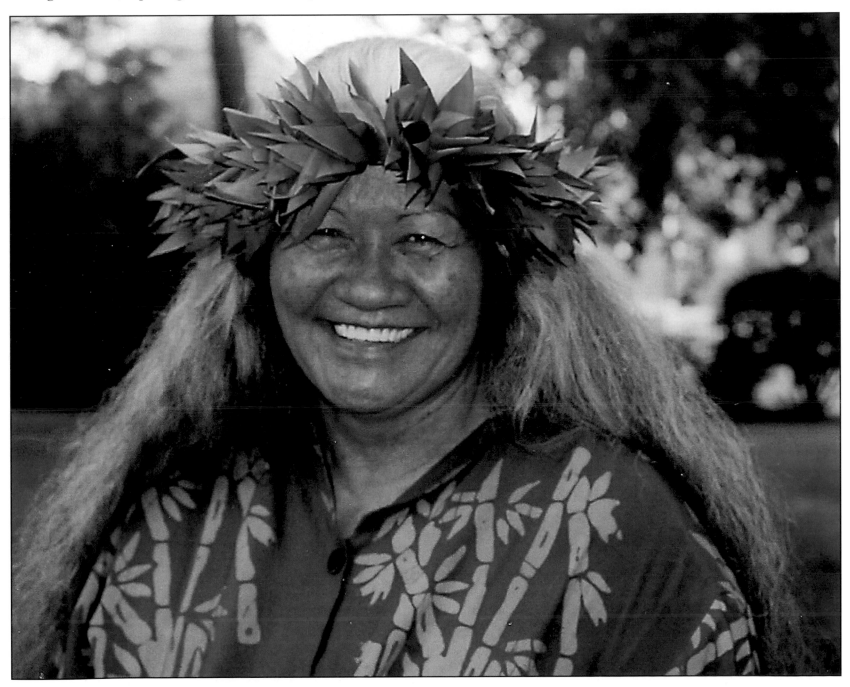

Beloved Hawai'ian kahuna Raylene Kawaiae'a.

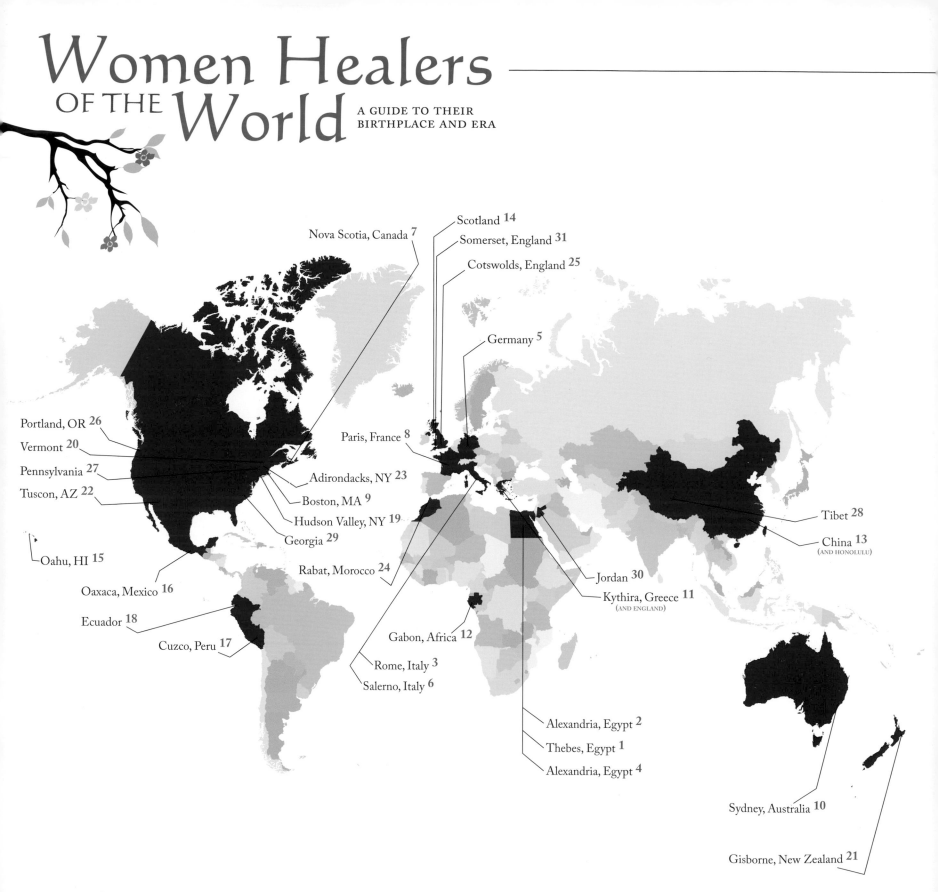

Women Healers
OF THE World
A GUIDE TO THEIR BIRTHPLACE AND ERA

Nova Scotia, Canada **7**

Scotland **14**

Somerset, England **31**

Cotswolds, England **25**

Germany **5**

Paris, France **8**

Portland, OR **26**

Vermont **20**

Pennsylvania **27**

Tuscon, AZ **22**

Adirondacks, NY **23**

Boston, MA **9**

Hudson Valley, NY **19**

Georgia **29**

Oahu, HI **15**

Oaxaca, Mexico **16**

Ecuador **18**

Cuzco, Peru **17**

Rabat, Morocco **24**

Gabon, Africa **12**

Rome, Italy **3**

Salerno, Italy **6**

Jordan **30**

Kythira, Greece **11**
(AND ENGLAND)

Tibet **28**

China **13**
(AND HONOLULU)

Alexandria, Egypt **2**

Thebes, Egypt **1**

Alexandria, Egypt **4**

Sydney, Australia **10**

Gisborne, New Zealand **21**

1	2	3	4	5	6	7	8
1508 – 1458 BCE	69 BCE – 30 BCE	? – 69 CE	c. 200 CE	1098 – 1179	c. 1200	1762 – 1860	1763 – 1814
Hatshepsut	Cleopatra	Locusta of Gaul	Mary Prophetissa	Hildegard von Bingen	Trotula of Salerno	Marie-Henriette LeJeune-Ross	Empress Josephine

9	10	11	12	13	14	15	16
1821 – 1910	1896 – 1966	1912 – 2009	1934	est. 1936	1938 – 2012	1939	1939
Mary Baker Eddy	Inez White	Juliette de Bairacli Levy	Bernadette Rebienot	Chang Yi Hsiang	Mary Beith	Auntie Velma Dela Pena	Dona Enriqueta Contreras

17	18	19	20	21	22	23	24
1949 – 2010	est. 1940	1945	1948	1949	est. 1950	1951	1952
Kia Ingenlath	Rocio Alarcon	Susun Weed	Rosemary Gladstar	Isla Burgess	Dr. Tieraona Low Dog	Kate Gilday	Zoubida Charrouf

25	26	27	28	29	30	31
1953	1954 – 2013	1959	1966	1967	1970	1972
Anne McIntyre	Cascade Anderson Geller	Dr. Jody Noe	Dr. Phuntsog Wangmo	Ada-Belinda DancingLion	HRH Princess Basma bint Ali	Zoe Hawes

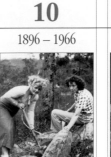
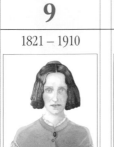
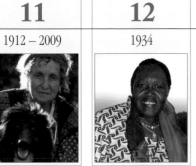
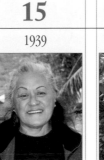
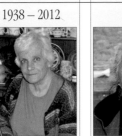
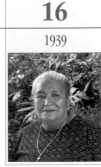
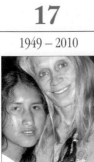
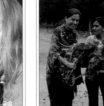
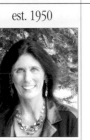
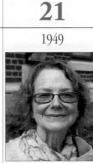
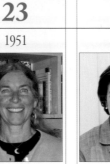
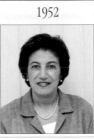
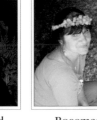
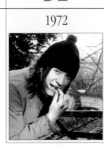

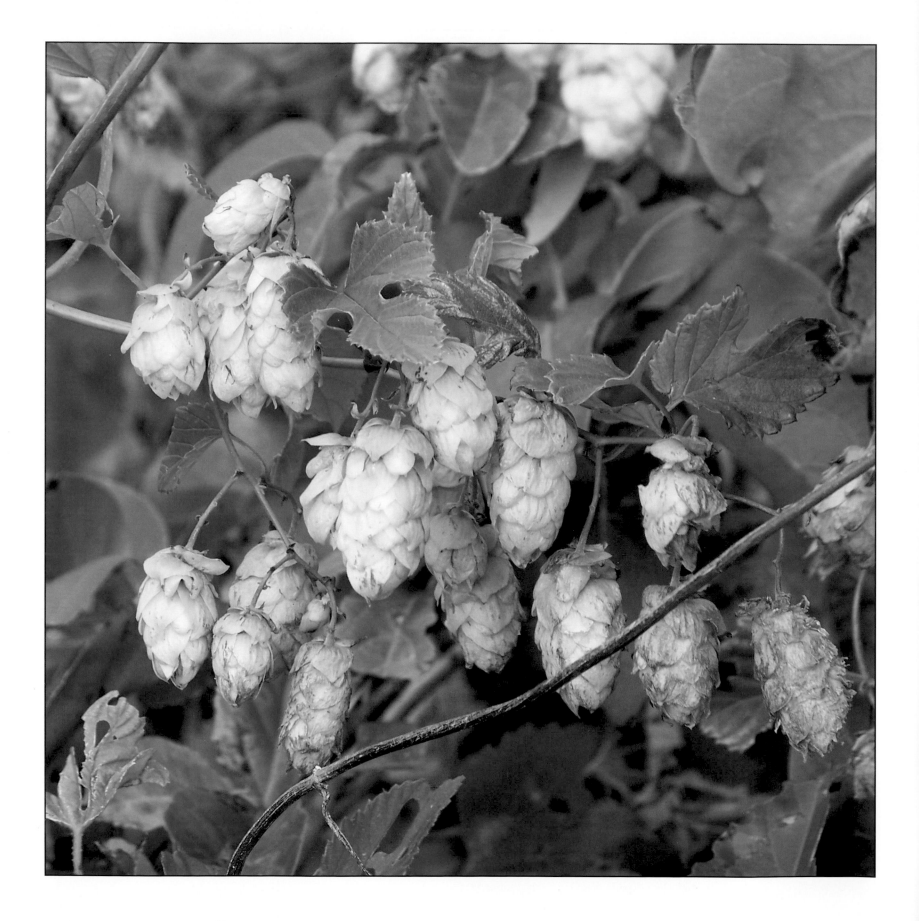

PART 1:
PLANT TRADITIONS

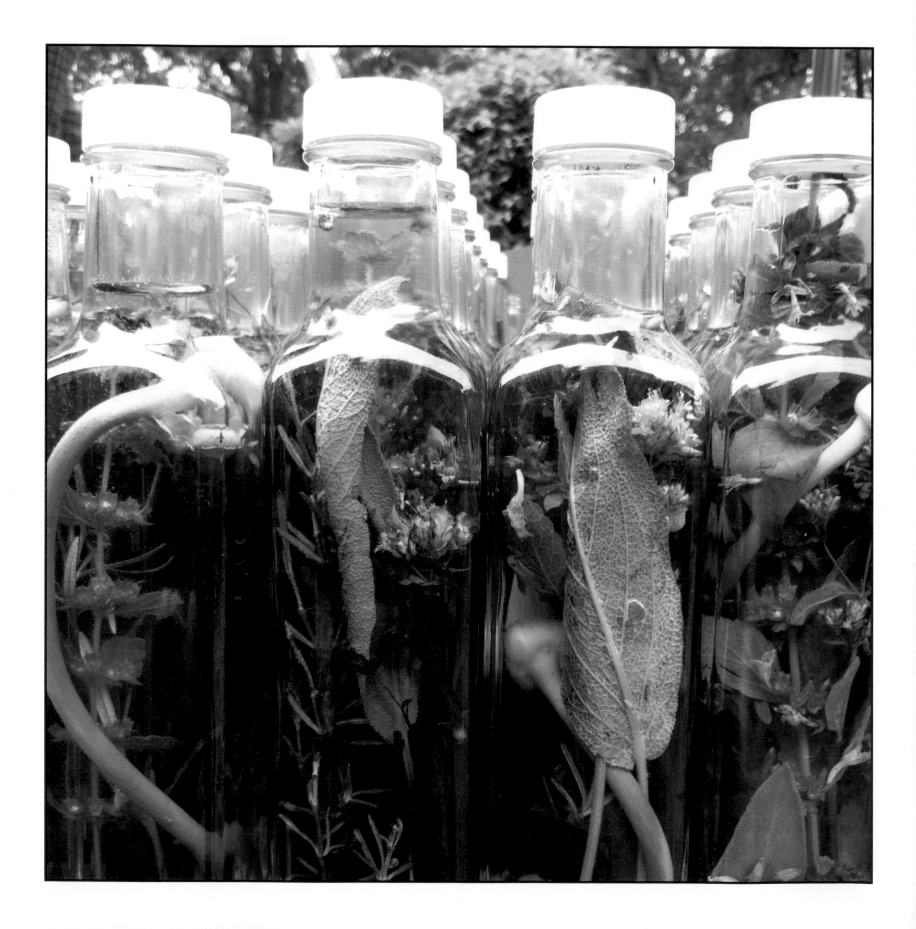

Chapter 1

WESTERN HERBAL TRADITIONS

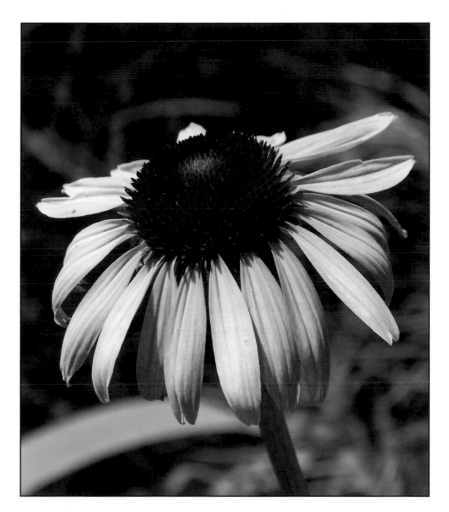

Western herbal medicine is a wonderful melting pot of international cultural, biological, and even astrological study. It evolved in concert with a wide variety of practices from around the world, including Eastern practices, shamanism, folk medicine, Arabic and Greek medicine, allopathy, and wise women and witch methods.

Ancient Egyptian medical practices originally centered on astrology and magic; Hippocrates and Galen later added anatomical and elemental views that formed the basis of Greek medicine. When Muslims spread across the southern Mediterranean in the ninth century, Arabic medical practitioners added Greek knowledge to their own advanced studies. Soon after, Arabs ventured into clinical, pharmaceutical, and botanical practices, stemming mostly from the Muslim belief that plants were Allah's gift for human health. (By contrast, Europe would not see separate pharmacists specializing in botany for centuries.)

Arabic physicians such as Rhazes (Ar-Razi, 869–925) and Avicenna (Ibn Said, 980–1037) passionately promoted botanical medicine so that their discoveries—along with older Greek Galenic knowledge—made their way north to Europe's Salerno School of Medicine in the twelfth century. Finally, Europe could access Arabic medical innovations and read Greek therapeutics in Latin. Western herbal medicine was born.

Today, western herbalism is generally considered to include European and North American methods along with some Russian methods, and it is distinct from Asian, African, South American, and other forms of practice. Western herbal medicine draws heavily from Native American traditional uses of plants and includes philosophies from Native American, Greek, British, European, and even North African and Middle Eastern traditions. It can be categorized by the use of common plants for creating and maintaining health without the inclusion of astrology, shamanism, astronomy, necromancy, or other folk traditions though it can include the use of intuition and even animal products such as beeswax and propolis.

Philosophies and schools of western herbal medicine have included the Doctrine of Signatures (based on a plant's physical features), Regulars (healing techniques based on purging the body violently), Thomsonian (based on Samuel Thompson's more gentle

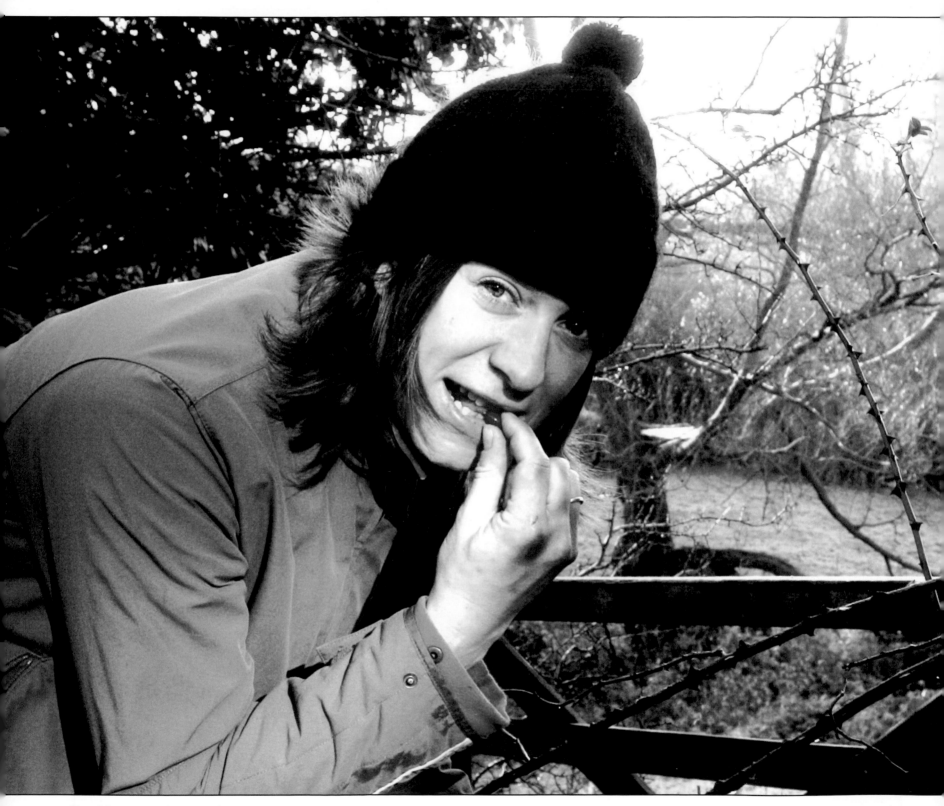

Zoë Hawes tasting rose hips
Photo credit: Vik Martin

criteria of healing), phytotherapy (a chemical-oriented approach to medicine), and the Eclectics of the United States (upscale reformist practitioners in the nineteenth century who included a variety of medicaments in their therapies).

Zoë Hawes

Apple orchards, bushels of freshly picked berries, and larders bursting with hot fruit pies: these are the fragrant childhood memories of English nurse and herbalist Zoë Hawes. Born in Essex and now living near Bath, Somerset, Zoë's back-to-the-land family grew vegetables, sailed, made functional hand crafts, and camped under the stars in a way that made active outdoor life her natural focus. Her grandparents were raised during the rationing of World War II, and they impressed upon Zoë and her parents the importance of providing for one's self.

Zoë's mother noticed a correlation between food additives and Zoë's wild behavior when she was a child, so they promptly became vegetarian—which greatly improved Zoë's behavior. Her eyes opened to the positive effects of foods and herbs on her behavior

Zoë in formulary
Photo credit: Vik Martin

NURSE

Many plants' liquids resemble breast milk (such as wild lettuce, figs, and milkweed) or they are named for their ability to stimulate breast milk production in nursing mothers (milk thistle). The Proto-Indo-European language (PIE) originally used *(s)nu* to mean "flowing," with natural suckling or breast milk connotations. Sanskrit *snauti* meant "she drips, gives milk," and the Greek *nao* meant "I flow." *Nu* led to *nutri* and *nutrix*, "she who gives suck," and French coined *nourir*. Latin created *nutricia* "nurse or governess." In the twelfth century, a *nurrice* was a wet-nurse or foster-mother.

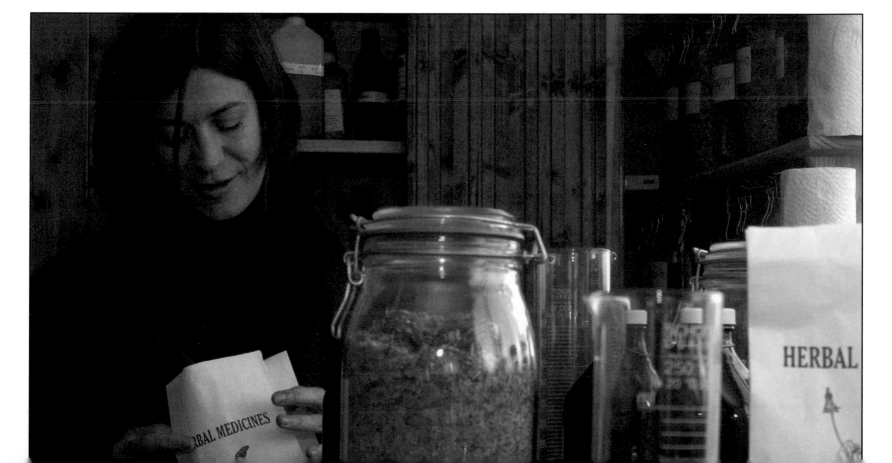

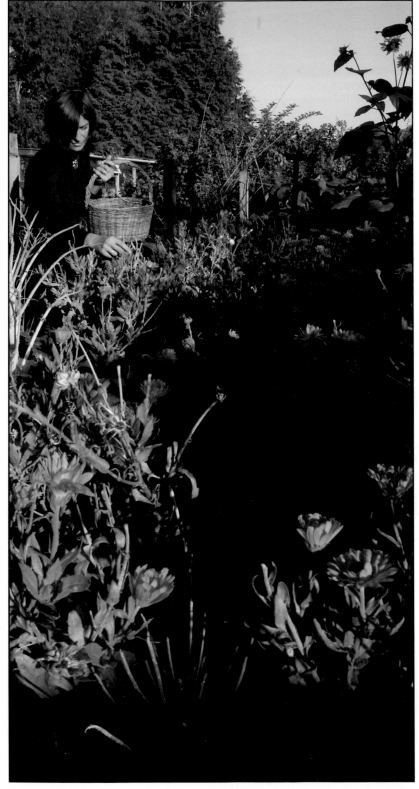

Zoë in calendula garden

and health, Zoë used homeopathic remedies, drank chamomile tea, and eventually found her path as a healer. She trained as a nurse and now practices in Frome in a multi-disciplinary clinic where she integrates her knowledge of allopathic nursing with botanical remedies, offering herb walks, classes and workshops on herbal medicine. She is also the nurse at a local boarding school where she introduces simple herbal remedies for many of the students' minor ailments. "I love giving the pupils insights about health and how the body works," she says.

While in nursing training, Zoë was struck that the medical personnel did not approach their patients with ideas of prevention or a plan for their overall health. "I remember seeing the causes of illness clearly in the people I was caring for in hospital," she recalls, "and I wondered why nobody seemed to be addressing fundamental basics like diet, stress, and lifestyle as a foundation for regaining health."

During a night shift at the hospital, Zoë found herself collecting the patients' magazines to read in the dark hours, and she discovered an article on herbal medicine written by a medical herbalist. "It was like a light bulb switching on, and I knew that was what I wanted to do," she says. She subsequently completed a four-year diploma at Britain's College of Phytotherapy and qualified as a Medical Herbalist in 2000. She is now registered with the National Institute of Medical Herbalists.

"I remember seeing the causes of illness clearly in the people I was caring for in hospital, and I wondered why nobody seemed to be addressing fundamental basics like diet, stress, and lifestyle as a foundation for regaining health."

She attended workshops by other herbalists and found Christopher Headley, who soon became an inspiring mentor. At his workshops, "we would all drink a mystery herbal tea and discuss its effects—it was very refreshing after all the science and medicine of the Phytotherapy diploma to do some really experiential stuff." Zoë credits Headley with a wonderful balance of spiritual, medical, and mystical insights and was "reassured to see a successful herbalist talk about [herbs] he had seen work, especially as I was still working in a strongly anti-herb environment like the hospital."

Her biggest challenges have been maintaining a belief in her herbal knowledge and not doubting herself, as well as learning to deliver information in an assertive, confident manner. "I don't have a colleague to turn to for reassurance or to hand over to at the end of a shift," she says.

And she is learning to be patient with the herbal remedies themselves, because they are very different from the "magic bullets" of allopathic medicine. "Having spent seventeen years working in orthodox medicine that aims to deliver instantaneous results, it took time for me to work at the slower pace of herbs, and also to slow the expectations of my patients and to tune them back into the slow adaptive processes of the body."

"Learn everything you can with your mind, then forget it all and listen to your intuition."

She published her first book, *A Forager's Guide to Medicinal Plants*, which extols the virtues of many of her favorite herbs including St. John's wort, plantain, oatstraw, milk thistle, calendula, and Oregon grape root. She also publishes the annual desk diary *Herbal Journal: Herbs, Healing and Folkways*. With a wise nod to her grandparents,

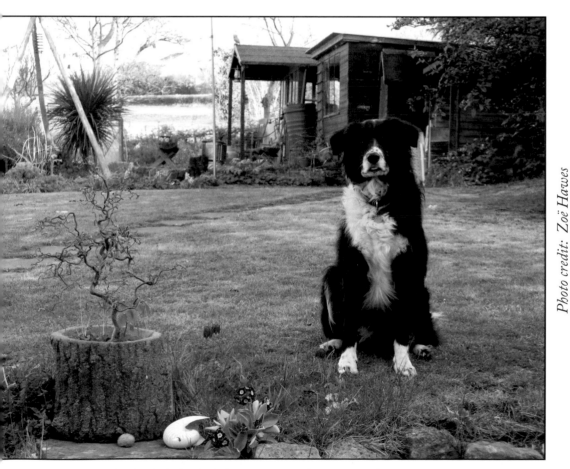

Photo credit: Zoë Hawes

Zoë Hawes's English herbal dispensary, well-protected

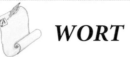

WORT

Wort is an ancient word for plant. Consider St. John's wort, pennywort, soapwort, and spearwort. Old English *wyrt* meant "root or herb"; Proto-Germanic used *wurtiz*, Old Saxon used *wurt*, Old Norse and Danish used *urt*. Old High German used *wurz*, but the word *kraut* won prominence; if this had won in English, we might refer to *Hypericum* as St. John's kraut.

Root, referring to the underground part, appeared in Old English and Old Norse, who used *rot*, and in German *wrot* or *vrot*, virtually indistinguishable from their words for plant. The Proto-Indo-European (PIE) *wrd* seems to have originated these, according to etymologist Douglas Harper. Eventually the anatomical parts of the plant separated linguistically to form separate words. The Latin *radix* derived from the PIE *wrad*, "twig or root," giving us radish and radical.

In Old English, *wort* "vegetable, plant, herb, or root" combined with *geard* "garden or yard" to form *wort-geard*, later shortened phonetically to *orceard*; hence, our modern "orchard." Today an orchard is a collection of fruit trees; in our past, an orchard was a garden of herbs.

she now owns three acres of meadow and orchard near her cottage and has adopted two children. She is teaching them the ways of straw-bale building, making and selling medicinal foods such as vinegars, fruit, berries, and leaf-herb-flower salads, and running a "pharmaculture orchard."

Zoë feels her biggest contribution is passing on the knowledge of medicinal plants to the children she works with at the school, to whom she says: "Learn everything you can with your mind, then forget it all and listen to your intuition."

SOMERSET, ENGLAND

Known as the Land of the Summer Farm Dwellers, Somerset in southwest England is known for its ancient Neolithic remains and its Old English, Roman, and Saxon inhabitants. First mentioned in 845 AD, "Sumursætum" is famed for apple cider and cheeses as well as archaeological treasures from local caves that include one complete skeleton known as Cheddar man, who dates from 7150 BC. The Somerset Levels and Moors are the swampy, sparsely populated wetlands drained by the Romans, and here the ancient practice of coppicing willow trees for fences and baskets continues.

Glastonbury, famous for its Tor and King Arthur lore, shares the county with Bath, a city founded upon the hot thermal springs and shrines built by the ancient Celts for the goddess Sulis. In 60 AD, Romans began building a temple and bathing complex here that took three hundred years to complete. They identified Sulis with Minerva, and the temple continued to be known as Aquae Sulis, "the waters of Sulis." The baths later silted up from neglect, but the hot thermal springs now support popular spas.

Frome, the small medieval town where herbalist Zoë Hawes runs her dispensary, is named for the River Frome and sits above a system of tunnels beneath the city; it is renowned for woolen cloth manufacture, weaving, cheesemaking, and arts. "Somerset is a beautiful rural county steeped in mystery, history and tradition," she says. "Magic still exists in hidden corners so strongly that it is tangible."

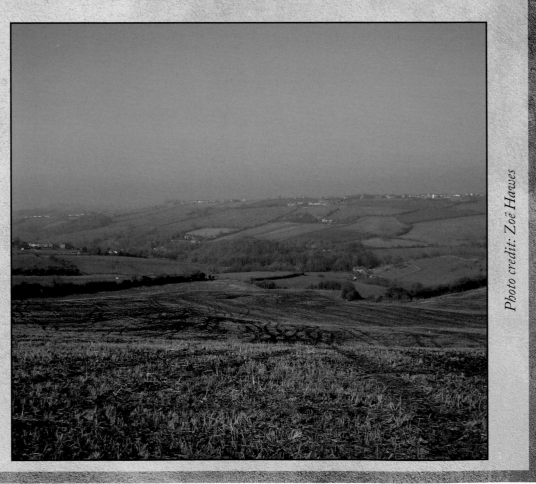

Photo credit: Zoë Hawes

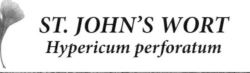

ST. JOHN'S WORT
Hypericum perforatum

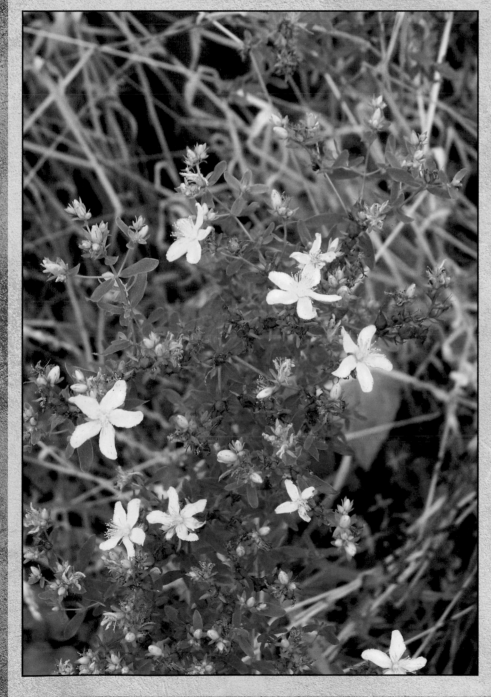

Used internally, St. John's wort is a cure for mild depression, anxiety, and nervous tension and is generally sold as a standardized extract at 3 percent hypericin, what chemists consider its "active" ingredient. St. John's wort contains glycosides (including retin), volatile oil, tannin, resin, and pectin, and Welsh herbalist David Hoffmann notes its slightly sedative and pain-reducing effect and classifies it as a nervous system tonic. It has been thought to be a monoamine oxidase inhibitor (MAOI) contraindicated with antidepressant drugs, but a 1999 study showed St. John's wort does not act by inhibition of monoamine oxidase as previously thought. Though St. John's wort demonstrates neurotransmitter activity, the study showed the herb to be "benign," saying possible harm with drug combinations is "remote."

Anti-inflammatory St. John's wort oil is rubbed externally on sore arthritic joints. When the herb is steeped in oil, the oil turns bright red, which indicated to early healers its use for hot conditions such as burns, sunburn, stings, and aching joints.

Maude Grieve suggests its use in pulmonary and urinary complaints, as well as for hysteria, parasites, hemorrhage, and nervous depression. The traditional German word for the plant is *hexenkraut*, or plant of the witches, as the herb blooms at the summer solstice and has been used in folk medicine to dispel evil spirits.

Mama Kia Ingenlath
(1949–2010)

It looks like a school: there are colorful flags waving, children running, yelling, and laughing, adults carrying tomatoes from the greenhouse with a teenager or helping a child with a skinned knee. There are picnic areas, art tables, and soccer games. Thirty-three children from ages two to eighteen are singing, playing, doing homework, harvesting in the garden, and preparing for a yummy dinner made with basil they grew themselves. It may look like a school, but it *feels* like—and is—a home. Many call it a miracle. Appropriately, it's named Casa de Milagros: Home of Miracles, and it is the brainchild and work of love of Kia Ingenlath, known as Mama Kia.

Mama Kia is a mother, grandmother, and director of the most visionary home in Peru; she is also a wise woman herbalist in the purest sense: it is part of her mission to introduce children to the world of plants.

Nine years ago, American-born yoga teacher Kia Ingenlath left Costa Rica and arrived in the fertile lands of the Urubamba Sacred Valley near Cusco, Peru. Kia had very little money, but with the help of several friends, including actor Woody Harrelson, she purchased and renovated a dilapidated two-hundred-year-old hacienda and took in orphaned children.

This was new for Kia; she had never raised a large number of children before, even though she was well past middle age. But she related to the orphans, partly because she'd been orphaned at the tender age of twelve: her parents, Seventh Day Adventist missionaries, and her brother all died (separately) within the same year.

"When I turned fifty," she told me in her incredibly quiet, gentle voice, "I did a midlife ceremony and dedicated the second half of my life to service." At Macchu Pichu, Kia gathered with friends and a powerful shaman in a ceremony meant to dedicate her life to a new purpose. "Everything flowed naturally," she told

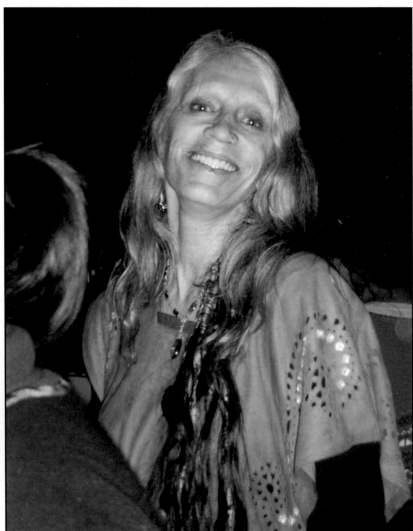

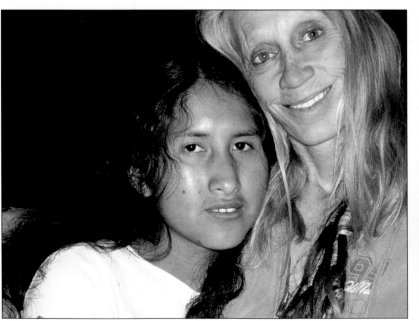

Kia Ingenlath with Luzma

me, "and it was very meaningful. It helped open up the second half of my life."

So many Peruvian children are without families. The country suffers a very high rate of child malnutrition and has no social service system, Kia says, and many children bear the brunt of the country's poverty. When children's parents die, the kids are passed from house to house within a village, and many are emotionally, physically, or even sexually abused.

Hearing the call to help, Kia created Casa de Milagros in memory of her grandson Chandler Sky who died as an infant. "I just received the calling," she says, "Everything has flowed together beautifully and I'm doing what I'm meant to do. It's been hard—but we usually learn best when we have to work hard. I have no regrets." She believes that preparing the children for a life of service not only helps them build character, but also creates sustainability. "We must start at the root of the problem, healing and educating children so they can give back to their community."

"Everything has flowed together beautifully and I'm doing what I'm meant to do. It's been hard—but we usually learn best when we have to work hard. I have no regrets."

She turned the decrepit hacienda into a colorful house and adopts each child as her own. Casa de Milagros does not operate the facility as an orphanage, where the children might go away to live with another family. Instead, they are their own family, and Kia raises each son and daughter with values for diversity, success,

CALENDULA
Calendula officinalis

Lovely calendula: the beautiful orange-yellow marigold so named because it was observed to stay colorful and vivid throughout the calendar year. Often called marigold (but not to be confused with proper marigold, *Tagetes*), calendula's vulnerary and antifungal petals contain saponins, carotenoids, bitter principle, essential oils, sterols, flavonoids, and mucilage, and calendula tincture is popularly used internally to remove parasites, kill bacterial infections, relieve sepsis, or kill *Candida albicans*. Used externally, the herb is an effective emollient for the skin. Many herbalists use calendula oil to heal wounds, scrapes, eczema and psoriasis. It is amazingly easy to grow and is profligate in its blossoms—the flower heads break off easily and can be used fresh or dried for tinctures or teas.

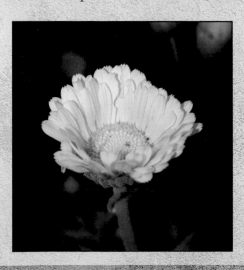

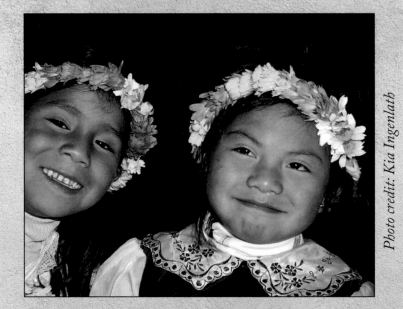

Photo credit: Kia Ingenlath

Girls wear calendula crowns at Casa de Milagros.

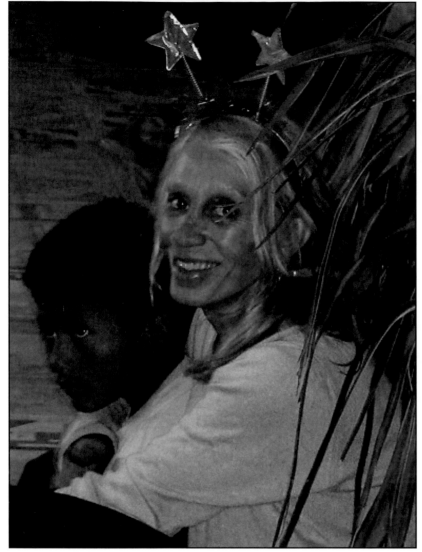

Photo credit: Rick Marquart

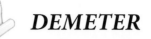

DEMETER

Demeter was the Greek's beloved goddess of grains. One theory of Demeter's name is that it derives from *da*, the Doric form of the Greek *ge* "earth" (see Earth sidebar). *Da* + *mater* (mother) is earth mother. Mythology historian W. Mannhardt argued that the first part of her name was derived from a Cretan word *deai* meaning "barley," so she was the Barley Mother. I propose it relates to the root of deity (god): the Proto-Indo-European word *dewos* meant god from the PIE base *dyeu* "to shine" and Sanskrit *deva* "god." Perhaps Demeter was "shining mother" or "god mother." It could even be our ancient ancestors considered barley itself to be divine, thus the words for god and barley were nearly identical.

Demeter's cult originated in Crete, and Homer dedicated a hymn to her. "My name is Dois," she tells the daughters at Eleusis when she is disguised as an old woman after the disappearance of her daughter Kore/Persephone. The Romans called Demeter Ceres, from which we derive cereal.

youngest to the oldest, learn Permaculture methods of planting, cultivation, and the medicinal properties of healing plants. The garden is not only a plot of land where vegetables are grown; it is a work of art. Terra cotta railings are intricately carved, child-high walls are festooned with colorful paintings of flowers and vines, and banners blow joyfully in the wind. The garden is a place of beauty, respite, food, medicine, and even income, since the orphanage strives to be self-sustaining. Though the not-for-profit accepts monetary contributions and rents accommodations to tourists, it focuses on maintaining its organic vegetable garden and greenhouse, cornfields, raising guinea pigs and rabbits, and using their herbs for medicine whenever possible.

"I just received the calling. . . ."

and kindness. She arranges their schooling, provides extracurricular activities such as music and singing, and encourages traditional Peruvian dancing so the children can study their own heritage. Moreover, at the heart of the home, Kia has created a thriving herbal Permaculture garden in which the children are active planters and harvesters.

A Children's Garden

At the center of Mama Kia's Home of Miracles is a charming and fully functional medicinal plant garden. All the children, from the

Looking beyond Casa de Milagros, Kia expands her services to include the broader community. She models proper nutrition for local men and women, teaching them how to grow a variety

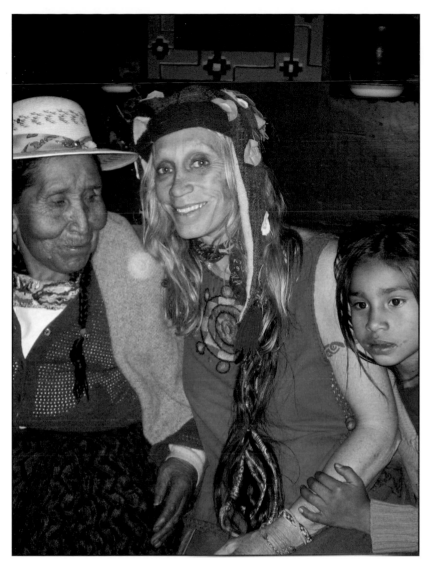

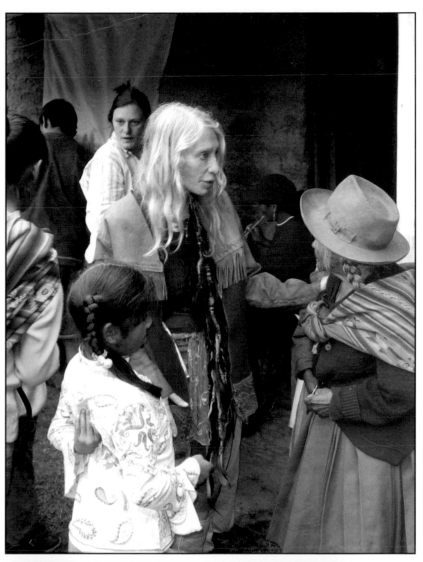

of food crops organically, which is a new concept for the residents of the Sacred Valley who have traditionally grown only corn and potatoes. As a result of this restricted diet, many children suffer from malnourishment. Kia wants the home to be an example within the community of variety, diversity, and creative expression; to this end, she encourages the children to learn about their heritage through art. "All the children at the Home know how to spin yarn and dye fabrics with plant dyes," she says proudly, and she invites children from the wider community to join their craft classes.

Beyond meeting the needs of orphans, Casa de Milagros and the Chandler Sky Foundation help conserve one of the world's most biodiverse rainforests. "Through teaching children methods of

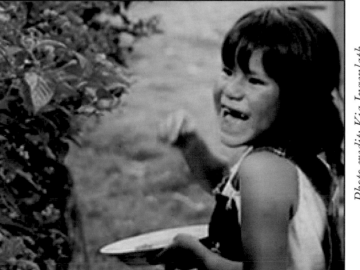

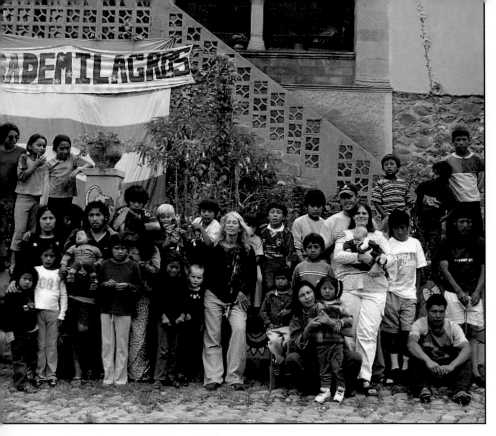

Photo credit: Kia Ingenlath

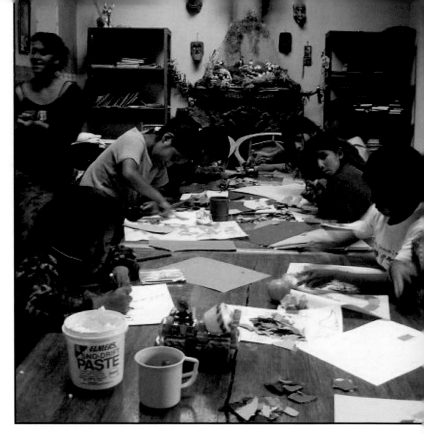

Casa de Milagros children's artwork
Photo credit: Kia Ingenlath

farming that allow the land to be used over and over again," Mama Kia says, "there will be a decreased need for migration into the precious rainforest reserves that we, as a planet, need for survival."

A typical day for Casa de Milagros children is to go to school, come home, play for an hour, do homework, and head to bed. Twice weekly they study music, singing, and original Peruvian dances. The boys love soccer, and once a week is movie night.

On weekends the children work in the Permaculture gardens, growing giant beets and kale. Mama Kia says the children "always respond with interest to the gardens and they love watching the seeds sprout. They know all the plants in the garden as well as the medicinal properties. They all have an active role in growing food and herbs in the organic gardens, with an emphasis on conserving water."

Among other culinary and medicinal herbs, the children grow comfrey, chamomile, fever few, aloe vera, rosemary, calendula, and lobelia to make medicine for what amounts to a very large family. Many orphans arrive malnourished or with bronchitis, tuberculosis, rickets, chronic intestinal infections, or infections of the skin. By combining an organic farming education with trade skills and an appreciation for the arts, Casa de Milagros and Mama Kia are helping to relieve Cusco of some of the 3,500 abandoned children as well as providing them a healthy childhood and prospects for a better future.

"The children always respond with interest to the gardens and they love watching the seeds sprout. They know all the plants in the garden as well as the medicinal properties."

Kia has pioneered outreach projects in the local pueblos, including a women's clinic, a midwifery practice, and a soup kitchen that feeds ninety-seven children and twenty elderly people daily. Kia spearheaded Hanaq Pacha Retreat Center ("Where Heaven Meets the Earth"). Since jobs are scarce in the Sacred Valley, the center is a place where the teenagers can work as they grow older; all profits from the center support Casa de Milagros. Kia is devoted: "When you're living your life and you love what you do, then it doesn't seem like too much. I love what I do; I never have a day that I don't love what I'm doing."

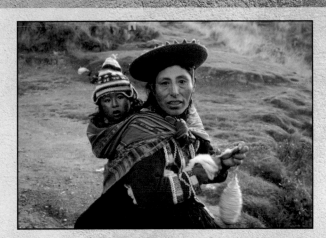

Quechua woman with child in Peru
Photo credit: Harry Beach

The gorgeous river Urubamba flows through the Sacred Valley of the Incas, winding around the base of Mt. Putucusi and Machu Picchu. Here, Mama Kia established her home for children, Casa de Milagros, near the ancient ruins of Yucay, as Cusco, Peru, was called by the Incas.

The Sacred Valley of Urubamba, north of Cusco, was considered sacred by the Incas for its fertility and beauty. Archaeological sites nestled between the towering mountains and rolling streams demonstrate the Inca's ancient irrigation systems and farming terraces. Palaces and sun-worship temples were built in Cusco to honor the god; constructed in the shape of a sacred Puma, one temple had a fortress as the puma's head.

In 1533, Spanish conquistador Francisco Pizarro arrived in Cusco with Vasco de Balboa; believing the Incan city of "Piru" to be "el Dorado," he and his soldiers plundered the city, desecrated its temples, and melted gold and silver artwork. Though most of the structures were demolished, some of the stone bases later became the foundations for houses and churches.

The community surrounding Casa de Milagros is very poor; most people have dirt floors, and guinea pigs eat food scraps from the floor (the guinea pigs themselves are eaten by the people and are considered a valuable food source).

Mama Kia's neighbors cook with wood, and though a few people in the province can afford electricity, Kia estimated the average income at only about $300 per year. Most children are malnourished. They have few clothes or shoes, so Casa de Milagros shares its surplus supplies with the community. Most people speak Quechua, the language of their Incan ancestors. Today, Casa de Milagros encourages its children to honor their ancestors through dance, music, handcrafts, weaving, and song.

After the fall of the Incan empire to the Conquistadors, most surviving Incans adopted Catholicism. Most Peruvians today are Catholic, and Kia noted there many religious celebrations honoring the Virgin Mary. Casa de Milagros raises the children at Casa de Milagros to make their own decisions regarding religion and she teaches that different cultures have different religions. This philosophy of tolerance and appreciation goes hand-in-hand with her community service work in the rich and fertile valley of Urubamba.

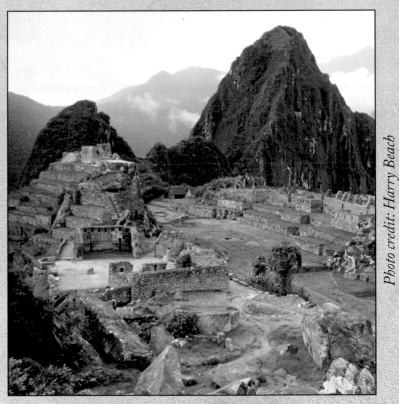

Photo credit: Harry Beach

Machu Picchu

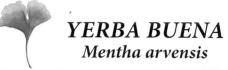

YERBA BUENA
Mentha arvensis

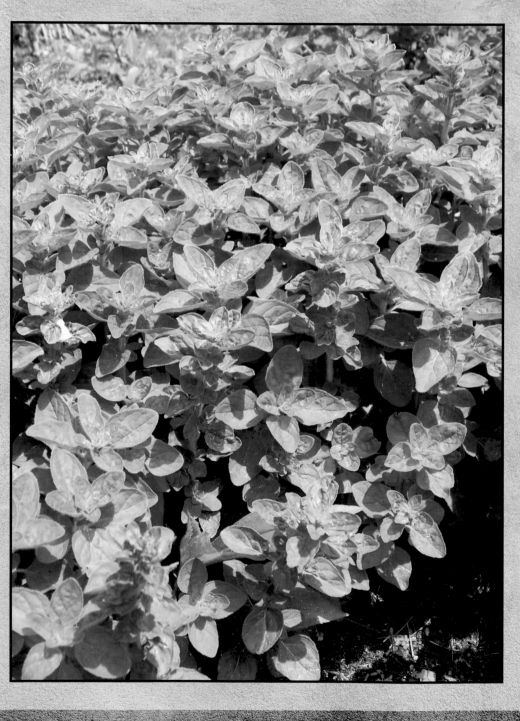

The "good herb," *Yerba Buena* is our familiar mint, native to Europe, Asia, and North America. The humble yet tenacious mint is circumboreal, thriving across Pangaea long before the continents divided. Mint boasts thirty species, some of which were brought to the New World with the colonists (to greet other mint species already living there), while additional species were introduced to the Philippines by Spaniards.

We enjoy many species of mint: peppermint, spearmint, water mint, chocolate mint, apple mint (with its fuzzy leaves resembling mullein). Mints will thrive in virtually any condition: poor soil, wet soil, dry fields, creek banks, gardens, and abandoned lots. *Yerba Buena* is most similar to *Mentha arvensis*, or field mint, and residents throughout South America chew its carminative leaves to aid digestion, oral health, and circulation; the scent and taste invigorate and refresh, making *Yerba Buena* valued worldwide for keeping one alert and awake.

Rosemary Gladstar

Often called the Mother of the American Herbal movement, Rosemary Gladstar is an icon in the field of herbal medicine. She is a bubbly, warm, enthusiastic advocate for herbal medicine and a champion for protecting our wild medicinal plants.

Rosemary's relationship with herbs began as a child in a farming community in Sonoma County. Her grandmother, Mary Egitkanoff, Rosemary's first herbal teacher, was an herbalist in the old sense of the word: she used plants simply because they were available, they made sense, and they were free. Mary and her husband had fled the Armenian genocide and she impressed upon Rosemary at a young age that it was Mary's belief in God and her knowledge of the plants that had saved her life. "She meant that literally," says Rosemary. "Without her knowledge of the plants, they would have starved to death and, without such strong faith and hope, they would have given up." Mary frequently took Rosemary into the fields around their farmhouse to teach her how to gather wild plants, which plants were good to eat, which ones were dangerous, and—especially—which ones were good for medicine. "Those teachings have stayed with me all my life, and most of my favorite herbs are still those I learned on those walks with my grandmother."

Since Rosemary was already very close to the land, the back-to-the-land movement of the 1960s did not inspire her to live on a farm. Instead, it germinated within her the desire to explore deep wilderness. After graduating high school, she backpacked across the mountains of northern California, Oregon, and Washington. In 1972, she returned to Sonoma County filled with the dream to journey to Canada on horseback. She needed money to buy horses and supplies, so she got a cleaning job at Guerneville Natural Food Store, scrubbing floors and sinks after hours. But her knowledge of plants quickly shone through and she was elevated to "herb lady," earning the money she needed to purchase horses. Her journey began the following summer when she took her toddler son and

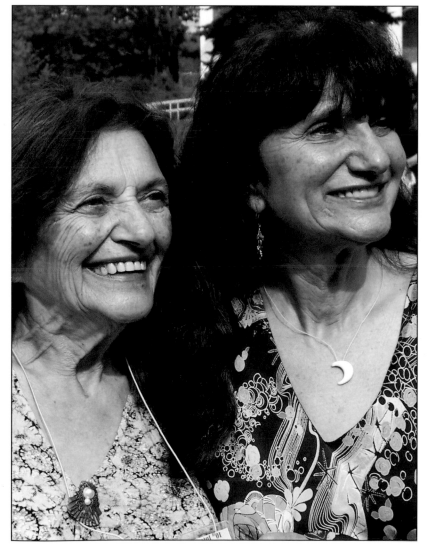

Rosemary Gladstar and her mother, Jasmine Karr

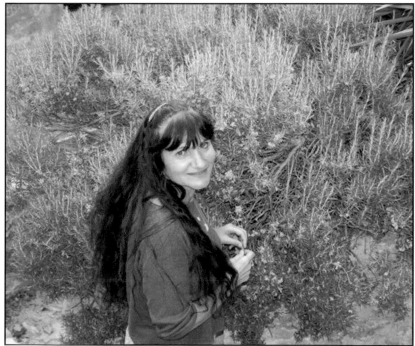

Rosemary with rosemary

a friend on the horseback ride of a lifetime: from Sonoma County to the Trinity Alps of Northern California. Amazingly, the two women wildcrafted all the food on their journey. "We ate greens, berries, and nuts we gathered along the way," she says. "We all kept fat and healthy the whole four months we rode, and I returned from that trip ready to give back. I felt so blessed by life and wanted to share what I was learning with the rest of the world!"

"Where we are seeded, planted and grown has a lasting influence in our lives, I'm quite sure. It certainly did for me."

Adept at herbal formulation and intuiting an individual's needs, she opened Rosemary's Garden in Sebastopol, teaching herb classes and facilitating gatherings to bring other plant lovers together. "It was an exciting, rich time as we woke up to the world of plants that were living beings right under our feet," Rosemary remembers. "There was so much to share and learn because herbalism had been resting peacefully 'under ground' for several decades and we felt we were just discovering it!" With friends, she opened Traditional Medicinals, an outlet for her original tea blends, and Country Comfort to produce salves, lip balms, creams, body powders, and baby products. Her life deepened even more when she opened the book *Traveler's Joy* by Juliette de Bairacli Levy. Enchanted, Rosemary wrote to Juliette via the publisher and, to her surprise, Juliette wrote back; they corresponded for years until Rosemary

finally visited Juliette in person, traveling to a small island off mainland Greece and cementing a lifelong friendship.

Rosemary helped open the California School of Herbal Studies in the late 1970s and, in 1987, she left California for the four-seasons climate of Vermont, where she cofounded Sage Mountain Herbal Retreat Center and Botanical Sanctuary on five hundred acres of pristine Vermont land. She is the author of nine herbal books, the founder/director of Sage Mountain, founder of the International Herb Symposium, and the director of the New England Women's Herbal Conference. Rosemary accepted the call to the conservation of wild medicinal plants by founding United Plant Savers, a nonprofit organization protecting native medicinal plants and their native habitats.

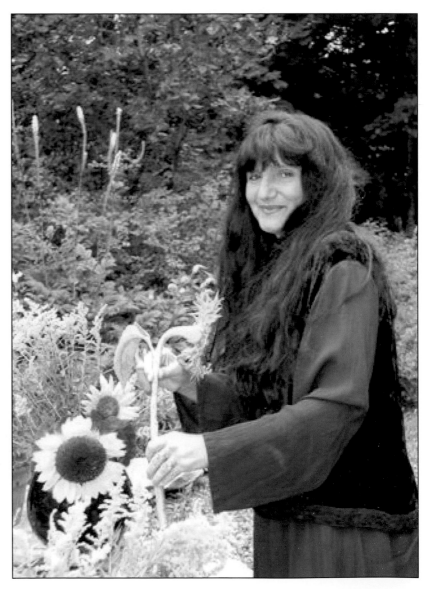

Photo credit: Rosemary Gladstar

ROSEMARY

The ancient people who lived on the north coast of the Black Sea, known as Scythia, called the River Volga *Rha*, meaning "flow." The ancient Hittites used *arszi* for "flow" and Proto-Indo-Europeans used *ras* or *eras* "to flow, wet or moisten." Sanskrit used *rasah*, "sap, juice, fluid, essence," and Latin used *ros*. Old Church Slavonic of ninth century CE of Slavic Macedonia and Bulgaria created *rosa*, referring in particular to dew falling from the heavens. French formed *rosmarin*, from *ros* "dew" and *marinus* "sea," to refer to the fragrant coastal plant. In circa 1300 CE, Latin coined *rosmarinus*, "dew of the sea."

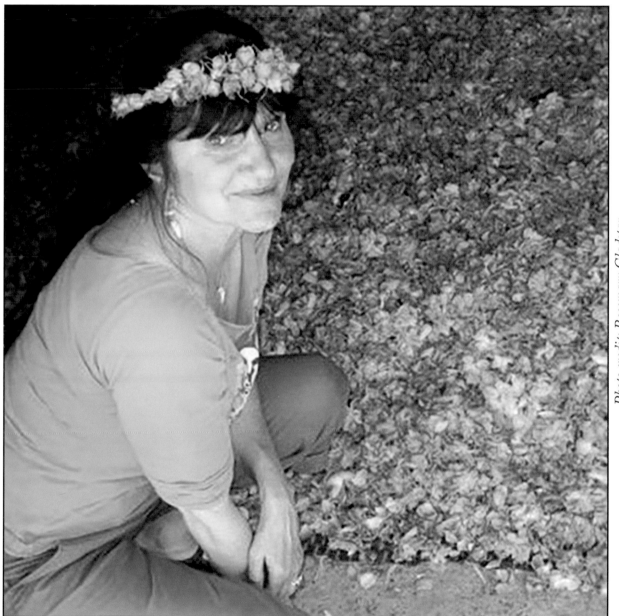

"Ever since I can first remember, the green ones have called me."

She is, of course, a visionary plant lover and an inspiration to women, but she would most especially like to be remembered for "saving" Hannah Hill, sixty acres of Vermont virgin woods that abut Sage Mountain, and for bringing Juliette de Bairacli Levy to America "for the first time in fifty years so that her fans could meet her, and so she could see the wonderful influence her work has had on so many. There's nothing nicer to know that your life has been of value, now is there?"

Rosemary advises, "Follow your heart. Always listen to the plants, spend as much time as possible with them—at least three times as much time with the plants than with your nose in a book. Then you'll know you know the plants, and they'll know you." This reciprocal relationship lies at the heart of Rosemary's legacy as an herbalist.

VERMONT

When most people picture Vermont, they envision downhill snow skiing, invigorating crosscountry skiing, and riding in romantic horse-drawn sleighs. This is a country of outdoor activity, even in the winter months when there is a great deal of activity in the rural Vermont countryside. A mountain wonderland, Vermont includes a portion of the Appalachian Trail as well as the Long Trail, a 270-mile footpath that links Massachusetts to Canada. Peaks on this trail reach 4,393 feet, a dizzying home for many native Eastern American woodland herbs.

Vermont is the leading US supplier of maple syrup, producing 450,000 gallons in 2008. The principal species tapped are sugar maple (*Acer saccharum*) and black maple (*Acer nigrum*); roughly ten gallons of sap are required to boil one quart of syrup, making this one of the world's most valuable plant products.

Rosemary's Sage Mountain is a 500-acre wilderness retreat center that abuts 26,000 acres of wilderness and is home to moose, deer, fox, coyote, bear, and wild cats. "I'm always in awe of the plants here," she says. "They live outside all winter where it typically gets thirty below zero . . . I marvel at how many plants not only tolerate such cold but thrive in it. . . . I am completely in love, deeply and forever, with the wild spirit of this place that called me, owns me, and has taken my heart as its own."

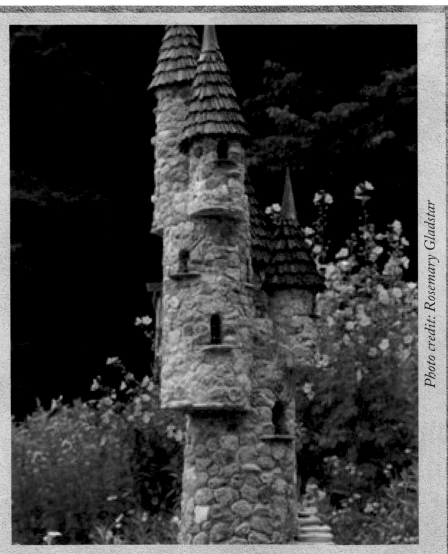

Photo credit: Rosemary Gladstar

Photo of where I live

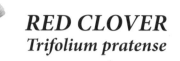

RED CLOVER
Trifolium pratense

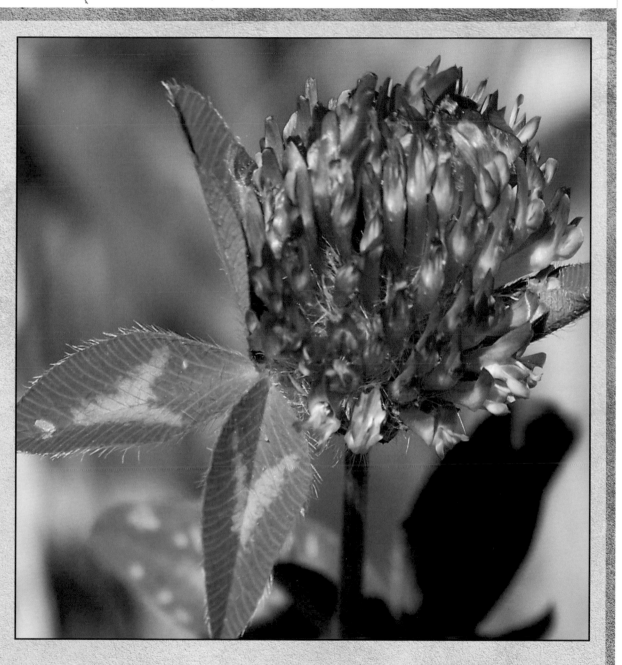

The genus refers to the three leaves under each blossom *tri-folia*, and the species reminds us it lives in the meadow. Red clover is a legume that can fix nitrogen in the soil. Valued both internally and externally to treat cases of children's and adult's eczema and psoriasis, red clover makes a useful compress for burns, weepy blisters, and rashes. Mid-nineteenth-century herbalist Samuel Thompson made it into a paste to treat skin cancers, and modern research suggests red clover has antineoplastic activity. Additional research centers on its benefits for the female hormonal system because of its phytoestrogens and phytosterols, compounds that make red clover valuable for menopausal women beleaguered with hot flashes.

Historically, red clover has been considered a "blood cleanser," draining fluid from the lymphatic system, improving circulation, and ridding the liver of excess toxins. Acids build up in the lymph and blood, and Chinese herbalists refer to these toxins as "heat" that contributes to "hot" diseases. As an *alterative*, red clover removes these toxins, dissolves external cysts, and aids in expectorant and antispasmodic formulas for bronchitis. It is so mineral-rich, many herbalists consider it a fertility tonic.

Cascade Anderson Geller

(1954–2013)

Cascade Anderson Geller came to herbalism by way of rebellion. Her grandmother and great-grandmother collected wild plants in the north Georgia mountains, though they would not have described themselves as "herbalists." Cascade's great-grandmother was a midwife, and her mother helped deliver babies, harvest herbs, and sell ginseng. Cascade credits her mother with instilling within her a deep trust in plants and their ability to provide. At her mother's side, Cascade learned to identify and harvest a number of wild plants, including sassafras, dandelions, wild grapes, and cherry bark.

In the spring of 1972, Cascade graduated high school and worked for the George McGovern campaign for political change. But the election was ugly and McGovern lost when incumbent Richard Nixon was re-elected. Cascade grew disillusioned and frustrated. "There were National Guard on the rooftops at colleges, the Vietnam War was going on, it was a stressful time," she says. "There were deep divisions. I felt like I needed something else. I was not enamored with the actions of the United States and I didn't have much confidence that things would change."

To clear her head and evaluate her idea of pursuing medicine as a career, she embarked on an adventure to the western United States, first backpacking in the Rockies and then in the mountains of the Pacific Northwest, where she and a friend foraged wild foods and explored the forest. She especially enjoyed building rafts, and one particularly frosty morning, she awoke with an epiphany. "I realized I had to join the world again, so I went out on my raft and dove into the lake. I baptized myself into never taking the straight road in my livelihood. I made a pact to become an herbalist instead of a medical doctor. I promised myself that as soon as I got down from the mountain, I would get busy with getting on that path. So when people ask me how I became an herbalist, I always thank Nixon."

The Professional Path

She sought herbal training from various sources, including Ella Birzneck of Dominion Herbal College, Iroquois herbalist Dr. Norma Myers (Dean of Green Shores Herbal College in Vancouver), and other elders now passed away. On a year's adventure out of the country, Cascade explored Ayurveda in Kathmandu and other healing modes throughout Asia. She trained as a midwife and served as the herbalist at a number of births. Throughout her early training, she nurtured the herbal knowledge handed down by her mother and great-grandmother, all while living in the deep woods

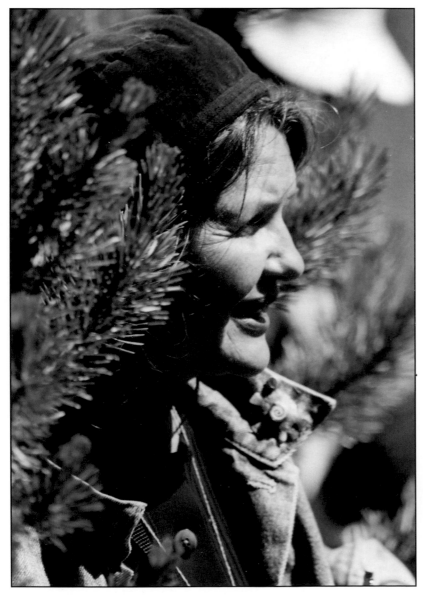

Photo credit: Tom Iraci

Cascade on Mt. Hood

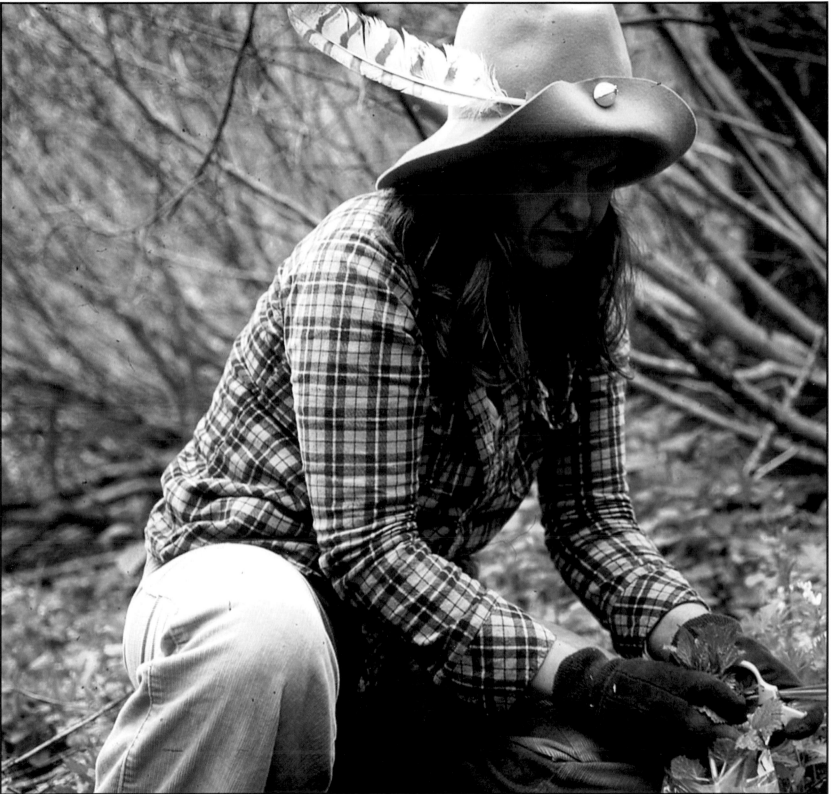

Cascade harvesting stinging nettles, c. 1980

of Oregon. As practicing resident herbalist, she was asked to join the founding of the Everest House Healing Center in Portland in 1979, a thriving center now known as Common Ground. That same year, Cascade was offered a job at the National College of Naturopathic Medicine teaching the Botanical Medicine Program. She taught there for more than thirteen years. She went on to establish the botanical medicine programs at Seattle's Bastyr University and at the Southwest College of Naturopathic Medicine in Tempe, Arizona.

"We owe every bit of our health to plants. We wouldn't be here without them!"

Remedies

A serene and down-to-earth woman, Cascade employed herbs primarily in the traditional western context of herbalism, subscribing to the "principle of enhancing the vital force using natural means of lifestyle, diet, herbs, and water."

When I interviewed Cascade, she had recently formulated a remedy for a young woman suffering from a urinary tract infection; the formula consisted of wildcrafted *uva ursi* and pipsissewa with organically grown marshmallow root as a mucilaginous corrective and spearmint as a cooling diuretic. She said she tries to make her medicines flavorful. "I always want to improve the beauty and flavor of formulas. This was something I turned my nose up at early in my career as I felt people should take their medicines, so to speak, no matter what they tasted like. But after working with people, I realized they respond better when medicines are gentler and more flavorful." Lemon balm (*Melissa officinale*) was one of her favorites. "It's balancing, it's a panacea, a good nervine. Latin American cultures and people in the Mediterranean consider it a powerful relaxing herb, good for the heart, for the soul, for babies, the elderly and everyone in between."

She also advocated the healing benefits of water. "I like to say, 'The best herb is the one you've got—if you don't have an herb, use water.' I would add to that now, 'Use salt water.'" Cascade learned about salt's healing powers from her travels across the Mediterranean and she says that salt water is purifying as a gargle, bath, soak, or scrub, relaxing and toning tissues at the same time. "I'm always looking for that kind of balance," she says.

REBEL

*R*ebel stems from Latin's combination *re* "against or again" and *bellare*, "to wage war," forming *rebellare*, which, in the twelfth century, became *rebelled* in French. Similarly, *reluctance* comes from Latin *re* "against" and *luctari* "to struggle."

The words *rebel* and *revel* have similar etymology. The same Latin *rebellare* gave Old French *revel*, but in this instance it meant to be disorderly. By 1300, *revel* meant riotous merry-making, and by 1754, it meant to take great pleasure in something.

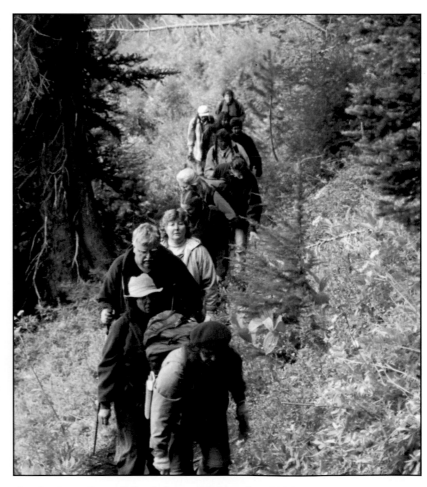

An herb walk on Mt. Adams, "Pahto," c. 2002

Photo credit :Tom Iraci

Bursting with evergreens and colorful deciduous trees, Oregon includes prairies, meadows, mountains, high deserts, and rugged Pacific coastline. It was originally settled by numerous native peoples who gave their tribal names to local geography: the Klamath, Chinook, Bannock, and Chasta, among others. The northern border with Washington State is the Columbia River, a huge river system that allowed for the development of the northern territory through trade, timber felling, and access to inner lands.

Oregon is home to the redwood tree, *Sequoia sempervirens*; its cousin the *Sequoiadendron giganteum*, or Giant Sequoia, thrives inland in central California. As the tallest trees in the world and with a life span ranging from 700–2,000 years, redwoods grow throughout northern California and the southern Oregon coastlines and provide shelter and habitat for the Northern Spotted Owl, the Bald Eagle, and various species of mountain lion, black bear, bobcat, and beaver. After 90 percent of the original old-growth redwoods had been destroyed (mostly for the development of San Francisco), the nation realized that salvaging what was left for posterity was important and preservation began in the 1920s.

The sea otter fur trade and later various gold rushes sparked emigrations to Oregon, prompting pioneers to traverse the dramatic Cascade and Bitterroot Mountains; the booming fur trade united such diverse cultures as Hawai'i, Canada, and England in the exploitation of local resources in the late 1700s, and by 1805, Lewis and Clark's Corps of Discovery Expedition alerted the country to the beauty of the western coast. In 1843, the first land claim by European/American investors created the city of Portland in the Willamette Valley near the Pacific coast, shortly before California's and Australia's gold rushes. Originally called the Clearing, later Stump Town, the city was christened Portland in 1845 and today is home to more than two million people and known as The City of Roses.

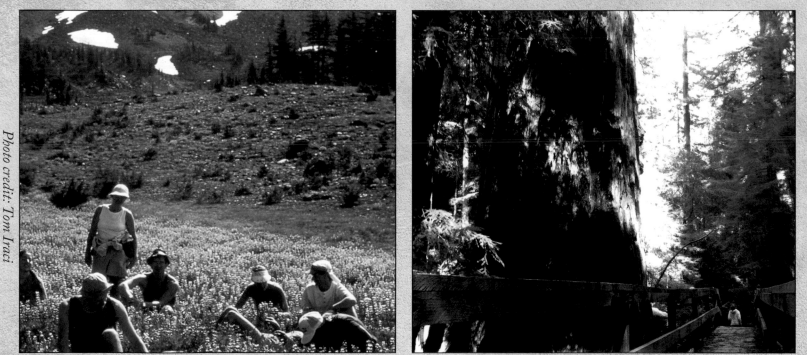

Photo credit: Tom Iraci

Cascade leads an herb hike in the Three Sisters Wilderness, Oregon, c. 1986

Oregon and California redwoods

BEARBERRY
Arctostaphylos uva-ursi

Native Americans introduced colonists to the lovely trailing *uva-ursi*, an already familiar European and Chinese ground-creeper botanists named *Arctostaphylos uva-ursi* (because bears love to eat the "grape"). Mountaineers call it upland cranberry or arberry. Favoring sandy soils, especially in gravelly exposed woods in the northern hemisphere, this perennial evergreen's shiny leathery leaves are oval and pointed at the stem joint, and its tiny white flowers produce dry red berries in winter.

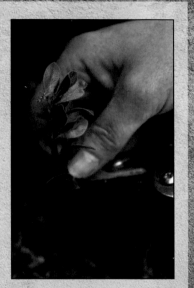

Uva-ursi
Photo credit: Tom Iraci

The leaves are collected in late fall and dried, then powdered to form teas or tablets. With its relatively high concentration of tannins (8 percent), it is approved as a urinary antiseptic in the United States, though use is restricted to one week due to its arbutin content. Tannin-rich bearberry is widely used to treat cystitis, urinary tract infections, urethritis, nephritis, gallstones, and kidney and bladder stones.

Jethro Kloss recommended *uva-ursi* for diabetes and excessive menstruation. He advised taking the remedy not only as a tea, powder, or tincture (as do earlier herbalists) but also as a douche, especially for ulcerations in the uterus.

"Being an herbalist provides many gifts," she says, "more than I could ever even add up in my life, and I keep discovering new ones. It brings me great joy to help nurture dynamic relationships between people and plants. Getting to know any plant, but especially wild plants, is a deeply enriching experience. Without direct experience with the plants themselves, it is difficult to develop trust in the healing power of plants." She said just looking outdoors and seeing plants gave her a sense of camaraderie "that I'm being cared for by those beings, especially by their beauty, resilience, abilities to adapt, feed and heal.

"We owe every bit of our health to plants. We wouldn't be here without them! I don't like looking at plants as just a medicine or a tool that I can use, I enjoy them for who they are. Plants have their own incredible reason for being that we don't really understand. The great mystery they offer is apparent if we take the time to think about it, even in the mundane things we do with them: we can make soup, tea, fabric, baskets, rope, build our homes, a fire, make a gorgeous bouquet. But we will never fully understand the mystery of that miniscule row of hairs that rotate up the stem of the delicious, nutritious, and healing little chickweed!"

Isla Burgess

Years ago, during her teaching career at her herbal medicine studio overlooking the Pacific Ocean near Gisborne, New Zealand, herbalist Isla Burgess met a *pohangar,* someone who would ultimately change her life. A pohangar is similar to a shaman and "fully grounded in local plant use, very much localized," she says. "In this part of the country, they wouldn't use a plant that grows only in the south island, for example. The pohangar was shamanistic in his abilities and had an extraordinary knowledge of the bush."

Intrigued by the pohangar, his psychic abilities, and especially his intrinsic knowledge of the bush, Isla decided she wanted to learn more, so she contacted him. "I phoned to ask if he would take me on and also have my students along." But he did not return her call. Again, she called and asked for permission to join him in the bush, to learn from him and give her students the same opportunity. Again, he ignored her call. Isla decided he was testing her, forcing her to prove herself worthy of his time.

"I think it took forty phone calls," she says, laughing. "Every week, he'd say, 'Phone back next week, phone back next week.' Eventually he said, 'Come tomorrow!' We had to drop absolutely everything and get in the cars and go. We weren't going to miss out on that experience."

Finally proving she was persistent enough to be taken seriously, Isla arrived at the meeting point in the desert with students trailing behind her. The shaman, however, was not impressed. He led the group into the bush and immediately, to Isla's surprise, stripped the berries off a well-known very poisonous plant.

"I knew the whole plant to be poisonous. But he looked me straight in the eye and he said hold out your hand." The shaman proceeded to squeeze the juice from the berries into her palm.

"Drink," he commanded.

Isla was astounded. "I knew that I was either stark mad to drink the juice, or this was another test. I decided it was another test. I drank it, and found out later the juice was the *only* part of the plant that was not toxic."

After her students left, the shaman set up yet another trial for her: this time it was a shape-shifting experience that profoundly influenced her thinking about western herbal healing and enhanced her entire relationship to plants. She embraced this new concept of looking at the world from the plant's perspective and continued to study with the pohangar for several years, a remarkable time for

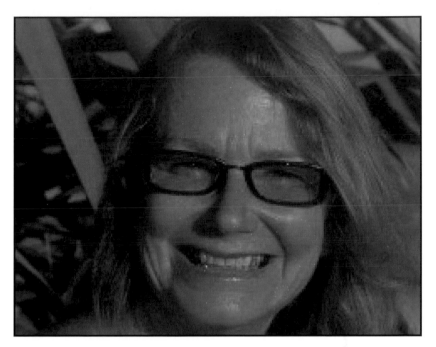

Photo credit: Isla Burgess

her. "He was both scary and amazing at the same time. He used to terrify me!"

Meet Isla

With her lovely, lilting New Zealand accent, Isla Burgess (pronounced like *island*) is spunky, enthusiastic, and charming. She is a beloved New Zealand herbalist, and, when I spoke with her, our conversation was speckled with laughter. Born in Dunedin in 1949, Isla is a tan, fit, and articulate ambassador for preserving and promoting herbal education in New Zealand and beyond. She directs the International College of Herbal Medicine, whose contemporary classrooms overlook flower-studded grasslands to the Pacific Ocean and beyond.

Her special interest in medicinal plants began after a friend gave her a copy of *Culpeper's Complete Herbal and English Physician* when she was a twenty-one-year-old high school biology teacher. "That just blew my mind," she says, "because at that time, there really wasn't herbal medicine. Well, you certainly couldn't buy herb plants from herbal nurseries and there weren't herbal manufacturing companies. That pretty much changed my life,

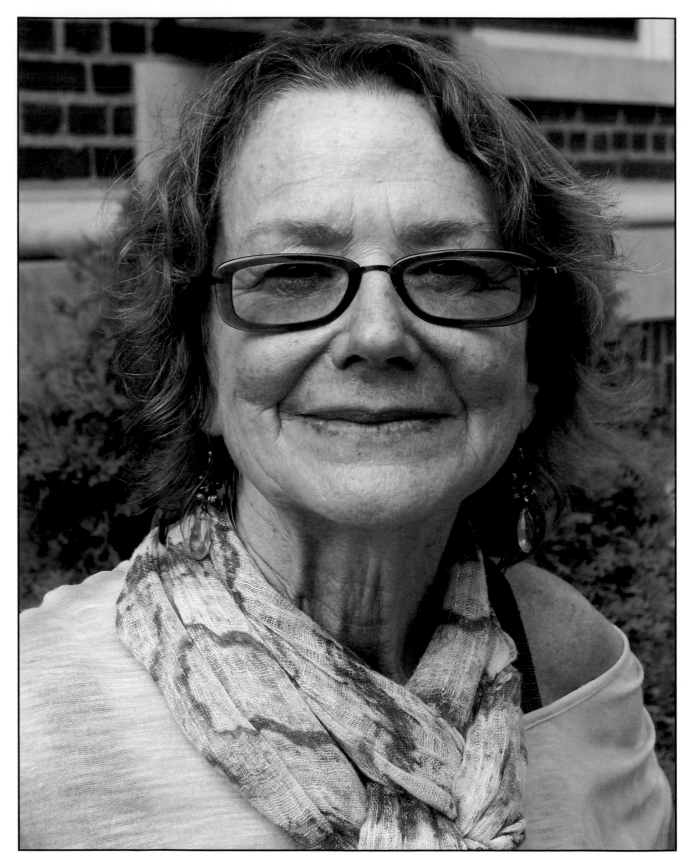

actually. It excited me that plants could also be used to heal, and so my search began."

"I really started looking at where I wanted to put my energy for the next decade or probably the rest of my life. I really wanted to give something back for the plants."

She discovered elecampane and valerian and enrolled in Dorothy Hall's correspondence course in Australia, but found it was only a few pages of reading. "I was hugely disappointed, because I was a science teacher at that point." She finally discovered Juliette de Bairacli Levy. "Her books were my mentor for quite some time," Isla says. She went on to study herbal medicine and naturopathy from an Australian college and engaged in some clinical practice, but she thought none of these approaches was truly adequate in terms of training people.

To remedy this, in 1990 she established the Waikato Centre for Herbal Studies, the first teaching college in New Zealand to focus on herbal medicine. For ten years, Isla served as director and principal tutor for the three-year course, and she spoke at international herbal conferences in Sydney and Auckland.

"I was seen as a bit of an upstart," she recalls. "I worked hard at putting plants back into the educational training here. I thought it was more important to have a *connection* with the plants that you use in medicine than it was to have anything else. That is still challenging some of the other educational institutes in New Zealand," she says. "And there was more talk about being less of a brown bottle herbalist and being more of an actual one."

In 2001, she established the International College of Herbal Medicine, an online two-year program of post graduate study for health professionals, and in 2003, she developed a three-year diploma in Clinical Herbal Medicine accredited by the New Zealand Association of Medical Herbalists.

Isla has also been a clinical practitioner for thirty-five years. "Even in clinical practice, I see myself primarily as an educator," she says. "I teach nutrition, taking care of yourself, herbal medicine. I primarily would say that teaching comes first and the other things follow." She teaches how to connect with the plants, which she now sees as the most rewarding aspect of her career. She published *Weeds Heal: A Working Herbal* in 1998 and educates others about mineral-rich herbs, such as nettle, oatstraw, St. John's

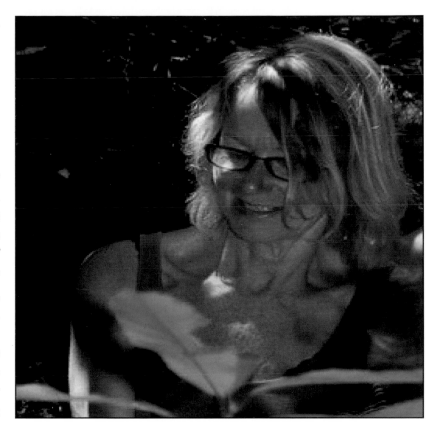

Photo credit: Isla Burgess

wort, ashwagandha, and rose hips. "These are the nourishing herbs," she says. "I see these as the staples. They're not perhaps herbs that I would use all the time as treatment approaches, but they're the underlying restorers and are wholly nourishing to the body."

After living what she calls a remarkable life for thirty-five years around medicinal plants, Isla began looking ahead to life after age sixty. "I really started looking at where I wanted to put my energy for the next decade or probably the rest of my life. I really wanted to give something back for the plants," she says. "I feel like we're in quite a serious situation in the world right now where we're losing medicinal plants every week because of the ransack. I wanted to focus my whole attention on the state of medicinal plants worldwide. How endangered are a whole variety of them? Can we develop a way of measuring the potential of that loss?" To this end, Isla enrolled at Schumacher College in Devon, southwest England, for a Master's Degree in Holistic Science, writing her dissertation on the sustainability of harvesting medicinal plants in the wild.

"For the first time in my life, I felt I really knew [plants] intimately. I feel like I've made another leap in that direction and that I am truly able to work from a plant perspective and get outside of myself."

Isla's most remarkable lessons came in the open bush of New Zealand, where she learned *Rongoa Maori*, the traditional medicine of the Native Maori tribal nations. She says there is some resistance from the tribal nations. "In the past, *pakeha* [Europeans] have come in and written books and not given respect to the sources from which they came." She says there are few who truly know the *Rongoa*, mostly those who are tribal-based or know someone in the tribe. Small Maori healing centers have been established with government support to work with local people in a primary health-care environment using only local plants in their practice.

A Plant's Perspective

Studies at Schumacher College led Isla to the philosophies of Johann Wolfgang von Goethe, a poet and playwright who died in1832. He researched plant development and embryology, teaching that the scientist is not, as previously assumed, a passive observer of an external reality, but instead participates with nature. Isla says her teacher helps her to "think plantly."

"For the first time in my life, I felt I really knew plants intimately. I feel like I've made another leap in that direction and that I am truly able to work from a plant perspective and get outside myself," she says, "I'm beginning to see that aspects of what [the shaman] taught me had dwelled in me in a way I wasn't realizing. I could pretty quickly shift now into feeling what that other being is like. I guess I'm on my way to becoming what you might call the shaman. I almost see it as the most important thing now, for which I am hugely grateful."

INNOVATE

Our word *new* is actually very old. The ancient hypothetical Proto-Indo-European language used *newos* for "new," while Sanskrit used *navah*, Persian *nau*, Hittite *newash*, Greek *neos*, and Welsh *newydd*. Old English speakers derived *niwe*, then *niowe*, then *neowe*, probably pronouncing each vowel. Finally, *new* became cemented in the English language. *Innovate* was first written in literature in 1548 and is a combination of *in* "into" and *novus* "new."

Isla is writing papers on developing plant–person relationships in healing and using an understanding of chaos and complexity science alongside a theory of co-evolution. She wants to establish that plants and people have an intimate connection in our evolutionary process.

"You have to make that plant connection if you're going to use its qualities, its parts, in the intimate plant–personal relationship in healing," she adds, "and I was looking at it from the perspective of restoration and maintenance of health. What we need to see is every single aspect of that plant is about energy—right from the electrons, every chemical constituent the plant has, everything. It's not so much that New Age way of saying, 'It's an energy relationship and something intangible.' This could be *tangible*. It could be what you see in an extraction of that plant, it's about every single aspect of that plant, right down to the particle level. That's why I think whole-plant medicine is very important. The essence of the plant, not the flower essence, but it's the whole plant that does this."

Her tutor at Schumacher College is promoting a scientific method to study this type of physical energy, and she is working with a colleague to publish their ideas. The whole plant is essential, she says—"no standardization, no isolation, no fiddling with the chemistry. I think if people pick it up, it will blow a few people's minds."

NEW ZEALAND

New Zealand is a country of water; it sports baths, hot healing mineral pools, spas, wells, crystal springs, beaches, glaciers, rivers, harbors, marine reserves, lakes, inlets, bays, and every type of water recreation imaginable. Its intimate population of only 4 million lives mostly on the North Island, leaving much of the South Island as wilderness preserves.

Polynesian Maori reached New Zealand in about 950 AD and the first Maori settled there around 1300 AD. In 1642, the Dutch East India Company sent Abel Tasman south from Java, Indonesia, to scout the territory, but his crew was attacked by Maori. The Dutch quickly abandoned the idea and Tasman fled New Zealand a mere three weeks after first seeing the "new" land. More than 120 years passed before James Cook arrived in 1769, and he smugly claimed the islands for England.

Many trees are sacred on these islands: the *Kauri* trees of northland once blanketed the region until they were logged. In Maori mythology, the *pohutukawa* tree was believed to be the conduit for the spirits of the dead, who descended down the roots of the tree to their homeland on *Hawaiki*.

The New Zealand Association of Medical Herbalists has been accepted for provisional registration under the Health Practitioners Competency and Assurance Act, which, says Isla, will both formalize and change the entire profession in the country. "Whatever we think of that (and there's huge debate about being licensed in the state and around the world) it will be interesting to see to what extent this changes the educational systems and programs, and to what degree there will be externally imposed procedures around the practice of herbal medicine in this country, and what will emerge from this."

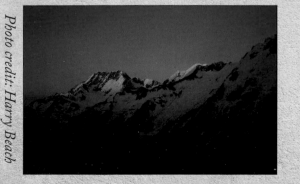

Photo credit: Harry Beach

Malte Brun Mountains in New Zealand's Southern Alps

ANGELICA
Angelica archangelica

A true favorite of drunken bees and other flying insects, angelica is an old-world plant that has been grown and enjoyed for centuries for its calming effect on the digestion. A biennial, it spends its first year close to the ground and sends up a tall, strong stalk its second year. The edible stems, leaves, and roots have a sweet, licorice-like flavor, and for this reason it has been candied throughout history for both pleasure and medicine. In addition to candies, the stem and seeds are used in liqueurs (notably absinthe, Chartreuse, Benedictine, and vermouth). Herbal medicine values the roots and seeds as carminative remedies for gas, bloating, and indigestion.

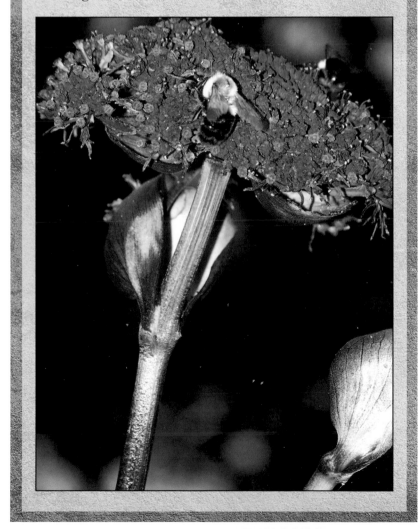

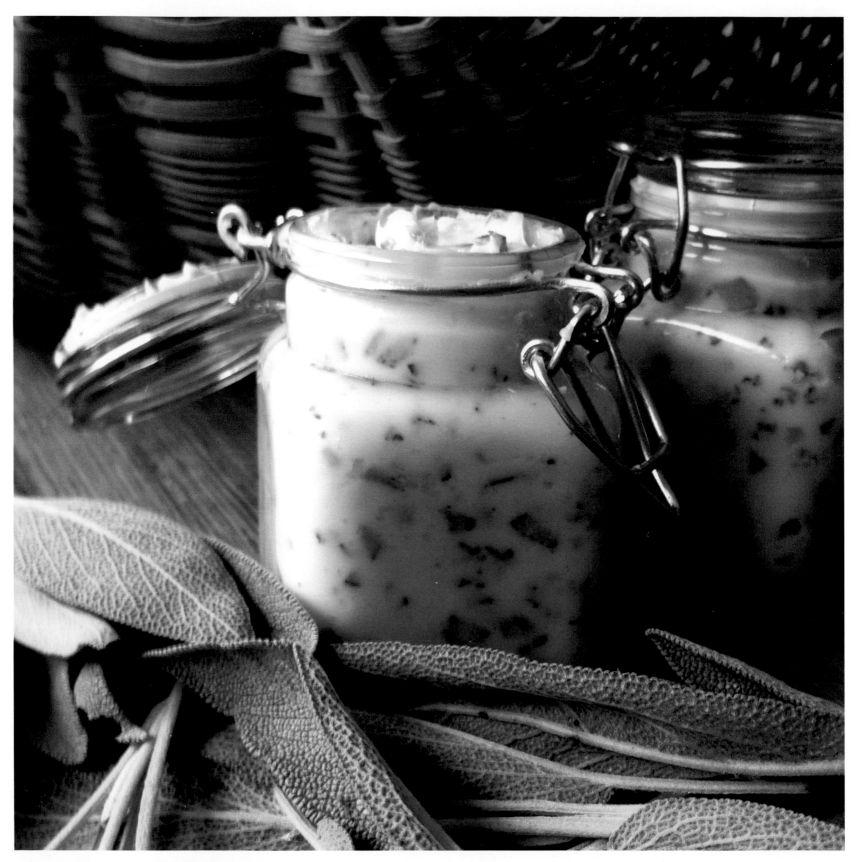

Chapter 2
NATIVE NATIONS MEDICINE

Today, 566 tribal nations call the United States their home—and since each region fosters its own kind of healing using herbs and trees endemic to its area, the broad collection that is native healing is rich and vibrant. While it's well known that native North and South American food plants such as corn, tomatoes, potatoes, cocoa, cranberries, ramps, juniper berries, squash, and pumpkins were new to European settlers/invaders in 1492, it's not so well known that North America has its own abundant healing herbs, as well.

Throughout history, native nations have used wild herbs as medicine to treat a wide variety of conditions, from headache and sore eyes to heart problems, skin issues, digestive disturbances, cancers, and more. Women's reproductive issues are commonly listed in books about native medicines and many plants were given monikers referring to their use for women, such as squaw vine (*Mitchella repens*).

Native plants include the bayberry shrub; the berberine-containing plants barberry, goldenseal, and coptis (goldthread); black cohosh and blue cohosh; bugleweed; boneset; chicory and dandelion; and the food plants cranberry and lamb's quarter. In addition to myriad edible and medicinal mushrooms, native people harvested bloodroot and other herbs to use as dyes and paints, and they used many grasses and barks for cordage and rope-making.

Sassafras was a popular herb when Captain Bartholomew Gosnold sailed the northeast seas in the late 1500s and early 1600s; its name is likely a corruption of saxifrage and the root was quickly shipped back to Europe as a potential cure for syphilis. The fragrant roots, twigs, bark, pith, and leaves of the tree were used by native tribes to treat fever, infection, nosebleeds, and to purify the blood.

Native healing methods are not restricted to botanicals; some tribes use fasting or cleanses before taking medicines, others include extensive prayer and spiritual shamanism. The sweat lodge is not only a place for stories and singing, but is a vital instrument for healing since letting go of waste products from the body and soul is required before healing can begin. Certain herbs are associated with this cleansing as well, including sage, tobacco, cedar, and sweetgrass.

Healing methods in the native Indian repertoire were more extensive than in European medicine; for example, one common way to relieve chest congestion was to inhale the smoke of burning herbs through a pipe; crushed leaves could be used as a snuff for headaches. These types of methods were seldom employed in other Western systems. Native medicine also included the widespread use of poultices, teas, rinses (eye problems were common), douches, and ointments.

Today there are roughly 5.2 million American Indians and Alaska natives living in the United States, which represents 1.7 percent of the US total population.[1] By far the largest tribal grouping is the Cherokee, followed by the Navajo, Choctaw, Mexican American Indian, Chippewa, Sioux, Apache, and Blackfeet.

Dr. Jody Noé

Jody Noé comes as something of a surprise: she says fun words like *moon-pauser* for women experiencing menopause and phrases such as *empower ourselves* in her popular herbal medicine lectures—and at the same time she conducts research and designs clinical trials in random comparison studies with prescriptive intervention in stomatitis. An anomaly for our age and a true inspiration, Jody is a fascinating and successful woman and role model who combines two identities not often found together: a traditional Cherokee and a nationally renowned naturopathic doctor.

Early in her career (as she would put it, in her "hippie days"), Jody approached her study of naturopathy with her arms held wide open: in addition to midwifery, she participated in California's gay pride movement, worked with Harvey Milk in San Francisco, "went a whole different way with my own civil rights movement," studied botany, ethnobotany, behavioral modification, psych nursing, plant science, exercise, nutrition, holistic nursing, healing touch, and worked with the disabled. She thought it would be a straightforward path from bachelor's to master's to medical doctor, but she received

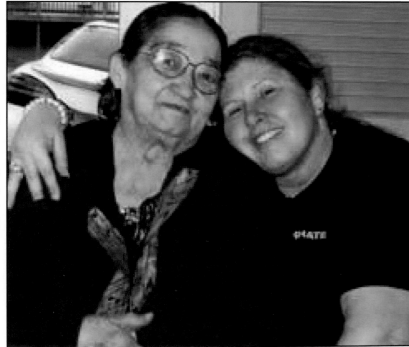

Jody with Mama Gene

a surprise soon after the completion of her studies that changed her life completely: the plants would not leave her alone. "I wanted zen in [my studies], I wanted all these things that didn't really exist in the eighties as an integrative degree. But I realized I really wanted to study the plants. They kept calling me, 'Just use me!'" Jody had to let go of her preconceived ideas of a mainstream career to heed to a spiritual calling. "I had a spiritual awakening because to go back to school, Spirit had to knock me over the head and say *this is not what you're supposed to do. You have to go back to school.* That's when I really started listening to Spirit; it was like a voice on the intercom, it was that clear."

Jody didn't want to listen at first; she tried to make outrageous deals, telling the Universe, *get rid of my credit cards and then I'll go back to school.* "And that happened!" she says. "My credit cards got consolidated, so I said, 'Alright I'll go back to school.'" At the time, she was living hippie-like on an organic farm growing produce she sold to a local food co-op; it was off the grid and very alternative. One night she had a dream where Spirit told her that school was really the Reservation. It was completely unexpected, as Jody had never had contact with a reservation, had not studied Native American practices or culture, and was only remotely aware that she might have Indian ancestry. She said to Spirit, "*What* reservation?!" But she decided to take a research trip to the Pamunkey and Mattaponi Reservations in Virginia. Intending her trip to be academic, she was surprised when she began cultivating relationships that led to spiritual education.

She was interviewed by Cherokee teacher Mary Chiltoskey (carefully interviewed, even *grilled*, one might say) and Cherokee teacher and pediatric nurse Mama Gene Jackson. These women took Jody under their guidance and instructed her to set up a campsite on a nearby mountain where Jody lived for the next three months, receiving counsel and learning. "It was very wholistic, not just studying. It was going out, walking in nature with the plants, the rituals of going to water, getting up at sunrise and going to bed at sunset." With these Cherokee elders, Jody studied herbal medicine and home remedies, considered the first line of therapy when sick. "The first medicines that all Cherokee women know are the helpful medicines. When you get sick in Cherokee fashion, you go home to the women—to the mother, the grandmother, the auntie—who will make you tea. It's a very indigenous tradition that was still in play in the eighties." But at the end of the year, Jody asked about the spirituality of the plants and the rituals of spirituality, and because she was not part of the tribe, she was sent to learn spiritual medicine in Oklahoma.

"I feel really connected to those South Carolina roots because I can totally understand giving up everything to stay with your landscape of memory, with your plants, with your land, with what you know and with those plants that talk to you and are part of your life."

To raise money for her journey, Jody called on her family and friends back on her organic farm; they held a giant potluck dinner, charged $5 per plate, and raised enough money to pay for the gas to get her to Oklahoma. She arrived in Tahlequah, the capital of the Cherokee Nation, and pitched her tent in the yard of the Cherokee Nation's spiritual leader Crosslin S. Smith; the elder returned from Stomp Dance to find Jody waiting for him "and I've been with him ever since. I'll train with him for the rest of my life," Jody says. "Traditionally, you study the Cherokee Way from age thirty to age fifty; at fifty you can become a teacher."

Jody had begun a little early, at age twenty-seven, after her year with Mary Chitolski in the Appalachians. With Crosslin and his wife, Glenna, Jody completed seasonal chores and worked in a medicine room in an old cabin. "It's his home," she says, "and people will come all hours of the day, and if we're eating dinner, even if they're strangers, they'll eat dinner with us and then they'll

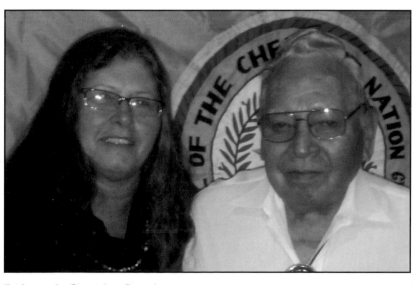

Jody with Crosslin Smith

go in and do medicine. It's very organic. It's a very different kind of concept of medicine, so the teaching too—you have to live there, you have to go through the chores of running a ranch to building a house, all that stuff is in the teaching. How to listen to the plants. I went through years and years of teaching with him on how to obtain the Good Mind, to put yourself into the Good Mind before you are able to go and collect medicine. The plants call you, and once you obtain that Good Mind, you can't talk from sunrise to sunset. The long and short of it is that it allows you to actually hear the voice of the plant, which I imagine is what many people would call the Spirit.

"We used to get up at sunrise and he'd say, 'Let's go get all the roots and plants that we'll need today because we'll have a large group of people,' and he wouldn't know, but they would line up down the block and they'd wait and they'd come one at a time and he would see them outside in his lawn chair underneath the tree, and they would do medicine. I would have the roots and would prepare them, all different kinds of roots. I asked him one time, 'How do you know what kinds of roots you need if you don't have the people there in front of you?' He said, 'That's what I'm trying to teach you, you gotta listen to the plants. I'm just going out and picking the plants that are telling me to pick them today. The people are going to come that need these plants. You're thinking about this all wrong!'"

Crosslin is the grandson of Redbird Smith, founder of the traditional Keetoowahs—the traditionalists of the Cherokee—and he is the son of Stoke Smith, the chief of the traditional Keetoowah.

Roots and Ancestry

The Cherokee Nation is a huge, prosperous, sovereign nation. "It's a city," Jody says, "it has courthouses, buildings, the high school gym is like a giant university. It's a big industry, a big nation." The Eastern band is much smaller, looks more Native American, and has a boundary—the top of the Great Smokies. The Nation is a boundary-less reservation and has many dilutes of blood since members are not required to meet a blood quantum or have direct lineage to qualify. Jody is a member of neither; when she began studying Native plant medicines, she was not aware of her Cherokee roots. She completed her bachelor's, wrote her master's thesis *Ethnobotany of the Cherokee People*, submitted her unique collection of 250 specimens of both Eastern and

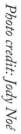

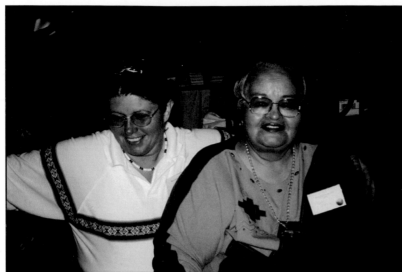

Jody with Glynna Smith

The Cherokee language is the only Southern Iroquoian language still spoken today. A reference to *Chalaque* first appeared in a Portuguese narrative of De Soto's expedition in 1557, then as *Cheraqui* in a French document of 1699, and finally in its current Anglicized form *Cherokee* in 1708.[1] Etymologist Douglas Harper also lists *Tsaragi* as an early spelling of Cherokee from the 1670s, though he lists no sources. The written form of the language was invented by Cherokee farmer and silversmith Sequoyah, or George Gist, in 1821.

Though Sequoyah's life remains largely speculative, he is believed to have been the son of a Cherokee mother and possibly a migrant German father, raised in the village of Tuskegee. He was a farmworker and also a silversmith,[2] and he began creating his syllabary in 1809. His loosely mixed alphabetical characters of Roman, Cyrillic, Arabic, and Greek letters, and his writing method was finally accepted by a wary and suspicious Cherokee public in 1825, a year after the General Council of the Cherokee awarded him a silver medal of honor and appreciation.

Western Cherokee botanicals to an herbarium collection housed at Dominion College, and moved to Seattle to attend Bastyr naturopathic medical school. It was here, of all places, that she finally discovered her Cherokee ancestry when, of all things, she met a man who had appeared to her in a dream years before: Robert Ward, White Cloud, a direct descendant of Nancy Ward, took one look at Jody and told her she must be related to him. They performed a big ceremony for Jody and when she later began genealogical research she discovered he was right: her grandfather's mother was a Martin Cherokee, a direct descendant of Nancy Ward. "That's the South Carolina Cherokees, those South Carolinians where my mother was born and raised, still living in the same spot where they've lived all generations as Cherokee. I feel really connected to those South Carolina roots because I can totally understand giving up everything to stay with your landscape of memory, with your plants, with your land, with what you know and with those plants that talk to you and are part of your life. In some way, that kept my people there. And they lost everything and had to hide their culture and hide who they were, but it's that connection."

Born in Norfolk, Virginia, in 1959, Jody was the first of her mother's family to be born out of South Carolina. She was also the first of her father's family born in America after he had emigrated from Sicily, Italy, to Ellis Island. Her parents moved to California, where Jody spent the first decade of her life in a close-knit, Italian, old-world community.

"The plants go on both sides!" she says happily. "The plant medicines go on both sides. My Italian *nonna* grew her own plants and would also smuggle plants from Sicily when she went to visit. She brought over a Sicilian jasmine, a fig tree, and other native plants to grow in her yard in California. She always used herbal medicine and cooked with herbs; she made everything from scratch like from old-world Italy. She never drove a car or became an American citizen, though she married an Italian American man after my grandfather was killed in 1939 in the war. All the herbal medicine I grew up with started with her because when we got sick, she would bring down jars of loose-leaf herbs and make herbal teas for us. She always used chamomile for everything, with lots of sugar to sweeten it up! I remember her boiling herbs in her coffee pot when we got sick. I'm not sure what those were but she grew them all in her yard."

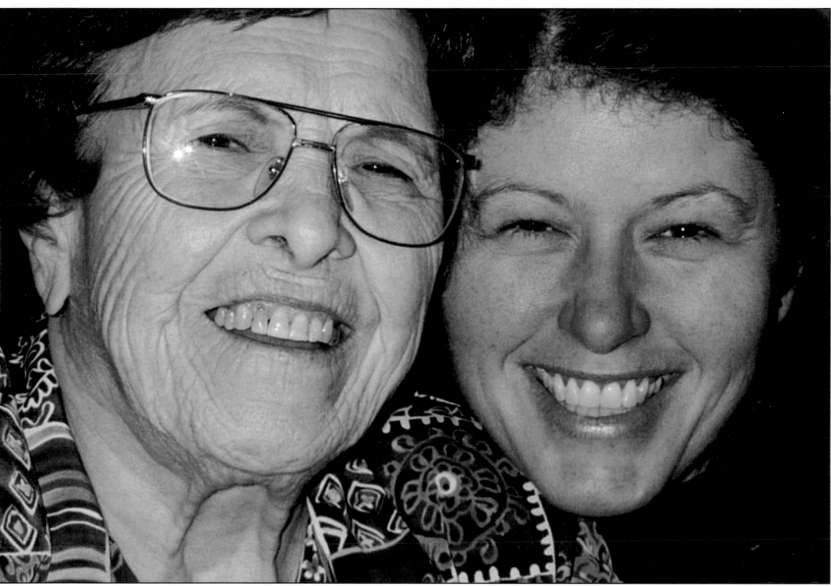

Jody with her Italian Nona Josephine D'Agostino Noé Satariano

When her parents divorced, Jody moved to Virginia with her mother and sisters. "At a 1970s family reunion in South Carolina, where the Cherokee branch was, my great Aunt Sally came up to me; since I'm pretty tall and big and she had tall girls, and everyone else in the family is pretty short, she tried to tell me things in a roundabout way about Indian people in our bloodline. I asked my mom about it but she said no way. I learned it was really taboo in a certain period of that family history to let your native bloodline be known, so it was hidden."

Jody's Practice

Today, the first thing Jody tries to do in her busy Connecticut naturopathic practice is make the patient feel like family. "It's very relaxed, sitting in comfortable chairs; we spend nearly two hours for the first visit and an hour for the second." For cancer patients that includes labs, diagnostics, pathologies, treatments, what they do, what failed. But, Jody says, integrated into that scientific medical approach is diet, lifestyle, spirituality, the "hygienes" (sleep habits, stress habits, elimination, and so on).

"It's a very wholistic old-fashioned approach. If we need to do a physical exam or test, we have time, and they also have time to talk to me, that's why they want to come. I put it together physiologically, biologically, with biochemistry, and I prescribe with the top layer of my intuition guiding that. The spirituality of the plants comes in through that way. I could be talking to a patient about their diagnostic imaging and a plant might pop up right there, so I've learned to listen and say, 'Oh that plant wants to be with this person, I've got to put this plant into their regimen.' We're blending the science and the spirituality. I call it spirit-mind-body medicine instead of mind-body-spirit medicine."

Jody's apothecary includes dried herbs, tinctures, essential oils, homeopathics, capsules, teas, whole herbs, combination therapies, aromatherapy, topicals, spirituals, ethnogens, and more, and she's created databases for intensive client education. Her book *The Textbook of Naturopathic Integrative Oncology* includes a large section on nutrition, diet, and medical botany where she looks at the constituents of the plants and their targeted effect on patients for cancer and their whole effect with the whole herb. "It's really fascinating because everything that my indigenous elders have taught me [about herbs] has proven true with science. Now that plant medicine is so abundantly studied across the world, it's easy to find that this plant was traditionally used for cancer and guess what—its constituent is now used for cancer! Periwinkle, your *Vinca* species, that's vincristine in chemotherapy. Sanguinarin from bloodroot . . . I can't tell you how many of those indigenous learnings are proving to be true. Mistletoe, that's *Viscum album*, that white mistletoe grown on oak is what isacadore is. It's amazing. That's been my whole life's work, using everything I've learned throughout all the levels and places."

Jody is a professor of oncology and family medicine at the University of Bridgeport College of Naturopathic Medicine, is the founder of the Integrative Oncology Clinic, and is the chair of Botanical Medicine. She's not nearly finished. "There's a lot more to [what I teach] than biochemistry, though I really think biochemistry is just the expression of Spirit. It works for me, the science of the Spirit. I tell my students and I tell my elders and my family: I have a lot to do in this lifetime, and I have to do it. It's like a calling."

CEDAR
Thuja spp. and Juniperus spp.

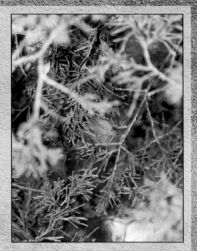

Many cedars and junipers share their names, making identification confusing. Red cedar, or *Juniperus virginiana*, grows throughout the Eastern and central parts of the United States and the poles made from its red wood (used as boundary markers by native peoples) were the inspiration for the naming of Baton Rouge by French traders. Known as White Cedar or Arbor Vitae (Tree of Life), *Thuja occidentalis L.* is used as a fragrance, ceremonial incense, medicine, and food. The lacy, flat-scaled leaves and the rough red bark contain the volatile oil *thujone* and, despite confusion, this tree is not the Juniper (*Juniperus Oxycedrus*) called prickly cedar.

The Ojibwe used the pith of the young white cedar to make a sweet soup, and the Iroquois inhaled the steam from a decoction of the leaves to remedy colds. Many nations used various cedars as a poultice to treat swellings and sores and burned the wood to purify sacred objects and ceremonial participants. Iroquois women valued cedar leaf infusion as a tonic during pregnancy and as a diaphoretic to increase a new mother's milk flow. The infusion made a type of "sitz bath" for the vaginal area postpartum.

Members of the Maliseet Nation used cedar as a burn dressing—drying the under-bark, pounding it to a powder and mixing it with grease. British Columbia nations burned cedar smoke or incense to clear bad emotions and to purify the air after an illness.

Often called red-dirt country, Georgia includes rural sprawling country, charming antebellum farmhouses, and inner-city metropolitan culture and business. The last of the thirteen colonies to join the Union (in 1733), Georgia seceded more than a hundred years later to join the Confederacy. The British attempted to empty their debtor's prisons into Georgia, though this was largely unsuccessful. Its neighbor South Carolina became a state in 1800, seceded in 1860, and was readmitted in 1868.

What *was* successful, however, at least from the white settler's point of view, was Georgia's removal of all eastern Native nations from its lands. When gold was discovered in 1829 near Dahlonega in Georgia's mountains, hoards of settlers moved in to claim the wealth. However, the lands were mostly Cherokee lands; in 1830, Georgia enacted the Indian Removal Act whereby it legally banished its Native American population (which had refused allegiance to Georgia's government and operated its own written constitution). Over the next eight years, first the Choctaw left Georgia and South Carolina, then the Seminole, the Creek, and the Chicasaw. By 1837, 46,000 Native peoples had evacuated their homelands, opening 25 million acres to white settlement and exploitation.

Most of those that remained by 1838 were forcibly relocated to Indian Territory (Oklahoma) during what came to be known as the Trail of Tears. "The Cherokee are very resilient people," says Dr. Jody Noé. "They were yanked out and stockaded and genocided along the way; some 6,000 to 10,000 people (underestimated at 4,000) died on that walk. [They moved] to a whole new earth-based place to live—and to thrive, to be successful and resilient and to now be prosperous says a lot about a people. I have a lot of respect for the Eastern band of Cherokee and their leaders and the Western band of Cherokee and their leaders. And the other bands—the Arkansas band, the Texas band, the state-recognized bands, the non-recognized bands like the South Carolina band, all these people are now successful at getting recognized, saying, 'We're here, this little part of our culture is still alive in this part of the community.' The Cherokee people are an amazing people."

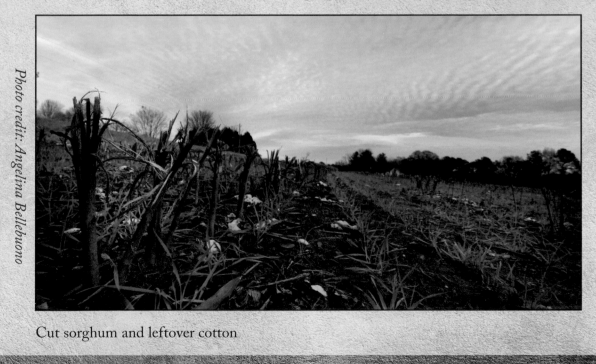

Photo credit: Angelina Bellebuono

Cut sorghum and leftover cotton

Ada-Belinda DancingLion

Born to parents of the Lakota Sioux/Blackfoot, and Anishinabe Nations, Ada-Belinda DancingLion also claims West African heritage and proudly refers to herself as a Black Indian. Tall and sporting long dreadlocks, Ada-Belinda has an easy laugh and a strong voice and is a vibrant, enthusiastic keeper of her ancestors' traditions. Her elders of the White Horse Warrior Mountain Lion clan named her She Walks With Lightning for good reason—Ada-Belinda is a powerhouse of historic information regarding women's traditions, healing ceremonies, and the importance of heritage.

At age eight, Ada-Belinda began apprenticing with her Lakota Sioux/Blackfoot great-grandmother. She later studied with Cameroonian healer and plant geneticist Tabi Orang and Master African Conga drummer Malik Del Mar.

"I carry a pipe and pour Lodge in Anishinabe fashion (though I'm of Lakota blood)," she says. "There aren't many women who pour in Lakota tradition. Anishinabe is more matrilineal." She is the youngest person in her nation to carry a pipe and facilitate the sacred "sweat lodge" ceremony as water pourer, an honor because water is Life. The meeting of water and stone during ceremony is a sacred occasion.

"When we sit in Lodge, we are literally availing ourselves of all elements—earth, fire, water, and air—to be reborn. We are in a womb-type structure shaped like a big pregnant belly," she laughs. "We go in with ails and worries, and we use herbs to release that which is causing us harm. We are renewed and reborn," Ada-Belinda says. "Plant your experiences into the earth and they'll bear fruit for future generations, which is why we say that for seven generations into the future we must consider our actions, words, and deeds."

"Every step upon the earth is a prayer."

Re-learning the Old Ways

Ada-Belinda believes it is important to archive knowledge for the use of future generations. "Information about the women's holocaust, herbal healers, the suppression of indigenous people—

this information was not available to us, which is why as a culture the wisdom of plants and natural healing was not there for us," she says. "There was a punitive energy that cautioned, 'If you reach for this, there will be terrible repercussions.' For a long time, humanity bore the brunt of this loss of information, suffering poor health and vitality, but as we mature as a culture, we find there is value in what the elders had to say. Now, we're consulting with them: 'What did you used to do?' It has new names: Permaculture, being green, living in harmony, but it's the indigenous way."

Plants are central to her tenets of healing. "We need to treat plants as teachers, as our elders and grandmothers, and respect them accordingly. Even if one plant becomes extinct, it affects everything else—the weather, the availability of medicine, air, and water quality. We have no right to wipe anything off the earth—if we do, we do so to our own detriment."

"Today's science is yesterday's magic."

Ada-Belinda uses abundant local foods as medicine, including nettle, oatstraw, and comfrey. "Start with food and toning plants such as motherwort and St. Joan's Wort. Then move to infusions, tinctures, to the really strong plants." In ceremonies, Ada-Belinda uses sage, cedar, sweet grass, tobacco, bear-root, and osha. "Use what is in season and grows near you," she advises. "Shipping plants across the globe is not natural. How much access did our ancestors have to Costa Rican lilies? We used to call it walking softly upon the earth—now it's called our 'carbon footprint.'" Ada-Belinda smiles: "Every step upon the earth is a prayer."

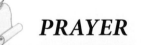

PRAYER

The PIE *prek* meant to ask, request, or entreat, just as Sanskrit *prasna* meant to question, and Lithuansin *prasyti*, to ask or beg. From this came Latin's *precari*, to ask earnestly. In the 900s, Old French used *preier*, which entered English circa 1300 as *prayer*.

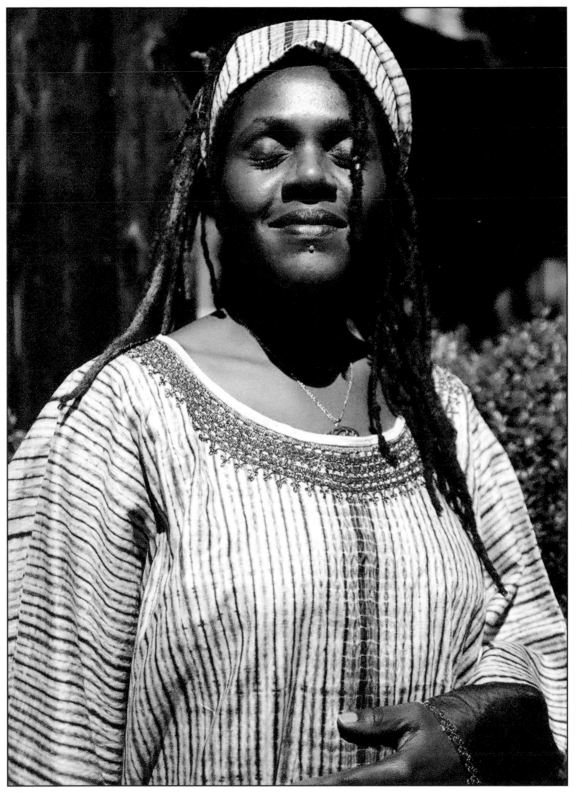

MILKWEED AND BUTTERFLY WEED
Asclepias syriaca and *A. tuberosa*

The cousins milkweed and butterfly weed have a very devoted winged fan club; both these perennials attract butterflies by the hundreds and are prized in colorful butterfly gardens. As the name suggests, milkweed exudes a milky latex sap from its stalk, though its young flower buds are edible and make a pleasant wild-food treat.

Named for the ancient deified healer Asclepius, the family *Asclepiadaceae* boasts more than two thousand species, one of which defies that characteristic that groups them all: butterfly weed has no milky latex sap but instead exudes a watery juice. This lovely orange wildflower is respectfully called *pleurisy root* because Europeans and Native Americans have both used it as an expectorant for lower lung congestion, pleurisy, and bronchial spasm. The bitter pounded root also has use as an external anti-inflammatory, a vulnerary for wounds, and as a laxative.

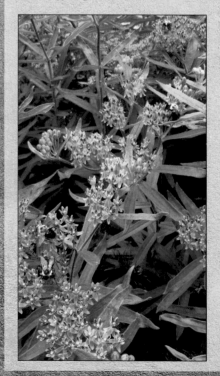

SAGE
Salvia officinalis

Sages are eaten, smoked, inhaled, smudged, dried, burned, drunk, and tinctured, as the plant is a source of great medicinal, culinary, and even shamanic value in cultures throughout the world.

White sage is a popular ceremonial herb, while *Salvia officinalis*, common garden sage, lends its unique flavor to grilled meats and broth. Medicinally, astringent sage treats fever, sore throats, mouth ulcers, and swollen gums. Nursing mothers wean their babies by drinking sage tea or cooking with dried sage. Rosemary Gladstar hails sage as a "yang" grounding herb for relieving menopausal hot flashes, and herbalist Ben Charles Harris praised sage for healing the liver and gallbladder and for removing kidney stones. Harvard scientists are researching the esoteric species *Salvia divinorum* as a hallucinogen with potential for treating schizophrenia and bipolar mood disorders.

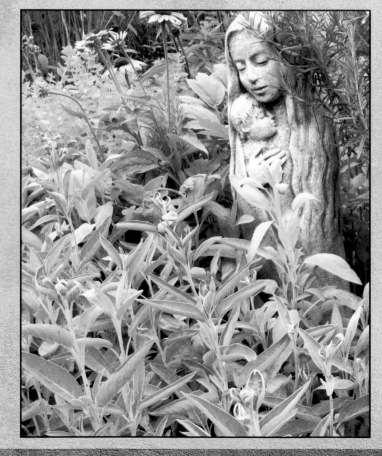

Chapter 3
POLYNESIAN MEDICINE

Polynesia is made up of more than one thousand islands in the central and southern Pacific Ocean, including Hawai'i, Samoa, Tonga, the Cook Islands, and Papua New Guinea. In Hawai'i, which means "the breath and water of God," many healing techniques and philosophies have withstood intense governmental and cultural pressure to cease to exist. In fact, much of Hawai'i's culture underwent a profound eradication campaign by the US government but, thankfully, it survived and is now experiencing a resurgence. Due to its history and locale, Hawai'i is strongly influenced by Eastern philosophies including Chinese medicine, chi gong, acupuncture, musical Qi gung, and other healing techniques that are not necessarily Hawai'ian. Between these Eastern influences and the crushing influence of modern Western medicine, traditional native Hawai'ian healing methods are fringe methods even in their home country.

At the University of Hawai'i at Manoa, Chair of Complementary and Alternative Medicine Rosanne Harrigan says that, unfortunately, "Ninety percent of local physicians and conventional health workers brush aside the *kahuna* and their work," unless a patient lives in a "Hawai'ian homeland" area. "Most [native Hawai'ians] are seen at the community health centers, but they really haven't set up a good model anywhere." Harrigan says integration of modern Western medicine with native practices is slow and is not a priority for white Western physicians, even though their patients are native Hawai'ians.

She adds, however, that a few physicians and hospitals will allow kahuna to come into their facilities and even practice their healing methods alongside the physician. "If you're from a Hawai'ian family and you know who to ask for, they just come marching in like they're your visitor," she says. "It's not like they do smoke signals in the room or anything weird. It's meaningful for the patients." But many hospitals are still hostile to local practitioners and decline the opportunity to integrate the philosophies. "For instance, at Waianai," says Harrigan, "it's very separate. I find that problematic because you have to integrate the two systems or nobody gets to enjoy the wealth of the other. [When I was] at Waimanolo Health Center, the kahuna there actually practiced [their traditional medicine] and wrote in the medical record. That's really much better: the *kahuna* knew what we were doing, we knew what he was doing, and everybody benefitted."

Other hospitals, such as the Queens Medical Center, allow healing touch for patients but don't charge for it, a vague practice that makes placing an economic value on healing impossible. "It's like it is really not allowed to be legitimate," says Harrigan. This may stem from the native barter tradition whereby healers don't charge but instead work out a system of exchange with their patients. Harrigan says there is now an undercurrent of exploration into placing a monetary value on the services provided by native healers within the modern hospital system.

Traditional Methods

Thanks to a strong cultural interest and the desire by native Hawai'ians to maintain their heritage (at a great cost), many native Hawai'ian techniques still exist today. They are being practiced not only by the elders (for whom many rituals are distant family memories), but also by young people excited by the reclamation of their ancient heritage that was precipitously close to extinction.

Of the many native Hawai'ian healing arts, the following stand out as emblematic of a proud, creative, and gentle culture: *lomi-lomi* (massage); *pale keki* (midwifery); *oli* (chanting); *hula* (dance); and *ho'oponopono* (mediation). The late healer Raylene Kawaiae'a said this means "to make things right with yourself and God."

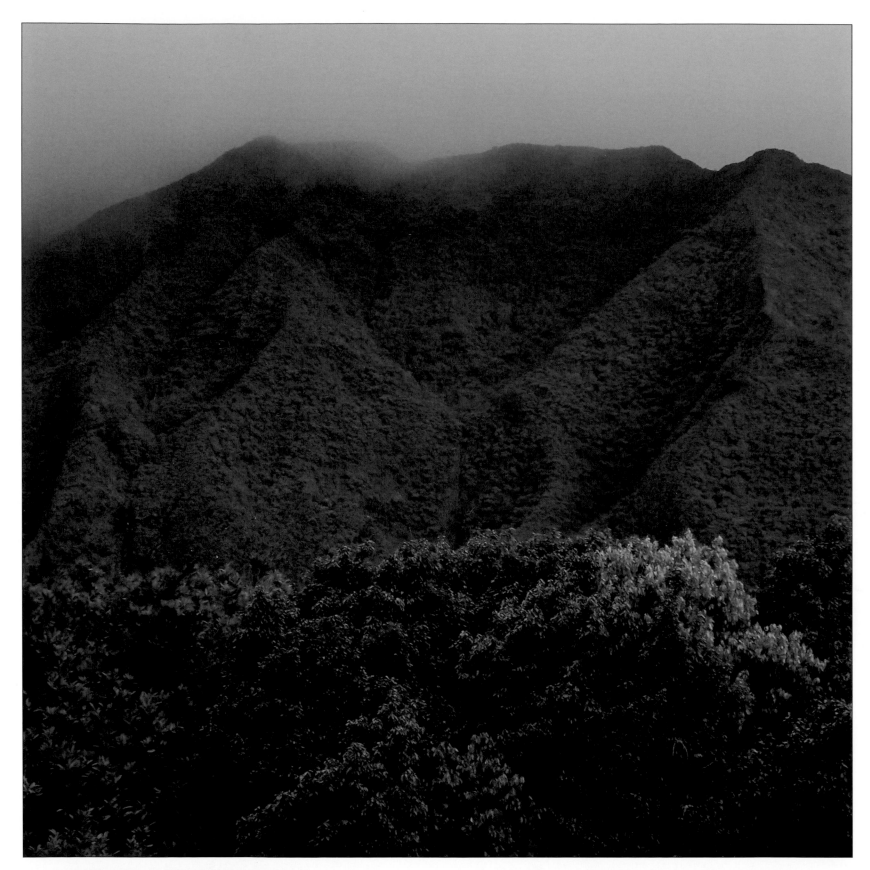

When healer Auntie Velma was growing up in the Kahuku and Kalihi regions of Oahu, her father was the *Kahu* (oldest member of the family) who presided over every meal with this very important ritual: before anyone could eat, they performed a blessing and practiced *ho'oponopono*. Her father asked everyone at the table, "Is there anything you've done wrong during the day? Any problems you've had? Misunderstandings? Hard feelings?" Auntie Velma's mother would confess any negative energy and clear out bad feelings. They would go around the table, each voicing his or her thoughts and letting the negative energy go—releasing it so everyone could eat peacefully. "It clears the energy in the house," Auntie Velma says. "He didn't miss it too many times. A few times everything was good so he just gave thanks."

La'au lapa'au

The medical practice of healing in ancient Hawai'i centered around the use of plants, a practice which became *la'au lapa'au*, or herbalism. Typically a child (usually male, but not always) was identified by his elders when he was young as possessing healing potential and gifts that would make him a successful healer. He would be trained throughout adolescence and would be given tests once he reached adulthood. If he completed these tests, there would be great ceremonies that solidified his status as a healer, and he would choose his specialty. He would become a *kahuna*, or priest.

The discipline was advanced and the areas of healing ability were very specific, though it must be understood that all healers were inherently spiritual priests, as well. The two disciplines of medicine and religion went hand-in-hand for the betterment of the patient and for the health of the community as a whole.

In the ancient Hawai'ian medical system—before Cook invaded the islands—new healers were taught the following skills, in this order:

> Learning all matters pertaining to the gods, "from whom all knowledge came."
> Learning prayers of thanksgiving and prayers to the gods;
> Learning the kinds of disease;
> Learning remedies for disease;
> Learning the art of killing;
> Learning the art of saving life. (Gutmanis, 15)

According to noted Hawai'ian cultural scholar George Kanahele, once indoctrinated as a priest and healer, the new kahuna could choose from the following specialties:

> *Kahuna la'au lapa'au*: a priest and trained expert in traditional Hawai'ian herbal medicine;
> *Kahuna haha*: priest or doctor who perform diagnosis by feeling with the fingers;
> *Kahuna 'ea*: specialized in treating congenital disorders in children;
> *Kahuna 'o'o*: treating infants to close the anterior fontanel;
> *Kahuna paaoao*: pediatricians for infants;
> *Kahuna ho'ohapai keiki* and *kahuna ho'ohanau keiki*: gynecologists and obstetricians;
> *Kahuna ha'iha'i-iwi*: bone setter;
> *Kahuna lomilomi*: physical therapist/massage therapist/osteopath;
> *Kahuna 'ana'ana*: priest trained in death prayers.

In Hawai'i today, especially on Oahu, there are many so-called underground healers, usually elders who have gained their knowledge through a lifetime of experience but who have not endured formal training at universities or hospitals. "They are the last ancient group," says Harrigan, "the old women healers. They haven't given their authority over to a newer group of younger women, and in some ways this is scary because they could actually cause their own demise. Their healing tradition could disappear. It concerns me because I sometimes watch people try to hold onto power. In Japan, they'll wait until some eighty-year-old has keeled over, but by then it's too late because the young person [who would have learned the skills had this master shared them] has already fallen behind." Part of Hawai'i's challenge is to integrate the knowledge of the elders with the new generation of healers who are anxious to keep this unique heritage alive.

Auntie Velma DelaPena

Kahuna Auntie Velma DelaPena is a Polynesian healer with a calm, comfortable demeanor that puts one at ease. When we met in Waimanola, O'ahu, Hawai'i, Auntie Velma welcomed me with a soft, merry voice to her home: a large tarp-tent with gravel flooring, a long table, a refrigerator, stove, television, and a healing/massage table. It is a chilly winter day on Oahu—70 degrees with a light rain blowing sideways into the tent. Auntie Velma brings me a mug of hot water, smiles, and sits in a folding deck chair.

At seventy years young, Auntie Velma finds happiness in her children, her twenty-three grandchildren, and fifteen great-grandchildren, many of whom visit her every Sunday. Born in 1939, Auntie Velma is a traditional Hawai'an healer, a *kupuna* (elder) and a *kahuna* (healer). She had no teacher ("I've never taken a class," she says) but she learned by listening to the spirits. "They were my teachers, my inspiration. The spirits are my mentors." She was born, she says gently, with the spirits guiding her. "When I was three, they'd show me things I needed to learn. I told them to go away and leave me alone. But they didn't! They taught me how to survive, how to look at things and see how to use them." Auntie Velma spent her life teaching *lomilomi* (massage), herbal medicine, spiritual healing, and leading workshops.

"It's not hard to do what I do," she says. "It's easy to let go, to release, to do what you have to do. I love to share what I know," and she notes that conventional medical doctors are fairly open to what she has to share, especially doctors who grew up in Hawai'i.

"I love helping people, it makes me feel good to see their faces with big smiles after I've worked with them. I work with the elders—the *tutus*, they like to be worked on and it makes them feel better. They love to vent," she laughs. "You have to be a good listener." She looks up at the giant mountains directly behind her, formed when the Koolau Volcano pushed the stunning steep peaks vertically more than three thousand feet, creating the thirty-seven-mile-long Koolau mountain range. "Do you want to see my spirits?"

While we shield our eyes from the light rain, she indicates features in the jagged cliffs that appear carved into almost-recognizable forms. "There," she points, "is Pocahontas. There is Kwan Yin. And there is the first Queen of Spain." The shapes resemble human features, and she looks tenderly at this mountain's resemblance to the world's brave women who serve as role models and spiritual guides. To Auntie Velma, I believe these spirits are more real than the mountain itself—they form the mountain, rather than the mountain forming them.

"I'm trying to wake everybody up—not to taste the coffee but to feel the energy!"

Auntie Velma is planning to establish a center below her beloved mountain where priests, healers, and elders can share their knowledge with "youngsters," where people can communicate, learn, and teach. "*Kahuna* love to share," she says, but she warns that a person's heart must be open to receiving. "*Kahuna* can tell your energy, and they won't work on you if it's negative. You must keep yourself open."

Auntie Velma has lived in this tent between the tall peaks of Waimanalo, on the eastern (windward) shore of Oahu, and the Pacific Ocean for twenty-five years. "I love it," she says. "I can feel the energies of the ocean and the mountain. It's awesome, when you're working on someone and feel that energy flowing. Hawai'ians believe you must go into the ocean to be healed; after that I'll work on them. You can feel the difference in their energy." She says mountains takes away negative energy and the ocean provides new energy. "Some people don't feel that energy, that's the sad part. You can heal yourself better if you can feel it. I'm trying to wake everybody up—not to taste the coffee but to feel the energy!"

She especially likes to guide children to feel that energy. "I like to teach the kids of today, but they have a different agenda," she says. "It's very hard. I work with them one day at a time. I like to tell them that there are better things out there in the world that we [the Hawai'ian elders] have to offer. But who knows? One day my dream will come true." Velma is a licensed Christian minister, and two of her sons followed in her path. "The girls are starting to get into it. I tell them, if you don't understand, ask the question. But they don't know how much work is in store for them!"

Hawai'i's History

Auntie Velma and her parents grew up in a strange, terrifying, and unfortunate time in Hawai'i's history, when the very

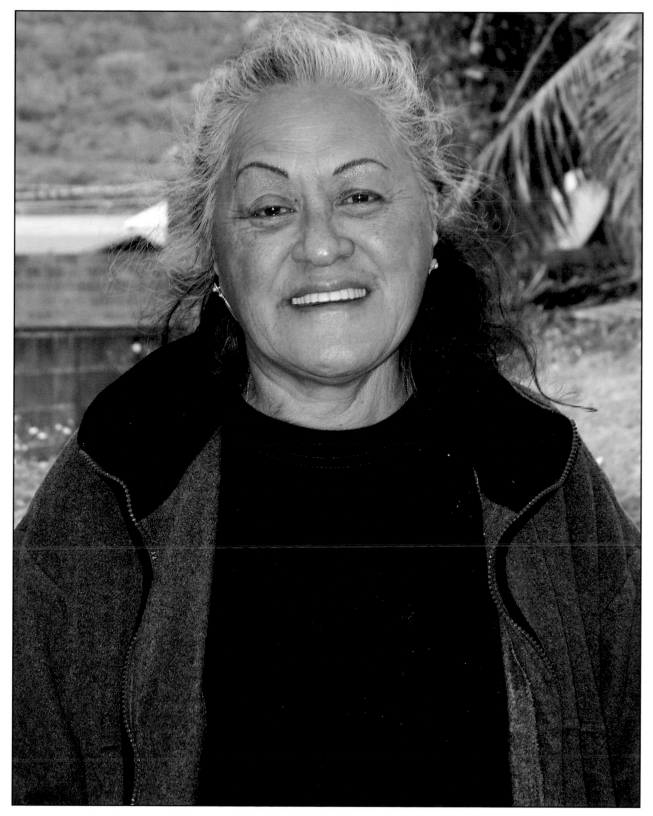

Auntie Velma DelaPena

knowledge of Hawai'ian language would land a family in trouble. The Hawaiian language, 'olelo Hawai'i, was suppressed and restricted from being taught in public schools when the Hawai'ian monarchy was overthrown in 1893. By 1896, the provisional government banned the speaking or teaching of Hawai'ian language in public schools, and complete annexation into the United States (as a territory) took place in 1898. Auntie Velma's parents were taught never to speak Hawai'ian, under threat of severe punishment. Many Hawai'ian families adopted Japanese names to avoid government notice. Later, she says, the Hawai'ian names were never recovered. "They were lost. Now Hawai'ian genealogy is full of Japanese names." Not until 1978 was 'olelo Hawai'i made an official language of the State of Hawai'i, and public schools were finally allowed to teach 'olelo Hawai'i in 1987. Not until 1990 (almost one hundred years after the overthrow of the monarchy) did US government policy acknowledge Hawai'ians' right to preserve and use their indigenous language and the ban was formally removed in 1993.

"The Hawai'ian language is a dangerous language," she says as the winds whip down from the high peaks and make the tent tarps slap loudly. "The word is sacred. I won't teach my children the language. I tell them if they want to learn it, they need to go take a class. In the older days, people were in-tune with each other, they could read minds" and understand the subtle ways of communicating. "Then, the words came and would be sung, not spoken. It was like a melody they had. The next generations learned how to speak the word, not sing."

"It's easy to let go, to release, to do what you have to do. I love to share what I know."

Auntie Velma wants to instill in the Hawai'ian people a love for their heritage and the pride and power that comes with honoring that history. "We want to bring back the strength we used to have," she says. "We need ho'oponopono." She wants to share with her fellow Hawai'ians her great love for her land and language, so that they can celebrate the ha "breath," wa "water," and i "life": the breath and water of life that is *Hawai'i.*

QUESTION

True healers say that if you don't ask, you'll never know. Auntie Velma DelaPena says, "If you don't understand, ask the question." Hawai'ian traditional healer Levon Ohai teaches that through *pule* (prayer), answers are received. "The best way to learn herbal medicine," he says, "is to ask the question."

Etymologically, *question* originated with *quærere*, the root of *query* and Latin's *quæstionem*. Old French coined *question* "legal inquest" and English adopted the word by 1300 AD. To *ask* the question, humans formed *ais*, a Proto-Indo-European (PIE) expression of "to wish, to desire." Consider Sanskrit's *icchait* "seeks, desires," Armenian *aic* "investigation," Old Church Slavonic's *iskati* "to seek," and Lithuanian *ieskau* "to seek." German coined *heischen* "to ask, demand," Middle Dutch used *eiscen*, and Old English *ascian*.

The PIE *sag* meant "to track down, trace, to seek." Latin used *sage* and *sagire* "to perceive quickly or keenly," and we can see the roots for both *seek* and *sage* or wisdom. Middle Dutch made *soekan*, Old Norse *soekja*, and Old English *secan*, meaning to inquire. Today we use *beseech* with a feeling of urgency or ultimate politeness.

She is now the matriarch—the *Kahu*—for her family of 156 people, including her siblings and their children. As a *kuma* (teacher), *kahu*, and minister, she performs healing touch for her family and community.

"It's healing work," she says of performing this traditional work for her community. "I go out and come home satisfied—anytime you do His work, it's worthwhile."

Polynesians began migrating to Oahu between 300–400 CE, later creating an intricate social system called *kapu*; its stipulated rules for male governance, basic hygiene, food preparation, waste removal, and seating between men and women at meals. The *kapu* system also allowed *la'au lapa'au*, the *kahuna's* sacred practice of herbal medicine and healing, but after Captain James Cook arrived in 1778 and missionaries brought western ideas, the system was renounced and western ways were adopted.

Once the island became financially viable, the five largest plantation (business) owners took the government by force from the native Hawai'ians to create a protectorate of the United States, which became a territory and then a state in 1959. This exploitation undermined the heritage of the native people since much native Hawai'ian tradition was banned, such as the teaching of *'olelo Hawai'i*, the Hawai'ian language, which was prohibited from being taught in public (and many say private) schools from 1893 until 1993. When it was renounced, local schools embraced the opportunity to teach native Hawai'ian heritage, which includes language, history, healing with medicinal herbs, songs, chants, artwork, pounding and weaving of *tapa* cloth, ancient games using kukui nuts, and mythology.

Oahu's diverse population comes from Pacific Rim countries: Japan, China, Philippines, Tahiti, Guam, Fiji, Thailand, and to some extent Mexico and mainland America. Asian immigrants arrived on Oahu for the sugar cane and pineapple harvests. Today the island is home to nearly a million people, most of whom live or work in Honolulu, whose skyline rests against the extinct volcano, Diamond Head.

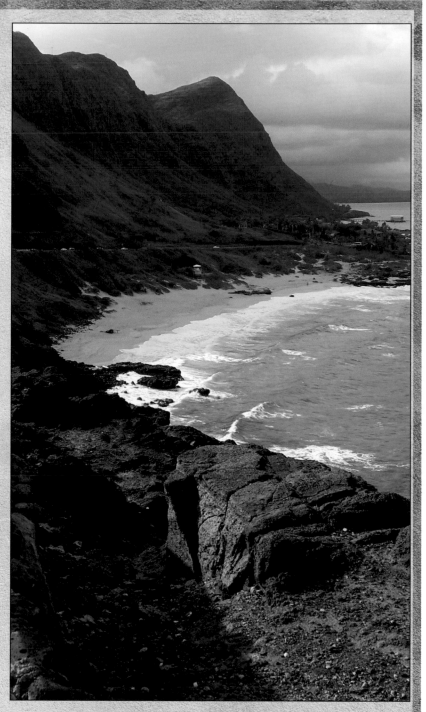

The mountains and seashore near Velma's home at Waimanalo Beach, Oahu, Hawai'i.

OLENA, OR TURMERIC
Curcuma longa

The lovely, golden turmeric (Hawai'i's *olena*) has been cultivated for so long (more than two thousand years) that its origins are unknown. Native to Polynesia, turmeric is widespread across the Polynesian islands, propagated only by root cuttings since it does not produce seed. The fragrant yellow rhizome is beloved for its heavenly scent and is used as a spice, condiment, dye, and medicine.

In India and across the South Pacific, turmeric rhizomes substitute for the precious and expensive saffron. The cooked root was traditionally used in Hawai'i to dye *tapa* cloth, and the dye was applied as a paint on newborn Hawai'ian babies and their mothers.

Medicinally, the root was used by Samoans and Tongans as an ointment for healing sores and rashes, and for medicating shingles. Tahitians used *olena* (called *re'a* in Tahiti) to cure gonorrhea, diabetes, and incontinence, and in the Cook Islands it is used externally to treat puncture wounds. Hawai'ians use *olena* for sinus infections and ceremonially for its sweet scent.

Long neglected in western herbalism, turmeric is now recognized as a first-class healing herb. Like its cousin ginger, turmeric is a remedy for digestive complaints (including salmonella poisoning), heart and liver disease, and especially rheumatoid arthritis. Its extract curcumin is anti-inflammatory and may offer alternatives to ibuprofen. In laboratory studies, turmeric has displayed anticancer activity, and the journals *Cancer Research* and *Carcinogenesis* report curcumin inhibits colon cancer and lymphoma. *Cancer Letters* reported a 2009 study revealing the antiproliferative properties of curcumin in chronic myelogenous leukemia.

Native Hawai'ian healer Auntie Velma DelaPena praises *olena* as one of the most sacred and scarce plants she collects.

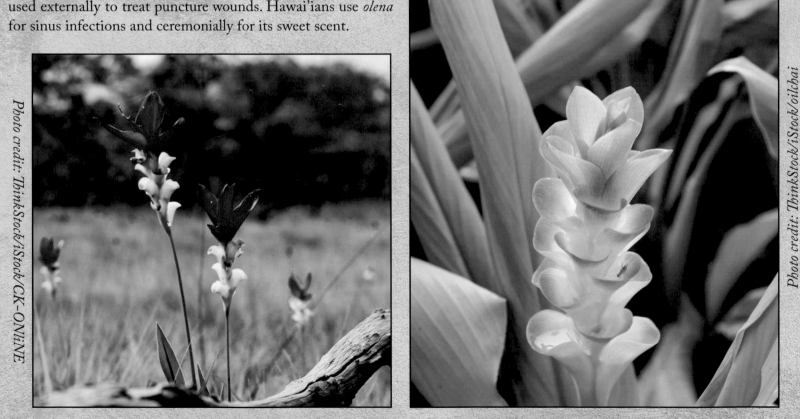

Photo credit: ThinkStock/iStock/CK-ONiiNE

Photo credit: ThinkStock/iStock/oilchai

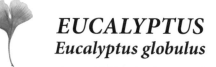

EUCALYPTUS
Eucalyptus globulus

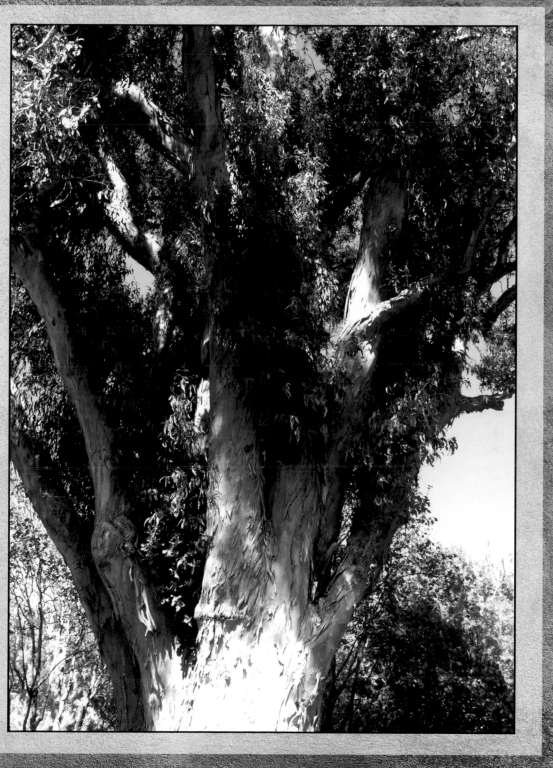

Native to Australia, the fragrant Eucalypt tree has charmed people into planting it all across the southern Pacific, so that most of the six hundred Eucalyptus species of the Myrtle family are found in the forests, swamps, and bogs of tropical and semitropical islands. Humans have collected the slender leaves, resinous gum, and essential oil of the Eucalypt for hundreds of years.

Western herbalism uses the fresh leaves as carminatives, for laryngitis, and as an expectorant, since its strong scent—like its cousins cajeput and Tea Tree—relieves congestion. The analgesic oil or gum is applied topically as a warming liniment to stimulate blood flow to sore joints. Eucalyptus oil is a favorite in saunas to ease bronchial airflow and as an antiseptic and disinfectant.

In Hawai'i, where the Eucalypt is the most frequently planted tree (for windbreaks, timber, and ornamentation), the tree is called *nuholani*. The aromatic leaves are boiled and applied as a "sweat bath" for aching joints and muscles, and the steam is inhaled for bronchial ailments and fever. In Hawai'ian, *nu* means "to cough or sigh," *ho* "to give," and *lani* "heaven," so a simplified and romantic interpretation of the name might be "to give the cough to heaven."

Chapter 4

FOLK MEDICINE, GYPSY, AND BEDOUIN TRADITIONS

Every peasant culture has a tradition of folk healing, from Bulgaria to Brazil. It is a heritage of simple people concocting simple remedies with simple—and deeply felt—beliefs, all with the good intentions of healing. Most times, these simple remedies are made with whatever is at hand, be it plant material (such as roots), animal material (such as dung), or household materials (such as combs, handkerchiefs, and necklaces).

The folk medicine tradition of the Scotch-Irish who settled the mountains of North Carolina is particularly rich with colorful and unusual remedies. These southern Appalachian mountains were settled first by the Cherokee, a native nation of fierce, proud, healthy, and intuitive people who flourished on the rugged land and pure waters. Later these remote and mist-covered 2,000 to 6,000-foot-elevation mountains were settled mostly by Irish, Scotch, and German immigrants who brought with them the music, stories, religion—and superstitions—of their homelands.

The Scotch-Irish heritage included a great number of do-it-yourself philosophies, which served these immigrants well in the rugged and isolated Appalachians. Most old-timers in the mountains today are creative and innovative souls who handcraft artistic yet thoroughly functional items for daily use. These men and women often create their household goods (for sale to outsiders) while spinning yarns and telling stories, many of which are lessons in basic healing.

Eliot Wigginton collected stories of survival skills and settler living in his documentary *Foxfire Books*. The men and women of the mountains subscribed, in general, to a system of healing referred to as Folk Healing, the roots of which extend deep into the psyche of the Old European country peasant of the Middle Ages. Folk Healing claims great miracles of healing with what are today considered rather odd means: for instance, the idea that one can cure a wart by rubbing the wart with a chopped potato, then burying the potato. Or that one can cure a cut by rubbing the offending knife (not the cut) with salve. Or that one can ward away evil spirits and sickness by hanging a clove of garlic on a cord about the neck. Common farm foods were often employed in folk healing, such as buttermilk, garlic, and onions—and not without a certain value, since raw onions and garlic do possess effective phytochemicals that stabilize bronchial respiration and kill bacteria when consumed.

Folk Healing displays the charming notions of a population at once innovative and uninformed. Without the knowledge of bacteria and germs, Appalachia's foremothers and forefathers blended common sense with an almost spiritual form of medicine to create a simple, obvious, and to-the-point healing system. An inherent belief in the supernatural was apparent in the folk cures, though such an accusation would have been staunchly denied by the Christian Scotch-Irish of western North Carolina. My own grandmother, for instance, lost her brother when he died at age four; her well-meaning Christian German parents blamed his death on the fact that he had played barefoot in a south wind.

Folk Healing, if nothing else, proves that mountain people were industrious, generous (they did not charge for healing or promote their cures as quack doctors did), and above all, hopeful. The reason Folk Healing persisted for so long was because people truly *believed* in the cure, despite any indication to the contrary. It was this strong faith, along with a neighborly system of care for one

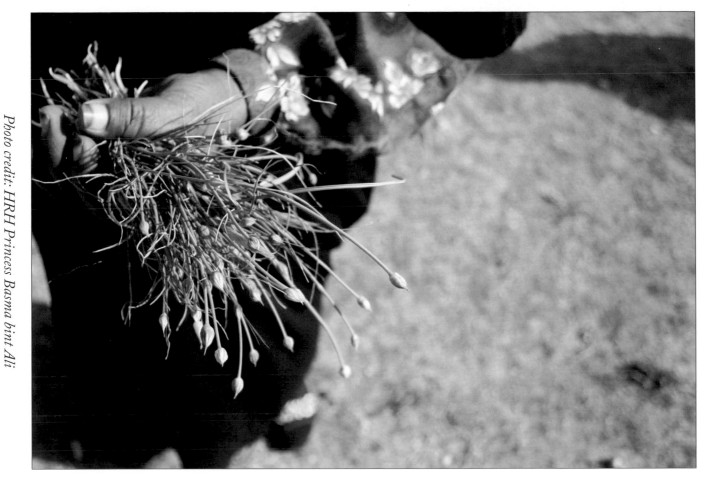

Photo credit: HRH Princess Basma bint Ali

A bedouin woman harvests Alliums at a Mushatta desert castle, 2009

another, that kept Folk Healing alive in the remote mountains for centuries before allopathic medicine, electricity, and paved highways swept into the forgotten corners of Appalachia.

Gypsy and Bedouin Folk Healing

The folk medicine of the wandering tribes of the desert is equally rich. Historically, bedouin communities relied on what was available in the scorching dry seasons or the promising rainy seasons: plants and animals. Shepherds carefully watched their flocks to determine which plants might offer remedies useful for humans—and they also used the bodies of the sheep and goats as medicines for themselves. For instance, among the many (mostly herbal) remedies for kidney problems, Bedouins will use sheep and goat gallbladder. Local fruits such as oranges contain vitamins that inhibit the build-up of fatty plaques in the arteries, according to a Bedouin anthropologist, and licorice root (native to Middle Eastern countries) will do the same thing.

Historically, charms, amulets, and beads have been hung on the body or draped upon the neck to ward away evil spirits that might cause illness; the "evil eye" that is so ingrained in Greece is a remnant of this superstition. Widely seen throughout Mediterranean cultures, the evil eye is believed to be an ancient form of a curse using nothing but the gaze of a malevolent person. Charms are made and sold that will protect the wearer. Other examples of superstitious folk healing include tying knots in string, adorning the fingers with symbolic rings, and creating glass charms and amulets that would be hung from the neck or affixed in the house.

Bedouins use fruit, vegetables, spices, herbal matter, seaweed, coral, and animal substances such as meat, fat, blood, and other tissues to ward off illness or cure any present disease.

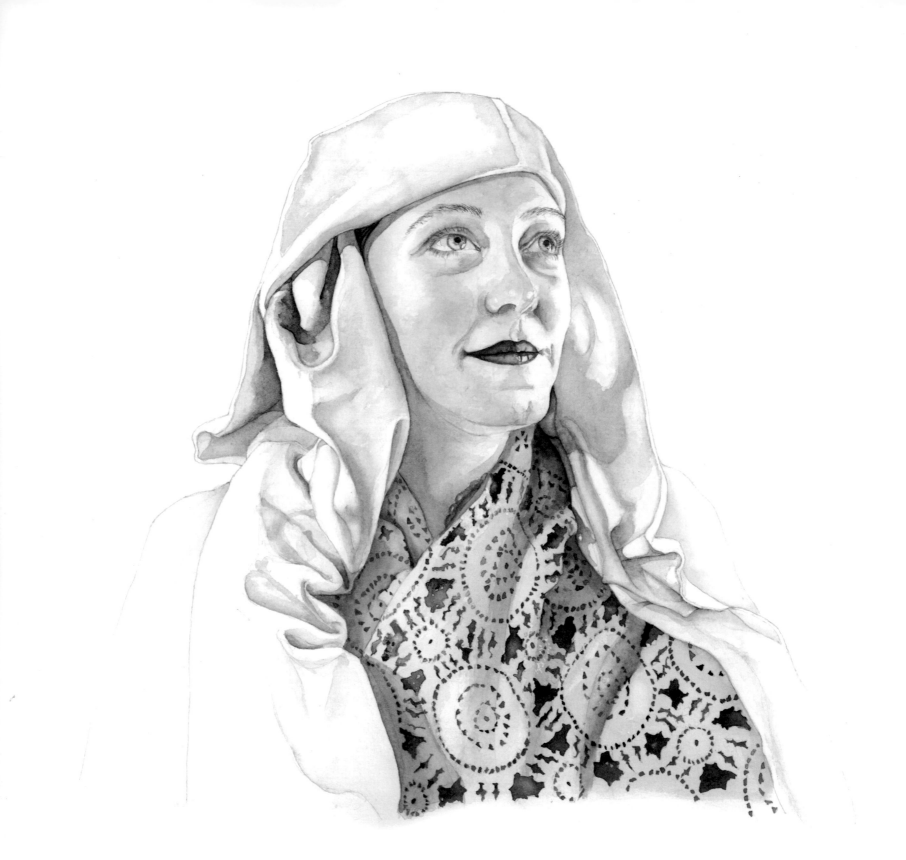

Hildegard von Bingen

(1098–1179)

The legendary Hildegard von Bingen has been identified multiple ways: as a victim of illness, a shaman, and a prophetic healer. History leaves us guessing as to the certainty of her abilities and accomplishments, but in twelfth-century Germany, Hildegard was widely regarded as a medical clairvoyant.

Poetically remembered as the Sybil of the Rhine, Hildegard was born the tenth child to a German family who subsequently gifted her to the Church ostensibly due to poverty, though she may have been tithed due to the visions she experienced as a young child. By age eight, the girl was a resident of the Disibodenberg Benedictine monastery.

Hildegard's early life at the convent was, by modern standards, harsh. She was mentored by the anchoress Jutta, an extremely reclusive nun who practiced strict aceticism and allowed no contact with the world outside the monastery. It was with this strict, isolated woman that young Hildegard learned Latin and listened to the songs of the convent through the walls, until Jutta died thirty long years later. Hildegard was soon elected by consensus Prioress of the cloister.

We assume Hildegard was utterly unprepared and untrained to lead a priory of nuns, yet she took the reins with enthusiasm. Finally free of her confinement, Hildegard could even leave the convent at times, and it seems she must have exhibited some degree of natural leadership. At age forty-two, she received a spectacular vision: a brilliant light appeared to her, which she believed to be God. The light spoke with a voice, imparting to her the meanings of famous historical religious texts and instructing her to record these meanings for the benefit of all.

But Hildegard did not write them down immediately. She was busy composing hymns and writing music for her priory, as singing was a chief method of worship. Persuaded by Pope Eugenius, Hildegard finally agreed to record the voices she heard and describe her visions. She wrote these (or had them written for her) in a text titled *Scivias (Know the Ways [of the Lord])*.

She made it clear that her visions were not witchcraft, were not mania, were not dreams. She maintained she was actually being spoken to by the Christian God, and to reinforce this (and to avoid punishment), she belittled her own abilities. How else, she argued, could a poor, uneducated nun know such things? It *must* be divine communication. Hildegard could have been a person with low self-esteem, as claimed by scholars today, or she was a shrewd visionary who desired to keep her head on her shoulders.

Between 1147 and 1150, Hildegard moved the convent to Rupertsberg at Bingen (later, in 1165, she founded a separate convent, Eibingen, nearby). As prioress, she wrote profusely—music, lyrics, and plays that were enacted by her fellow nuns. In 1158, she completed and published her primary medical text *Subtilitatum Diversarum Naturarum Creaturarum (Of the Simplicities of Various Natural Creatures*, or alternatively *Subtleties of the Diverse Qualities of Created Things)*. Her works focus on using simple plants (and other ingredients) as medical solutions and are presented pragmatically yet with compassion: *Physica (The Book of Simple Medicine)* and *Liber Compositae Medicinae* or *Causae et Curae (The Book of Compound Medicine)*. Interestingly, Hildegard relied on her previous acceptance as a mystic to publish a medical text. She was not a physician, nor a monastic nurse, nor did she possess any medical training or advanced Latin. In her favor was her status as a Christian visionary and the fact that the Church, and therefore the community, believed her.

It was here that Hildegard went out on a limb—no longer was she just a nun, or even a nun who wrote creative lyrics and songs, or even a mystic. Now Hildegard proceeded, in a text she called *Subtleties of the Diverse Qualities of Created Things*, to examine and advise on medicine—and this time she did it from a medical perspective with few claims of prophecy or divine intervention. Later titled *Physica*, Hildegard's text was the first book on natural physics written in German and is generally assumed to reflect some monastic medicine as well as Hildegard's own observations of local folk customs.

Her book was organized into nine sections, or books: Plants, Elements, Trees, Stones, Fish, Birds, Animals, Reptiles, and Metals. Author and translator Priscilla Throop notes that the title's word *Subtleties* "refers to secret powers hidden in natural creatures for the use of human beings and revealed by God."[1] With her opening line in the book, Hildegard hints at the respect with which she holds the earth, saying, "With Earth was the human being created." She clarified why the earth, its elements, and its plants might have been created: "The earth gave its vital energy, according to each person's race, nature, habits, and environment. Through the beneficial herbs, the earth brings forth the range of mankind's spiritual powers and distinguishes between them; through the harmful herbs, it manifests harmful and diabolic behaviors."[2]

While Hildegard may have had experience with medicinal plants, it's doubtful she had direct experience with sexual intercourse, orgasm, or reproduction, though she did not hesitate to describe in frank and straightforward terms how a woman achieves orgasm:

"When a woman is making love with a man, a sense of heat in her brain, which brings with it sensual delight, communicates the taste of that delight during the act and summons forth the emission of the man's seed. And when the seed has fallen into its place, that vehement heat descending from her brain draws the seed to itself and holds it, and soon the woman's sexual organs contract, and all the parts that are ready to open up during the time of menstruation now close, in the same way as a strong man can hold something enclosed in his fist."[3]

She may have gleaned this information from the many community women who approached the nunnery for information and assistance, or it may simply have come from her creative mind. Since she often advised moderation, her reputation for temperance probably allowed her to get away with describing in flowery prose a sexual subject that otherwise would have been taboo. Thus Hildegard became one of the first women in the twelfth century (along with Trotula, her Italian contemporary) to discuss the medicinal properties of plants, medical treatment for women, and, in particular, the details of a woman's orgasm and neonatal conception.

The Mystic Medic

Hildegard based her medical writings on the standards of the day: Galen and Hippocrates. She did not stray far from the Greek cosmology of earth, fire, water, and air with their respective humors in the body—black bile, yellow bile, phlegm, and blood. She stressed the use of a plant based on its ability to affect the humors: "Reyan (tansy) is hot and a little damp and is good against all superfluous flowing humours and whoever suffers from catarrh and has a cough, let him eat tansy," she wrote. "It will bind humors so that they do not overflow, and thus will lessen." She even appreciated what we would today term *aromatherapy*, saying of lily, "The odor of the first buds of lilies, indeed the odor of the flowers, makes a person's heart joyful and furnishes him with virtuous ideas."[4]

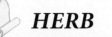

HERB

Latin speakers referred to grass or green plants as *herba*, Old French *erbe*, and in 1290 English referred to grasses and flowers as *erbe*. Old French formed *erbier*, and in the thirteenth century, English coined *herber* to convey "herb garden." Eventually *herber* meant a grassy plot or shady nook: today's arbor.

She asserted that all herbs were either warm or cold, and that warm herbs were to be used for healing a person's soul and cold herbs were useful in treatments of the body She explained the virtues of many grains and pulses (oats, wheat, barley, millet, rye, lentils, etc.) and many herbs and spices (lavender, rose, cinnamon, nutmeg, licorice, ginger, cumin, pepper, nigella, galingale, thyme, gentian, horehound, fenugreek, butterbur, coltsfoot, mullein, calendula, germander, and more). Hildegard emphasized moderation in all things, even in the eating of eggs, which she considered "like poison": "They are harmful to eat since they are sticky and slimy, and are almost like poison. A person should not eat them since, if eaten, scrofula and the bad worms that eat a person grow on the person easily. But it is possible to eat the eggs of domestic hens. Nevertheless, let them be eaten moderately . . ."[5]

She went to great lengths to liken plants and their physical natures to humans and their physical natures, sometimes comparing people to plants:

"And the earth sprouted greenness in accordance with the race, nature, customs, and ways of humans. For the earth has many useful herbs that reach out to people's spiritual needs, and yet they are distinct from people. In addition, the earth has useless herbs that reflect the useless and diabolical ways of humans. Certain herbs are nourishing, and a person is willing to eat them. They are light and do not weigh the person down. These are assimilated into his or her flesh. The sap of fruit-bearing trees, newly engendered and flowing, can be compared to a person's blood."[6]

She likens stones of the earth to a person's bones and recommends using "herbs of the air" for body parts that are exposed to air, such as the hair.

Was She a Healer?

Despite her renown and her published works detailing the use of plants, we do not know if Hildegard was really a healer—did she consult with patients, or work to directly cure the sick? Or did she observe and report? She wrote extensively of properties and folk medicine, but it is unclear whether she applied this knowledge in a clinical setting or if she was simply recording what she observed or heard. She was certainly a creative writer and enjoyed playing with words; indeed, once she was established as Abbess at her new priory, Hildegard created for her nuns a secret and mystical reality, even crafting an entire language she called Lingua Ignote with more than nine hundred unique words and its own alphabet of twenty-three letters. Indeed, Hildegard may be due praise from a number of contemporary herbalists for her creation of the now-popular and enchanting word *viriditas*, which meant "greenness" and was "construed as the blossoming creativity found not only in the botanical world, but also in the intellect of each virgin monastic."[7]

Generally, Hildegard is accepted today as an eccentric mystic, or as the victim of migraine headaches that could explain the visions and the lights. Few scholars today consider her a true healer, though she is remembered for her tenacity and her courage to write about women's bodies and experiences without fear of monastic retribution and with what seems to have been a genuine interest and concern for humanity's welfare. She also explored the vast pharmacopeia of herbal medicine and offered her own perception of the complex relationship between people and plants.

GERMANY

Hildegard lived at Disibodenberg in the Palatinate Forest, now Germany. Today, this forest borders the Vosges Mountains of France and together these regions form the UNESCO Biosphere Reserve, one of the largest temperate deciduous forests in Europe. The town where Hildegard established her nunnery was named after Saint Disibod, a monk and hermit about whom Hildegard composed a *vita*.

Today, Germany's population is the largest in the European Union, and it is the top user of herbal medicines. Germany's herbal extraction industry is the largest in the world, supplying Europe, the United States, and Japan. It comprises 49 percent of the European market's licensed herbal sales (France 17 percent, Italy 9 percent), with its top-selling raw materials being ginkgo, valerian, and horse chestnut.

Governed by the Federal Institute of Drugs and Medical Devices, the herbal industry is much more complicated than even Hildegard might have prophesied. The Germany Commission E Monographs of more than 230 plants can substitute for a manufacturer's testing and trials, but other plants are heavily restricted. Herbal remedies are strictly considered medicines and are prescribed by doctors and covered by health insurance. Contrast this to the Netherlands or Spain where most herbal remedies are classified not as medicines but as foods.

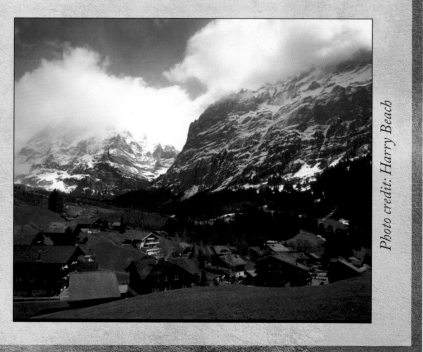

Photo credit: Harry Beach

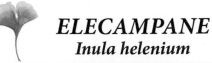

LAVENDER
Lavandula angustifolia

Prized for its heavenly scent, lavender has adorned women, houses, cribs, carriages, and closets since time immemorial. Lavender earned its name from the Latin *lavare*, meaning "to wash," but smell-good plants whose flowers could be infused in precious oils were called *nard* in the Bible, and the spikenard in the Song of Solomon is likely lavender. Even in 1653, Nicholas Culpeper referred to oil of lavender as "oil of spike."

Common or English lavender (*Lavandula angustifolia*) is renowned for its soothing effects. Its scent is therapeutic, sedating, and calming to the nervous system. Lavender essential oil reduces scar tissue formation from burns and is often used in toiletries such as bath salts, perfume, and soaps. The distilled essential oil of lavender contains linalyl acetate and is antibacterial and antiseptic: listed in the US Pharmacopoeia and the National Formulary since 1820, lavender kills diphtheria bacilli, typhoid bacilli, streptococcus, and pneumococcus.

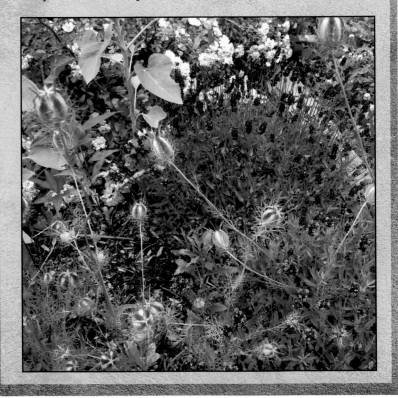

ELECAMPANE
Inula helenium

The queen of any garden, elecampane, *Inula Helenium*, is named for Helen of Troy and has been used throughout history for its sweet medicinal root. Far beneath its towering yellow flowers, its thick root holds the dietary fiber inulin and strong sesquiterpene lactones that are valued as expectorants and antispasmodics. I value elecampane to ease cough, bronchitis, asthma, and to calm spastic lungs enough to allow children to sleep. The root has been candied, made into a tea, a tincture, and a capsule, but by far the most enjoyable way to take this medicine is as an electuary in honey.

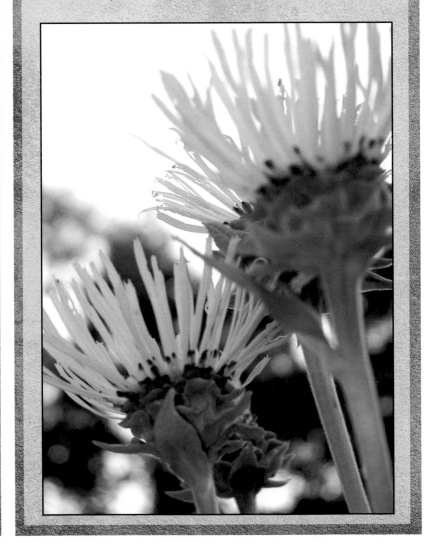

Juliette de Bairacli Levy

(1912–2009)

To be vigorous and young! Juliette de Bairacli Levy inspired generations of men and women not only with youth and enthusiasm, but also with her grace, adventurous spirit, and veterinary genius. And—to be vigorous and old! She equally inspired us with her great passion for life even well into her nineties. Born November 11, 1912, in Manchester, England, Juliette packed her extraordinary life full as an accomplished and world-renowned veterinarian, author, herbalist, mother, traveler, poet, and—though not credited as such—a folk ethnobotanist.

Raised in a loving and affluent family, Juliette and her three sisters and two brothers were indulged with a nanny, chauffeur, maid, and gardener, and Juliette was sent to study at Lowther College, a well-to-do girl's school. She then attended the Universities of Manchester and Liverpool but abhorred the schools' practice of vivisection and cruel animal experimentation; after two years she left in protest to pursue her own education in veterinary health.

Smart and stylish, Juliette established a distemper clinic in London in the 1930s, writing her first book *The Cure for Canine Distemper*. She raised Afghan hound puppies and competed in Crufts and Westminster Dog Shows, winning Best of Show in both. She soon developed a retail line of herbal supplements for dogs under the brand Natural Rearing Products which "were the only products of their kind on the market. Today these supplements are still distributed world wide."[1] Her book *Medicinal Herbs: Their Use in Canine Ailments* came out in 1943.

During World War II, she worked in the Women's Land Army, gathering sphagnum moss to be used as bandaging material on soldier's wounds. After the war, she continued her veterinary study and work, gaining attention in Yorkshire where, in 1947, she treated and cured a huge flock of three thousand very sick sheep using herbs.[2] Her inquisitive nature and "travel bug" led her to explore widely, and she traveled throughout Europe, Turkey, Northern Africa, Israel, Greece, Mexico, and America. She often lived with gypsies and Arab farmers, acquainting herself with their local cures

and home remedies, which she recorded, tried, and often published alongside riveting stories and tales about her adventures in the country. The peasants and nomads taught Juliette how to cultivate plants, dry fruits, preserve olives, and make medicines from herbs, leaves, roots, and tree barks. "I also learned their simple laws of honesty and morality, and health, hardiness, how to live rough, to be happy every day," she wrote.[3]

Finally in 1951, Juliette published *The Complete Herbal Handbook for Farm and Stable* and soon after compiled several earlier articles into *The Complete Herbal Book for the Dog* (now called *The Complete Herbal Handbook for the Dog and Cat*), the first veterinary herbals. These were the first texts directed to an audience of trainers and breeders that specifically called for herbal and natural treatments, foods, and cures—and they were taken seriously, being quickly translated into German and other languages. Levy's books mandated strict adherence to a raw-food diet, fresh air, plenty of exercise outdoors, natural-habitat kennels without concrete, and herbs for healing rather than vaccinations or pharmaceuticals, which were becoming all-too-prevalent in the 1930s, '40s, and '50s. Of the herbs she recommended be included in a dog's daily diet was mineral-rich kelp, which acts in a dog's body much as it does in a person's: strengthening the hair, bones, teeth, and skin.[4]

In addition to her revolutionary "natural rearing" method for dogs, Juliette espoused groundbreaking yet completely traditional philosophies for people. Plants can heal, she taught. Be self-sufficient. Fast when you are sick. She advocated laying leaves directly on wounds—a soon-to-be primitive method in the fast-growing age of science and sterilization.

Somewhat reluctantly, Juliette detailed her knowledge of herbal remedies in books for people, including *The Natural Rearing of Children, Traveler's Joy, Nature's Children*, and *The Complete Herbal Handbook for Everyone*, plus many more, each one feeling more exuberant and joyful than the last, as if she had finally broken through her hesitation about being a world-renowned herbalist and the risk of pulling away from a veterinary focus. Her books were instant successes: throughout her travels she gathered information primarily from Berbers, peasants, gypsies, nomads, and gatherers— and not only does she credit them in her writing (with a respect

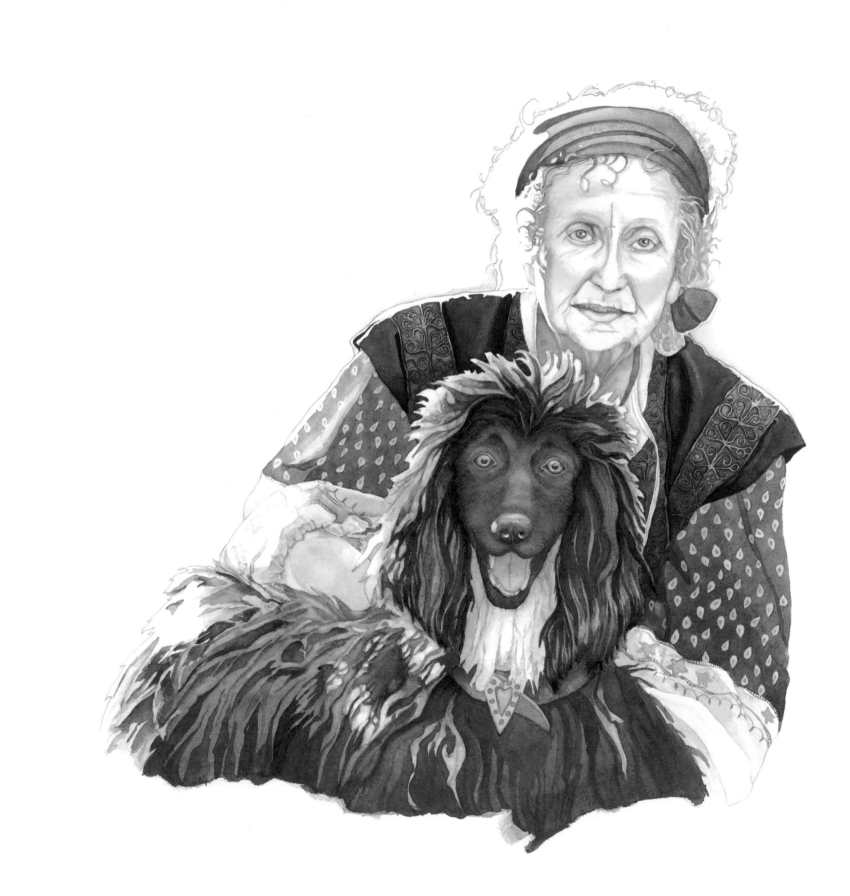

and admiration previously lacking in healing literature), she also names them as friends, which is especially noteworthy considering her affluent upbringing and education. Perhaps what makes Juliette such a beloved mentor to so many around the world is that her writings are full of lively stories about her children, Rafik and Luz: the reader escapes into their adventures in the wild areas, creeks, deserts, and farmlands of Europe and the Middle East, relishing in tales of bright-eyed, pink-cheeked children breathing hard, running fast, and loving life. Reading Juliette's herbals is like indulging in a private diary, and we feel comfortably connected to her ruggedly healthy children and inspired to raise our own children in the open air and warm sunshine just as Juliette did.

Her zeal for live plants comes through in every protocol; two of her favorite plants were rosemary ("beloved by the bees," she said) and southernwood, an Artemisia: "What is beautiful about southernwood is it is a protector of women and the newborn infant, and I have done miracles with it giving it to animals which have been unable to pass their young ones and placentas, giving them a drink of southernwood and honey and ivy leaves."[5] She strongly advocated using fresh herbs and not processing them at all; rather, most of her protocols involve chewing fresh leaves or plant parts or placing fresh leaves directly upon the body: she seldom used oils, ointments, or extracts, though she taught how to make them and gave very specific indications for their use. "The most healthful way to use herbs is to gather them fresh from the countryside, or fresh from the herb garden."[6] Her second most common method was to make a water extract or "standard brew," today referred to as an *infusion*.

Reading her books is a type of armchair travel—an educational jaunt into distant and exotic lands. And since her writings are based entirely on her own observations and experience (they are not second-hand research!), the reader is treated to a very unique type of study. Her colorful writing about the Andalusian region of Spain is picturesque and dreamy and her children's strength and vigor shines through in every passage, making Juliette one of the foremost and beloved writers of her time. Always prolific (even on her typewriter), Juliette wrote novels and three books of poetry in addition to more than a dozen professional books; near the end of her life, she lived and gardened on Kythria, an island off Greece, with her beloved Afghan hounds. She died peacefully in her sleep in Burgdorf, Switzerland, at age ninety-six.

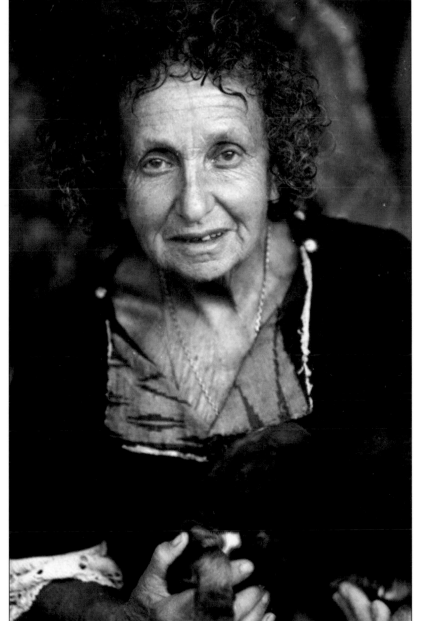

"If every hospital had its garden growing these plants," she said, "instead of shelves and shelves of chemical medicines, there would be so much less pain in the world, and successful healing. And it's promised in the Bible! It says, 'I've given you the plants of the Earth to heal you and keep you healthy.'"[7] Juliette ends one of her books as an herbalist and a mother: "Every family with a bit of land should plant a herb garden. It will bring them closer to Nature, and that is always a good thing for Everyman."[8]

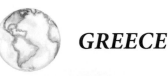

Under sunny skies, Mount Olympus gazes down as the highest peak in Greece to look at thousands of Greek islands that dot the Aegean, Ionian, Crete, and Mediterranean Seas. From this lofty mountain and its colorful countryside, Greek myths and mythic characters were born, growing over the millennia to perhaps the most intricate and influential mythical system in the world.

Herbs and this seaside landscape fit together naturally and complemented the culture's creative myth-making: rose and myrtle became the beloved plants of the sea goddess Aphrodite, and rosemary, parsley, mint, and hundreds of other herbs developed characteristics of myth as well as medicine. Even fennel gained fame as the lucky herb in whose hollow stalk Prometheus hid the burning embers of fire as a gift to humanity. Watching over all this was Zeus's son, Apollo, god of the sun, music, and medicine.

Most of Western medicine (both herbal and allopathic) can trace its genesis to Ancient Greek physicians and healers. The earliest of the celebrated physicians was Hippokrates, who, in about 450 BCE, taught the use of simple food-based remedies using vinegars, honey, herbs, and water treatments. His philoso-

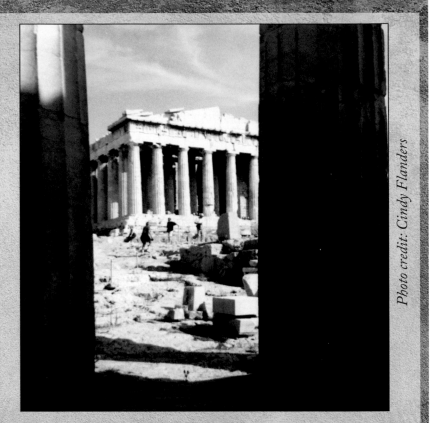

Photo credit: Cindy Flanders

phies celebrated the natural health of the body and the person's ability to heal if given fresh food, time, and common sense (as opposed to intervention through witchcraft, sorcery, astrology, bleeding, purging, or complex chemical formulas). Hence, Hippokrates is considered the first to promote "rational or scientific" medicine, and the Hippocratic philosophy is now a major branch of healing.[1]

Pedanius Dioscorides emerged from Greece as the most famous writer on pharmacy and herbs, writing the five-volume *De Materia Medica* which became the most influential resource on herbal medicine for more than a millennia. As an army physician under Emperor Nero, Dioscorides traveled widely and recorded the use of various substances and especially plants for treating wounds and illness. His vivid descriptions of herbs and their healing uses were wildly popular and his writings were the basis of natural healing for more than 1,500 years.

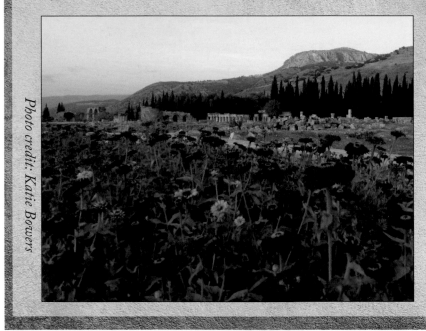

Photo credit: Katie Bowers

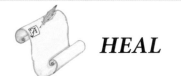

PLANTAIN
Plantago major, P. lanceolata

HEAL

The common weed plantain is a treasure-trove of food and medicine. Nearly all yards in North America harbor *Plantago major*, a broad-leaved herb with wide scalloped thick leaves forming a rosette at the base, from which a tall, slender seed stalk emerges. *Plantago lanceolata* sports long, thin linear leaves with fine, downy hair; the leaves can be used interchangeably. Nicknamed Englishman's Foot or White Man's Foot, it spreads everywhere the colonists went.

In the spring, its small, tender leaves make a fine addition to salads and may be steamed and sprinkled with vinegar. The ripe seeds can be sprinkled on oatmeal or baked in bread, adding calcium, iron, and potassium. Laxative in large doses, these fiber-rich seeds form the basis for many over-the-counter preparations that contain *Psyllium* seeds. They work by forming a bulky mucilaginous mass in the gut that stimulates peristalsis and pushes food material through the intestines.

The mucilaginous leaves make a pulpy mass when chewed and swallowed, soothing burning ulcers. Externally, they are vulnerary and have the ability to draw liquids and objects from beneath the skin. A poultice, compress, salve, or oil infused with chopped plantain will literally pull from under the skin toxins, bee, and insect venom, poison ivy oils, and more, similar to the traditional use of poke root—drawing out cancers, polyps, and cysts from breast and other soft tissues.

Heal shares its origin with health, whole, and holy. The Proto-Indo-European (PIE) language used *kailo*, "whole, uninjured, of good omen." Later Proto Germanic coined *khailaz*. Other ancient cultures used similar words for "heal":

Old Saxon	*helian*
Old Norse	*heila*
Old Frisian	*Hela*
Dutch	*heelen*
German	*heilen*
Old English	*hal*

Old English used *haelp*, *hal*, and *haelan* "being or making whole, sound or well, or hale" from the PIE word *kailo*. Our greetings *hail* and *hello* came from wishing someone health or wholeness. Old English *halig* meant health; Norse *heill* meant "healthy" and *helge* meant holy or sacred.

Ancient Greeks used *akos* "cure" and *pan* "all," creating *panakes* and *panakeia*, all-healing. The Greek Goddess Panacea was the source of healing; she was the daughter of Asclepius, god of medicine, and the granddaughter of Apollo, god of healing and strength. The Greek *althein* "healing" contributed to *Althea officinalis*, our familiar marshmallow. This came from an even more ancient PIE word *al*, "to grow and nourish."

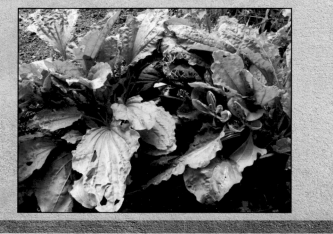

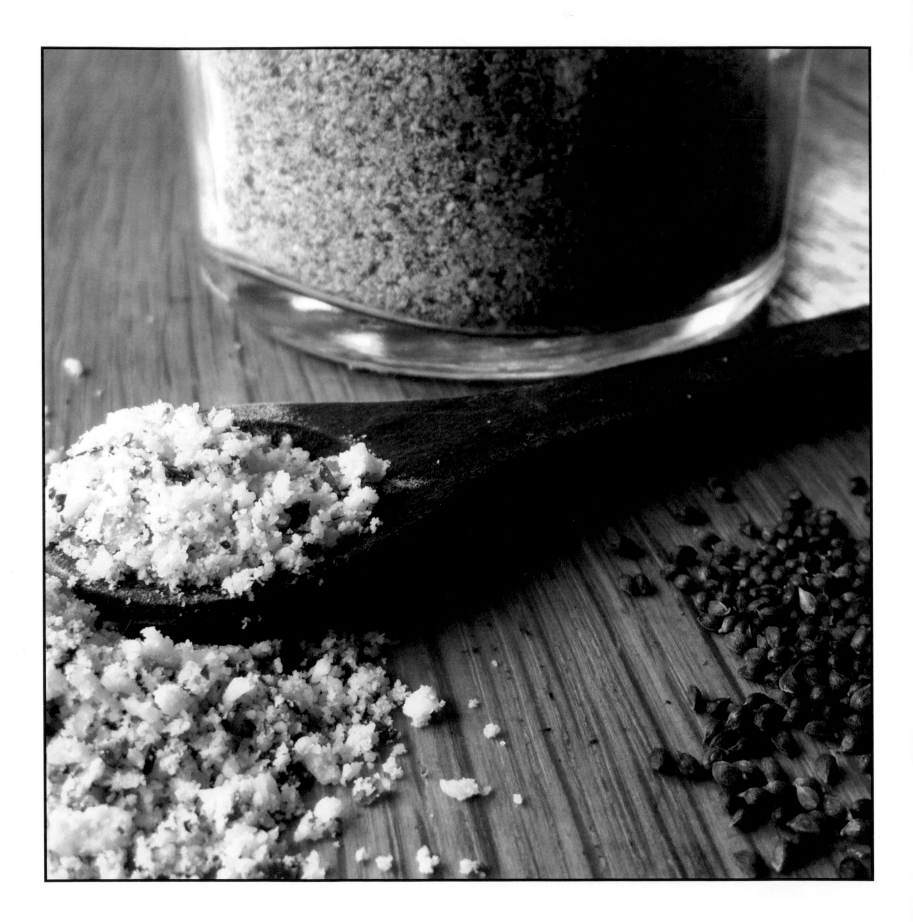

Chapter 5
ALCHEMY AND AROMATHERAPY

In the early part of the new millennium, humanity was consumed with thoughts of creation. Spiritual people questioned the origins of existence (and early Christianity was born), at the same time curious scientists explored the possibilities of creating—or extending—life from minerals and substances. While Judaism began its slow divergence from the new forms of Christianity, science entered into a new realm that combined spiritual practice with a unique form of experimentation: chemistry.

Between the first and third centuries CE, Alexandria, Egypt, was a vibrant playground for philosophers and scientists, many of whom worked tirelessly to determine the origins of life and even tried to re-create those origins. Ultimately, alchemists wished to achieve two similar results: secular alchemists wished to create perfect gold from imperfect non-gold substances such as lead, under the right conditions; and Gnostic alchemists wished to experience immortality and a release of the soul from sinful matter. Gnostics believed that, like gold, the human spirit was perfect and that the imperfect body (like lead) could be transmuted into a more perfect state (i.e., immortality) under the right conditions. In each instance, the "right condition" involved a catalyst that would tip the balance in favor of the more perfect state of being. In their fervor, Gnostic alchemists gave this elusive catalyst a variety of intriguing names, including The Philosopher's Stone and the Elixir. The search for the catalyst consumed alchemists for centuries and in the process led to many useful inventions that transformed early medieval life.

While searching for the catalyst, alchemists relied heavily on words and philosophies related to birth: a copper "seed" was placed into the steam distiller called "the womb," and the resulting steam was likened to amniotic fluid. The resulting fragrant essential oil is said to have been described by Maria Prophetissa as "an angel." Arguably the most famous alchemist of Egypt, Prophetissa's inventions and discoveries included hydrochloric acid, distillation of alcohol, equipment to distill steam, proper laboratory heating and cooling methods, and the collection of hydrosols and essential oils. (See the profile Maria Prophetissa, this chapter.)

Alchemists gifted later herbalists with a wealth of knowledge for medicine-making; monasteries learned early to distill fragrant and healing skin hydrosols and even to distill beverages from aromatic plants. Carmelite nuns created scented cosmetic waters using lemon balm and angelica, and European liqueurs such as Fra Angelica, Benedictine, and Chartreuse are all results of the distillation of herbs and flowers begun by monks at monasteries throughout the Middle Ages.

The second desire of the alchemists, however—the quest for immortality and the release of the soul from the body—was harder to achieve. Alchemists applied all sorts of yellow colored substances to the distillery, since the mineral gold was considered perfect. Flowers such as fennel, ladies mantle, melilot (sweet clover), and other yellow flowers were likely used simply because of their color. Alchemists also likely used the clay yellow ochre and arsenic in their experiments.

Alchemy represents a great shift in the medical philosophy of ancient Egypt. It has nothing to do with the study of the body, which, from the Ebers Papyrus of 1550 BCE, focused on folk remedies and showed that ancient Egyptians considered the heart as the true center of the body:

> "The beginning of the physician's secret: knowledge of the heart's movement and knowledge of the heart. There are vessels from it to every limb. As to this, when any physician, any surgeon (lit. Sachmet-priest) or any exorcist applies the hands or his fingers to the head, to the back of the head, to the hands, to the place of the stomach, to the arms or to the feet, then he examines the heart, because all the limbs possess its vessels, that is: it (the heart) speaks out of the vessels of every limb."[1]

By the first and second centuries, however, anatomical knowledge of the body seemed secondary as alchemists moved beyond folk medicine to chart new ground using mineral substances and inventing technology they believed would coerce a complete transmutation of substance from far-flung materials; in the process, they unwittingly combined a complex system of religious and medical beliefs into a fascinating new science that led directly to today's study of chemistry and our institution of laboratory science.

Aromatherapy

Part of the allure of the alchemist's lab was the smell—certainly much of the smell was atrocious as these early scientists combined poisons and base metals in their small, enclosed chambers. But other scents—such as those created when distilling aromatic plants—must have been highly rewarding. These scents occur due to the volatile oils present in the stems, leaves, flowers, bark, roots, fruits, and even zests of certain plants and, thanks to alchemists such as Maria Prophetissa, we know how to extract or isolate these oils and put them to use.

Volatile oils are also called essential oils; they are typically extracted from the plant using steam distillation, but they can also be commercially extracted using chemical solvents or mechanical presses.

Modern herbalists generally use essential oils in dilutions upon the skin (in crèmes, salves, oils, and baths), and professional aromatherapists in France typically teach patients to use essential oils internally. When distilled, essential oils generally float on top of the lighter hydrosol that is produced along with the oils; this hydrosol is approximately 1/1000th as strong as the essential oil, lending a gentler and more consumable remedy for a variety of conditions. The hydrosol (also called a flower water) can be used as a refreshing facial wash, a douche, a bath, and even as a drink or in cooking. Typical doses of hydrosols are small—a tablespoon or so daily, whereas doses of essential oils are minute—a drop or two, at most, daily, and only under professional guidance.

Aromatherapy as an art and as a clinical practice arose in the 1960s and '70s as a result of healers wishing to return to more natural substances and to take control of their own health. As a branch or wing of herbalism, aromatherapy uses natural substances (essential oils) to pursue health, often stimulating the immune system and fighting pathogens, since essential oils are extremely antiseptic. And, of course, their fragrance can stimulate certain moods or feelings in the person who smells them. The aromatic component has created an entirely new branch of medicine called aromatherapy, which provides relief and balance based simply on the scent of the oil.

Because these oils are highly potent (more fragrant than simply smelling the flower, for instance), they can be applied by the drop to diffusers, handkerchiefs, clothing, cleaning supplies, light bulb rings, and candles to permeate the scent through the air. Depending on the fragrance, the person in question might find their anxiety reduced, their depression relieved, or a childhood memory reawakened by a certain scent. Many teachers find that using essential oils of stimulating plants (such as peppermint, spearmint, rosemary, or lemon balm) can create an uplifting atmosphere in the classroom and even enhance student's memory and recall of subjects, especially when the subject is taught with the smell of a certain plant and then the test is given with the same smell permeating the room.

Today, clinicians worldwide use aromatherapy to calm patients at the clinic and also as remedies given to the patients to use at home. Though they are natural, essential oils are not necessarily gentle or safe; careful use is required to ensure safety for pregnant and/or nursing women, children, and on sensitive areas of skin or mucosa.

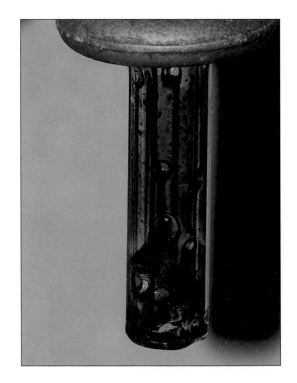

Queen Cleopatra

(69 BCE–30 BCE)

Today we know Cleopatra VII as the famous Greek queen of Egypt, but it seems that, in addition to her avocation as a stateswoman, she was also skilled in the art of perfumery. According to folklore, Cleopatra specialized in the pleasurable arts of cosmetics, and it has even been suggested that Cleopatra VII operated a type of early spa or perfume factory near Ein Gedi by the Dead Sea, complete with what appear to be seats in a waiting room, possibly for students or massage clients. She is rumored to have recorded her perfume recipes in a book titled *Gynaeciarum Libri*,[1] the original of which has never been found but which has been referred to by historians.

If Cleopatra was indeed skilled in the use of perfumery, she may have been one of the first proponents of what we today call aromatherapy. We can guess that she directed her knowledge of spices toward the treatment of wounds for Egypt's armies (as did Achilles in Greece) and in the care of her four children. Heavily bejeweled and smelling wonderful, Cleopatra was certainly crafty in the ways of flirtation; historian William Stearns Davis states that "Plato admits four sorts of flattery, but [Cleopatra] had a thousand. Were Antony serious or disposed to mirth, she had at any moment some new delight or charm to meet his wishes."[2] One way she charmed Antony, in addition to playing at disguise, playing dice, drinking with him, hunting with him, and cheering him in his exercises, was surely anointing herself with intoxicating fragrances and ornamenting her body with priceless jewels. She is said to have spoken many languages (including Ethiopian, Troglodyte, Hebrew, Arabian, Syrian, Medes, and Parthian[3]), and surely she spoke the language of scent. Davis records her first meeting Antony by

"sailing up the river Cydnus, in a barge with gilded stern and outspread sails of purple, while oars of silver beat time to the music of flutes and fifes and harps. She herself lay all alone, under a canopy of cloth of gold, dressed as Venus in a picture, and beautiful young boys, like painted Cupids, stood on each side to fan her ... The perfumes diffused themselves from the vessel to the shore ... while the word went through all the multitude, that Venus was come to feast with Bacchus for the common good of Asia."[4]

KORE

Before Persephone became Queen of the Underworld, she was Kore, Ancient Greek for girl or maiden, that which is growing, or she who is nourished and becoming larger. The ancient Proto-Indo-European (PIE) *ker* meant "to grow," or according to etymologist Douglas Harper, to "come forth, spring up, grow, thrive." This certainly applied to a young nubile girl about to reach womanhood under the guidance of her strong mother Demeter. The base word applied equally to either sex: Greek *kouros* was "boy" and *kore* was "girl." (Greeks nicknamed their girls Korinna, a diminutive form meaning "maiden," giving us Corinna.)

The Latin *Ceres* sprang from *kor* or *ker* and referred to the Goddess of agriculture and grains (pronounced with a hard C); this led to *creare* "to bring forth" (from which we derive *create*). Ceres's daughter was Proserpina; the equivalent of Demeter's daughter Persephone, her name means "creeping forth" as vines in a garden (think "prosper").

Old French took Latin's idea of growth (*crescentum* from *ker*) and applied it to the moon's waxing phase, as *creissant*, which in 1399 Anglo-French became *cressaunt*: our crescent moon. When shaping breads (Ceres's nourishing grains) into a crescent, the French call them *croissants*. Finally, we use *ker* in the musical crescendo. From this one root word, we refer to girls, the moon, music, deities, agriculture, bread, and prosperity.

Legends grew about Cleopatra's famous barge, from tales of rose petals knee-deep, to the intense fragrance of camphire wafting from the barge, to the enchanting artistry of henna upon Cleopatra's skin. In *Antony and Cleopatra*, Shakespeare described the lilac-colored sails of her barge as "so perfumed that the winds were love-sick with them." Much later, as their love blossomed and they became a family, Antony gifted Cleopatra with lands throughout Palestine, including the fragrant groves of balsam and persimmon trees used at Ein Gedi for making perfume.[5] These balsam plantations of the Dead Sea area were surprisingly powerful tools in the arsenals of royal rulers at the time. "The methods of cultivation and products were a closely guarded secret and a powerful political tool," say

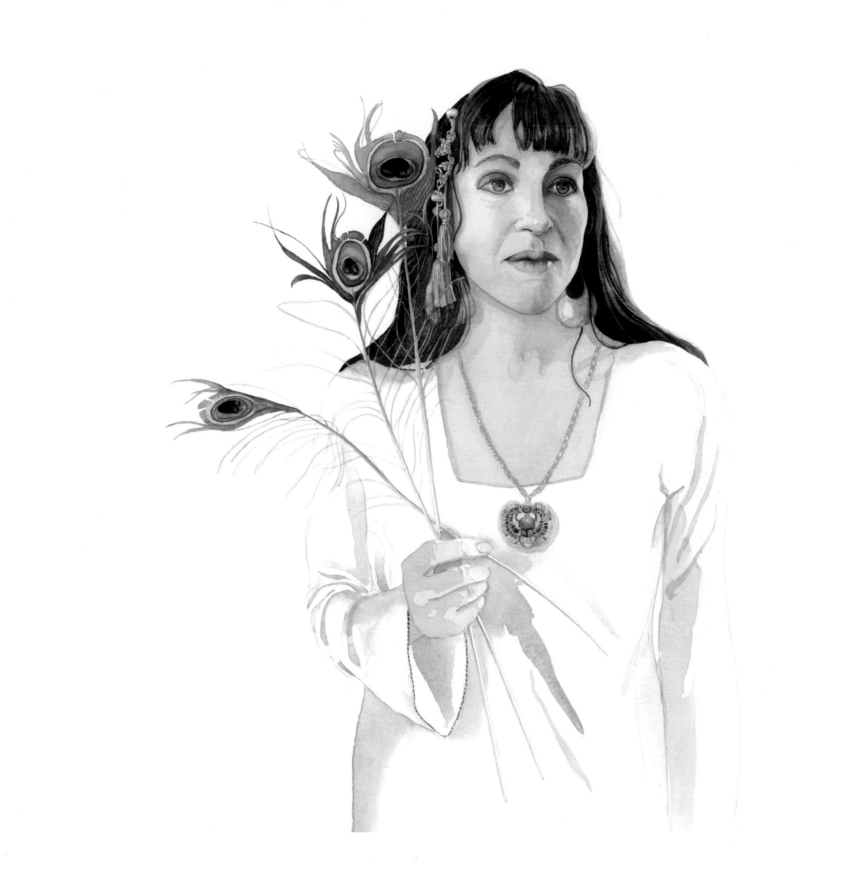

modern-day professors who are interested in reviving the plantings, which died centuries ago. "For example, the balsam groves in Jericho became a bone of contention between Cleopatra of Egypt and Herod the Great. During the Bar Kokhba Revolt, in the second century CE, Jewish fighters uprooted the plants so they would not be captured by the Romans."

Today, these historians and scientists are attempting to replant the balsam, identified as *Commiphora gileadensis*, a task that has proven difficult since transplants have died and seeds have failed to thrive. If successful, however, it is hoped the plants will once again yield their fragrant sap from which Cleopatra's legendary perfume can be made.[6]

ALEXANDRIA, EGYPT

In 331 BCE, Alexander the Great visited the thousan-year-old town Rhacotis and, determining that its port was precisely what he needed for his military, he established a new base for his operations there, renaming the city Alexandria. He left and never saw the city again, but upon his death his burial-ready body was stolen by Ptolemy and taken to Egypt. Alexander's golden coffin was a pilgrimage site until its destruction in the thirty-century riots.

It was under Ptolemy, not Alexander, that Alexandria became a center for learning and arts. Ptolemy created the university (called a museum), a library of seven hundred thousand volumes representing the greatest collection in the ancient world, and a highly technical lighthouse constructed on nearby Pharos, which was listed as one of the Seven Wonders of the World by Herodotus. Ptolemy welcomed Jews, Greeks, and philosophers from all over the world to contribute to the city's art and scholarship.

Massive earthquakes and subsequent tidal waves struck the city four centuries after Cleopatra's death, destroying palaces and cities throughout the coastlands. Many ancient relics of Alexandria now lie submerged in the Portus Magnus, or Great Harbor. Lost for millennia, the ruins have now been discovered by archaeologists and Cleopatra's own palace has been found.

In 1992, French explorer/marine archaeologist Franck Goddio, working with historians, geophysicists, archaeologists, and divers, discovered the ancient Queen's palace beneath the modern bay of Aboukir, Alexandria's Eastern Harbor. He located treasures such as a statue of the Greek god Hermes; a coiled serpent; a sacred bird of Egypt; and the head of a Roman empress. Goddio discovered that precious ivory decorated

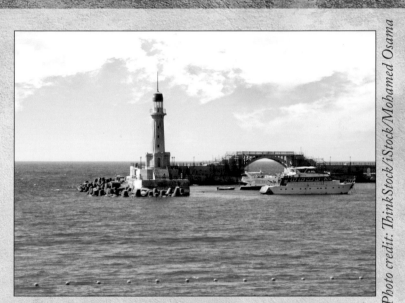

Photo credit: ThinkStock/iStock/Mohamed Osama

Alexandria, Eygpt

Cleopatra's entrance hall and that Indian tortoise shell and emeralds were inlaid on her massive palace doors. Numerous obelisks, sphinxes, and other statues have been found in the harbor, belonging to a wide span of pharaohs, kings, and queens, as well as turn-of-the-millennium Greek and Italian shipwrecks at the harbor's entrance.

Today, the area around ancient Alexandria is a vital part of Egypt and the religion is Muslim and Coptic. Women are generally segregated in public and on buses, and women and men who are not acquainted refrain from speaking to each other, following cultural mores. More than 80 percent of Egypt's imports and exports (mostly cotton, grains, sugar, and wool) still pass through the famous ports of Alexandria.

CINNAMON
Cinnamomum zeylanicum

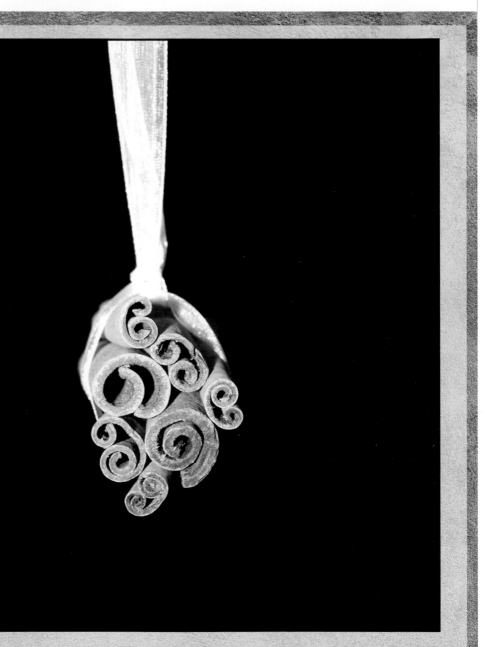

Valued as a spice in the Bible and by ancient Greek and Latin historians, heavenly-scented cinnamon, *Cinnamomum zeylanicum*, was mentioned in Chinese herbals as early as 2700 BCE. Variously known as *kinnamon* in Arabic, *kaju manis* in Malaysia, *Cinnamo'mum* in classical Greek, and *ginnamon* in Hebrew, it is often confused with similar species, especially Cassia. The Greek root *kassia* meant "to strip off the bark," as the thin fragrant bark of young trees was gathered, cut, peeled, and rolled in layers to be sold as sticks or powder.

Cinnamon and its cousin cassia were among the most highly prized spices in ancient world markets. In Ezekiel 27, cassia was exchanged alongside wrought iron. Exodus instructed Jews to "take the following fine spices: 500 shekels of liquid myrrh, half as much (that is, 250 shekels) of fragrant cinnamon, 250 shekels of fragrant cane, 500 shekels of cassia—all according to the sanctuary shekel—and a hin of olive oil. Make these into a sacred anointing oil, a fragrant blend, the work of a perfumer."

Near the frantic end of her life, Cleopatra stashed Ptolemy's most important treasures inside the Temple of Isis at Alexandria (Cleopatra's intended mausoleum): she hid gold, silver, emeralds, pearls, ebony, ivory—and cinnamon.

Cinnamon is prized today in cuisine and medicine. It is used to flavor hot cocoa and apple pie and is especially popular in Indian cuisine. Medicinally, cinnamon is aromatic, pungent, fragrant, carminative, and astringent, used as a glandular system stimulant, as a stomach antacid, and for colds and flu alongside elder and thyme. It is rubefacient—stimulating blood flow when applied topically in arthritis salves. Some herbalists use the tincture to stop bleeding from the uterus.

In the US Pharmacopoeia since 1820, cinnamon is valued for its high concentrations of volatile oils (distilled from twigs of *Cinnamomum cassia*). The trees are grown today in Ceylon, China, Vietnam, Laos, Java, and the West Indies. The genus includes the Camphor tree (*C. camphora*) and cassia (*C. aromaticum*), used as an adulterant of the true cinnamon (*C. verum*).

HENNA
Lawsonia inermis

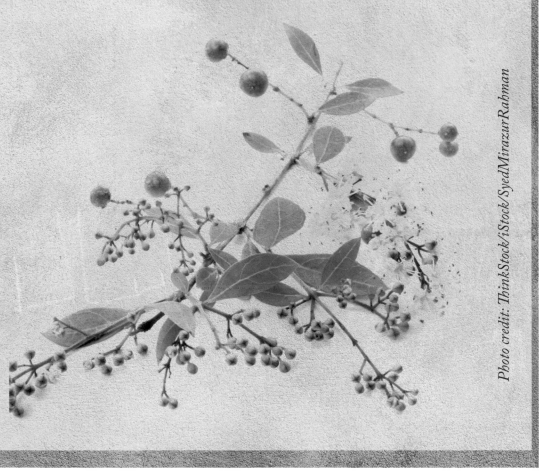

Women of ancient India and Egypt traditionally applied the natural dye henna, an ancient plant of North Africa and the Arabian Peninsula, to color their hair, hands, and feet. Teenagers today indulge in henna (or Bindi) treatments on their hands and feet, and traditionally Indian women celebrate the night before their wedding with women friends painting floral and fertility-symbol henna swirls, circles, and dots on their hands and feet. Today, thick henna flower attars called *Gulhina attars* are produced commercially in Uttar Pradesh, India.

But Henna is much older than this. The Biblical Song of Solomon (Song of Songs, or Canticle of Canticles) extols the virtues of Henna, or *Camphire*, a thorny shrub planted as a protective border around vineyards. The shrub produces many tiny and extremely fragrant blossoms, the scent of which did not go unnoticed by the Song's lovers:

"My Beloved is unto me as a cluster of
Camphire in the vineyards of En-Gedi,"
—Song of Solomon, I, 14.
"I am my Beloved's,
and his desire is for me.
Come, my Beloved,
Let us go into the open,
Let us lodge among the henna shrubs,
Let us go early to the vineyards,
Let us see if the vine has flowered,
If its blossoms have opened,
If the pomegranates are in bloom."
—Song of Solomon 7:11-13

Regarded as a deodorant, anti-irritant, antiseptic and, in Ayurveda, for the treatment of heat rash and skin allergies, henna is also considered aphrodisiac. Though safely used as a skin dye for tens of centuries, the US Food and Drug Administration forbids the sale of henna for use on the skin.

Photo credit: ThinkStock/iStock/SyedMirazurRahman

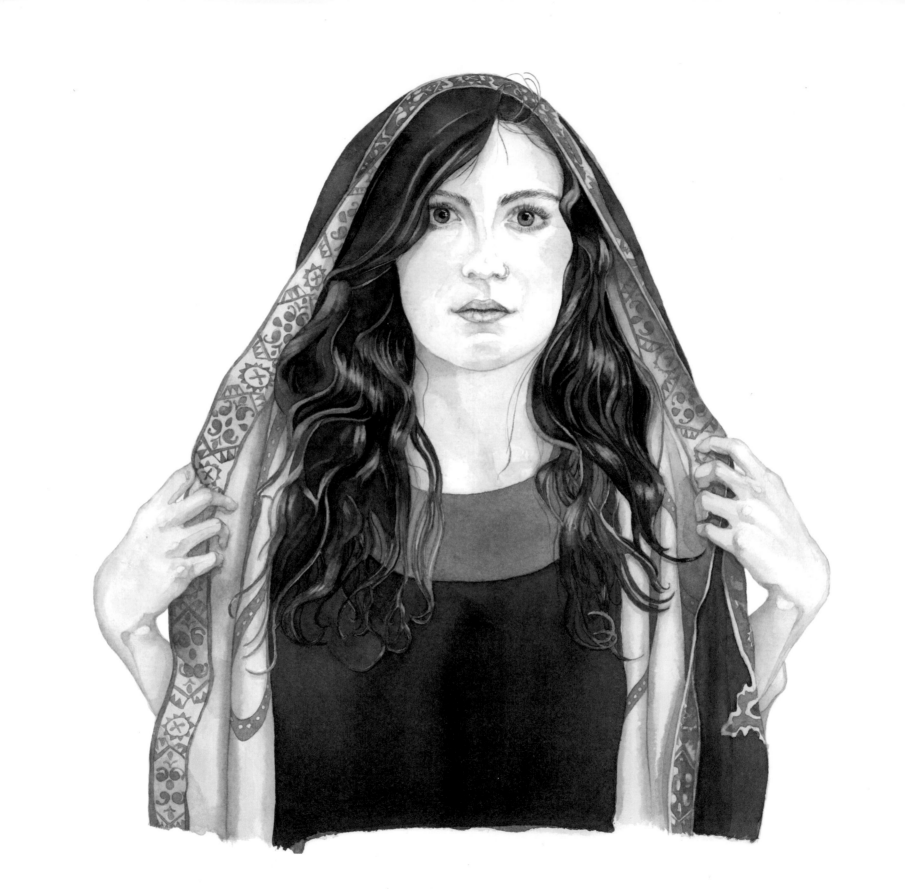

Maria Prophetissa

(c. 200 CE)

Nearly two thousand years ago, Alexandria was a bustling multicultural city poised on the port between Spain and the Near East. Its Egyptian citizens welcomed scientists from Greece, Italy, and Arabia, and Jewish and Gnostic philosophers studied and taught here.

In the first or second century CE, Cleopatra has long gone and the Ptolemaic dynasty has been replaced by Greek militaristic rule. Constantine won't be born for another 200 to 300 years, so early Christianity was colorful, diverse, and creative. Amid this melting pot of ideas, science, and religion, one woman was hiding.

We know little about this intriguing woman. Legends abound and theories about her identity may never be proven. She may have been a native Egyptian or a Greek immigrant, or possibly an Arabic raised in Alexandria. She is known today by various names, including Miriam the Jewess, Mary of Cleofa, and Maria Prophetissa (or Prophetissima), but it is not clear whether she was branded by others or whether she developed these aliases to protect her own identity. It's doubtful that she secreted herself away because she was being persecuted, since it appears women's contributions to society were accepted rather openly. And she wasn't hiding because of politics or gender discrimination or even for her own safety. Most likely, Maria Prophetissa kept herself—and her work—secret because her competition wanted to learn what she was inventing.

Alexandria was, at that time, a hotbed of creativity and invention. In this one city, people produced for the first time the steam engine, the piston, the water organ, and the medical syringe, and Maria Prophetissa would not be outdone. As a brilliant Gnostic chemist, Maria was renowned in second-century Alexandria for her explorations in chemistry and alchemy. Like most alchemists, she sought to transform common elements into gold, and like most Gnostic Christians, she likely desired to find the "elixir" that would give immortality and end what Gnostics considered the suffering of life.

To this end, Maria is credited with the invention of machines and the writing of texts that greatly impacted the way modern pharmacy and our cosmetic's industry function. In the early twentieth-century, she was back-credited with the discovery of hydrochloric acid, now called Mary's Black, and she is widely regarded with inventing devices that control and gauge heat. Specifically, she created a heating device that kept liquids in a chamber above a lower heating element: our now-common kitchen double boiler (or *bain de Marie, baño-Maria,* or Mary's Bath), used to gently heat liquids without burning them, allowing scientists and chefs to keep

MER, MARY

Mary Prophetissa is credited with the "black art" of alchemy and the discovery of liquid hydrochloric acid, sometimes called muriatic acid, "pertaining to brine or salt." *Mer, mar,* and *mur* all pertain to salt, or specifically, to the sea. Mariam, a popular ancient Hebrew name, meant "bitter sea," and some speculate it recalled tears and sadness. (Consider Miriam, sister of Moses, and the Israelites' tearful oppression in Egypt.)

Merlin Stone, in *Ancient Mirrors of Womanhood,* suggests sea and horse share etymology; the crests of waves were seen as horse heads, and, she notes, both the ocean and the animal were used for transportation. "This connection of sea and horse might help to explain the double use of the word *mare,* meaning 'sea' in Latin and Russian (and the root of the English word *marine*), while at the same time used to designate a female horse."

liquids at the constant temperature of 212 degrees Fahrenheit (100 degrees Celsius) to produce steam.

Maria also invented what she called a *tribikos,* a distillation machine that radically changed the way aromatherapy, perfumery, and ultimately herbalism would be practiced for the next two millennia. She devised a contraption of copper tubing, ceramic pottery, and metal that collected the mysterious steam and re-concentrated the vapors back into liquid, which was deemed essential to the understanding of other-worldly physics. Accordingly, this distillation and re-collection seemed a quasi-religious function for alchemists who considered steam akin to the release of soul from matter. Following Gnostic theories, Maria's distillery may have symbolized the womb of creation; future distillers would place a tiny copper "seed" in the "womb," which would be bathed in the recondensed liquids, possibly symbolizing amniotic fluids. Whether this was Maria's concept or not we do not know, but her skill in capturing steam was genuinely new thinking. It took another 100 to 200 years for Chinese and Arab scientists to begin distilling essential oils, followed much later by scientists of Japan and Europe. Maria's invention allowed herbalists to distill alcohol, essential oils, and scented waters (hydrosols) later valued by medieval women for cosmetics and medicine.

Maria is believed to have documented her work in *Maria Practica,* now lost. *The Dialogue of Maria and Aros on the*

ALCHEMY

Where the waters of the Nile deposited silt for their crops, ancient Egyptian men and women worshipped the god Khem. His cult originated in the fourth millennium BCE; since he was the god of reproduction and fertility, he was often depicted with an erect penis held in his left hand and a flail in his right, which is why, though he governed the harvest of food and medicinal herbs and is sometimes viewed as a god of healing, he more accurately symbolized reproduction. Rowdy festivals honored his "coming forth" with the milky, semen-like latex of wild prickly lettuce (*Lactuca virose, Lactuca serriola*) and cultivated *Lactuca sativa*.

Khem meant "black" and may have referred to the life-giving black soils of the Nile or to the skin of his people; their country was called *Khem* or *Khemit*, the "Black Land." Egypt's Arabic conquerors adopted this name as did the Barbary Moors, and according to W.E.B. duBois, when the Biblical authors wrote *Ham*, they meant the Egyptian *Khem* (DuBois, 21).

Later, in the fiery distillation laboratories of Alexandria, many substances turned black, thus the Black Art was named for the Black God Khem: *Alchemy*—and modern *chemistry*—had begun.

Magistery of Hermes is a fictitious conversation between Maria and Aros likely written centuries after her death. These texts describe her obscure Gnostic-inspired formula and hint at the genius behind the technology: she endeavored to manipulate a substance through four stages she called *nigredo*, *albedo*, *cinitritas*, and *rubedo*. Presumably, once a substance passed through these stages, it would transform into the Stone, or the substance of immortality. Maria famously coined the axiom, "One becomes two, two becomes three, and out of the third comes the one as the fourth," which can be symbolized as a circle inside a triangle inside a square inside another circle. To Maria, this complex symbolism may have addressed immortality and the concept of infinity, and it certainly conveyed mathematical grace.

Her ultimate goal of immortality (presumably) failed, but her legacy to the industries of perfumery, herbalism, cosmetics,

LADIES MANTLE
Alchemilla mollis

Astringent. Soothing. Toning. Ladies mantle is cherished as a gentle firming aid for the skin, the uterus, the perineum, and more. Named because the scalloped leaf resembles a woman's cloak, the herb is circumboreal, being found in North America, Europe, Asia, and even in the high mountain ranges of the Himalayas, according to herbalist Mrs. Maude Grieve. In Britain, the common and showy Ladies Mantle shares space with two more inconspicuous relatives, Field Ladies Mantle and Parsley Piert.

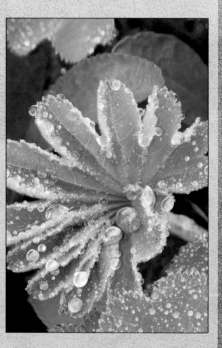

The leaves are harvested when wide, full, and fresh and can be tinctured in grain alcohol or witch hazel. The fresh or dried leaves can also be made into a strong water infusion with other astringent herbs such as sage, cranesbill, goldenrod, or yarrow and used in sitz baths, a very useful method for healing torn tissues for new mothers post-delivery. Some herbalists prize ladies mantle as a drinkable water infusion to reduce heavy menstrual flow.

aromatherapy, chemistry—and even culinary arts—are invaluable. Her quest for religious truth led to two thousand years of culinary and medicinal applications and the betterment of industries today that span hearth, home, restaurant, and laboratory.

TANSY
Tanacetum vulgare

Early alchemists worked with yellow flowers and sun-colored substances in an effort to create metallic gold. In ancient Latin, *auripigmentum* was a gold sulfide pigment used in art and alchemy, which the people of Syria, Middle Persia, and Old Iran called *orpiment*. Later, Greeks called orpiment *arsenikon*, our current *arsenic*. The yellow tansy flower was likely used in the process of gold transmutation because, like arsenic, it was toxic in large doses.

Pungent wild tansy grows across Europe and North America in disturbed areas and along roadsides. Since its bright yellow flowers form a patchwork of buttons at the top of the stalk, its names include bitter buttons, parsley fern, and scented fern. Strong volatile oils can be isolated from dried tansy leaves and flowers: thujone, borneol, and camphor, as well as resins. Thuja, wormwood, and sage also contain thujone and are powerful anthelmintics (worm expellers).

In folk tradition, women made a face lotion with tansy flowers steeped in buttermilk for nine days. The seventeenth-century physician Nicholas Culpeper advocated tansy for nearly everything: as a bitter, a carminative for upset stomach, as a powder for expelling worms, and especially for pregnant women. He claimed tansy was much safer than those nasty poisons hellebore and mercury, and he prescribed tansy for everything from ruptured appendix to toothache. Culpeper felt passionately that people's superstitions were keeping them from eating the healing tansy leaves, and he blamed this on the pope. Culpeper writes of tansy:

"Dame Venus was minded to pleasure women with child by this herb, for there grows not an herb fitter for their use than this is; it is just as though it were ordained for this purpose. This herb bruised and applied to the navel, stays miscarriages … Let those women that desire children love this herb, it is their best companion, the husband excepted."

Today, however, herbalists recognize tansy's toxicity and the herb is considered a powerful abortifacient—tansy oil has been used to induce abortion and in the process has proven fatal. Tansy tea and tincture can induce abortion even when the menstrual cycle is weeks overdue, according to herbalist Susun Weed, and she lists it among the strongest emmenagogues.

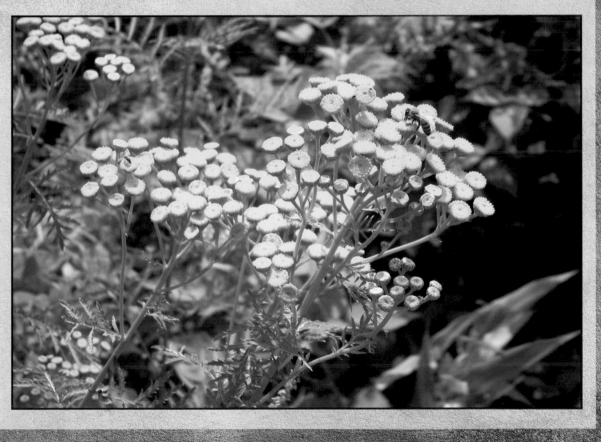

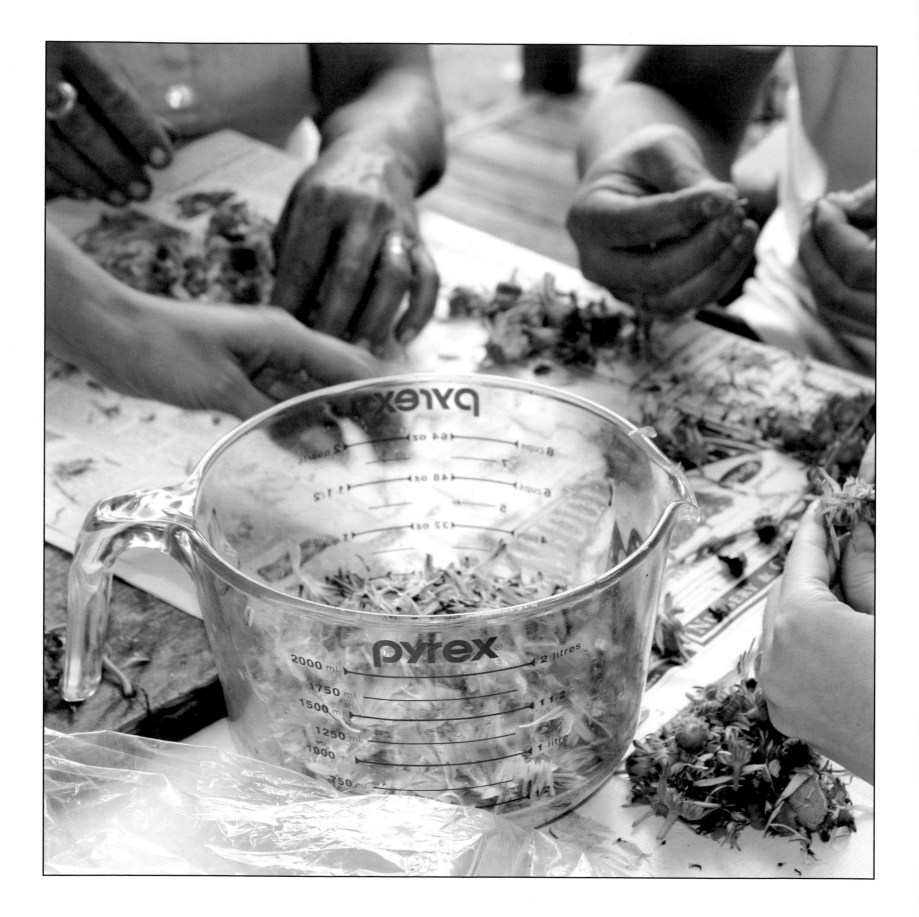

PART II:
BODY TRADITIONS

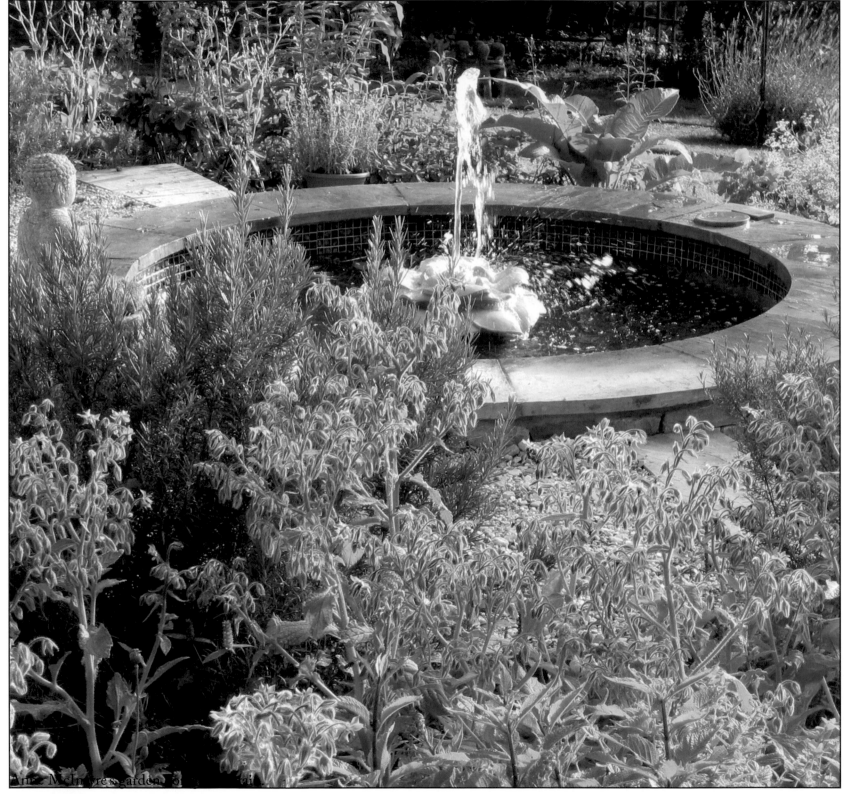

Anne McIntyre's garden

Chapter 6

AYURVEDA

yurveda is believed to be the world's most ancient system of natural healing, having been practiced for approximately 5,500 years in India and Asia;[1] the Sanskrit *Ayurveda* means "Knowledge of Life" and its remote Himalayan concept of simplistic healing maintains that suffering is disease but contentment is good health. Body, mind, and spirit naturally work together for harmony and longevity.

Ayurveda holds that the human spirit is the intelligence of life, and that physical matter (body as well as earth) is the spirit's energy or manifestation. Ayurvedic practitioners follow simple guidelines for maintaining physical, mental, and spiritual balance: deep breathing, meditation, yoga, diet, remedies, and guidance toward self-control. The primary focus of this healing system is on balance, harmony, and equilibrium, and rather than isolated people individually pursuing happiness, we're collectively moving toward a deeper understanding of life.

One of the earliest sages celebrated for founding Ayurveda was Atreya Punavarsu, who, according to legend, traveled thousands of miles to convene with other great healers in an effort to relieve human suffering. His student Agnivesh was the first Ayurvedic physician to collect wisdom that would place Ayurveda among the top medical systems for millennia.

In the first century AD, this oral tradition was recorded by Charaka, Ayurveda's third physician. Today, much of this original information is still revered as central to the philosophy; the system still teaches balance but tempers what could be misconstrued as "stagnant" with the important flow of energy, or *prana*.

Ayurveda consists of eight branches, of which *Rasayana* involves therapy, rejuvenation, and the building of strength. Herbalism has much to offer in this respect, and Ayurveda promotes the use of herbs and the inclusion of a healthy diet in this process. There are also eight tissues of the body, the eighth being *ojas*, the essence of life, which is a partly physical/partly spiritual product of nutrition and digestion that serves as an energy reserve.

In addition to the *ojas* are the three *doshas*, or vital energies, which comprise every person's makeup (*Prakruti*). The doshas must work harmoniously for a person to maintain health. Kapha represents earth and water and governs phlegm, mucous, and obesity. A majority of kapha results in a voluptuous, strong, calm, grounded—but often sluggish and overweight—person. Vata represents ether and air, and an excess of vata can result in a high-strung, fast, agitated, creative, nervous, and restless person. Pitta governs fire and water and affects the digestion; an excess results in a passionate but ordered, precise, and often pushy person. Every person contains all three doshas; the goal is to maintain their flowing balance.

Digestion is of utmost importance; this is where the outside world is assimilated into the inner. If assimilation is inadequate, or if the nutrition is toxic, then health is impossible. Ayurveda governs proper digestion through a variety of mechanisms, including detoxification and rejuvenation.

Detoxification clears *Ama* (toxins) and is employed before a period of rejuvenation, so as to begin "with a clean slate." Cleansing diets include kitchari (brown rice, mung beans, spices, and ghee); fasting; and herbs such as ginger, black pepper, cinnamon, clove, cumin, myrrh, and asafetida.

Rejuvenation can begin after *Ama* has cleared; this stokes the digestive fire or *Agni*. Rasayana tonic foods and herbs are nourishing for the body and the mind as well, resulting in longer life, better mental agility, and a livelier spirit.

Rasayana includes eating meat, milk, honey, ghee; indulging in brisk oil massages (the vitalizing kind, not stupefying); and comforting baths. Rasayana herbs include ashwagandha (*Withania somnifera*); shatavari (*Asparagus racemosus*); pepper; gotu kola (*Centella asiatica*); tulsi or holy basil (*Ocimum sanctum*); and amalaki (*Emblica officinalis*).

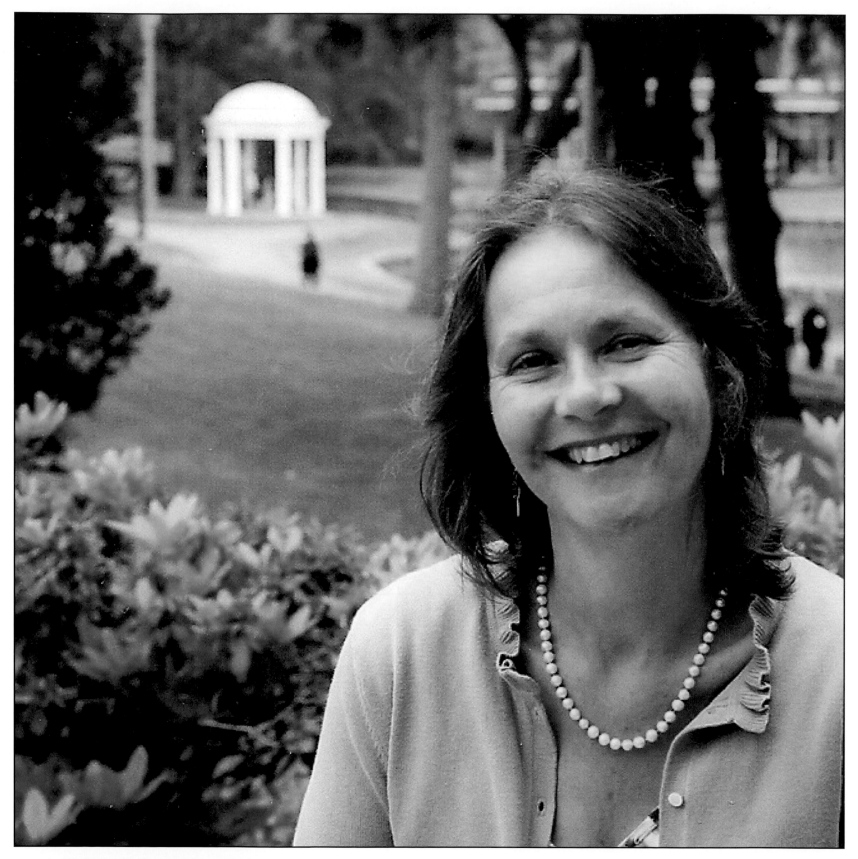

Anne McIntyre

Anatural herbalist, and intrigued at age sixteen with the poetry of India, Anne McIntyre now blends the ancient wisdom of Ayurveda, the "Knowledge of Life" of India, with the home-and-hearth wisdom of European women healers and gardeners.

As a teen, Anne was enamored with the ancient hymns and poetry of India: the Upanishads, the Vedas, and the Bhagavad Gita. "I was amazed by their beauty, and really inspired. I thought, 'This is incredible and I want to know more.'" Anne attended Buddhist meditation classes, becoming engrossed in the sacred process of clearing energy and remaining pure—even to the extent that she would refuse to go out to dinner with her parents or to attend the cinema because she felt it was an indulgence of the senses. "I was very young and idealistic, and seriously thought that if I worked very hard and really delved into this, I would probably achieve enlightenment . . . because it's all about enlightenment, love and liberation, pure bliss, and moksha, and so on. I was so inspired that I thought maybe by age thirty, which was a long way away, I might be an enlightened being!"

Anne laughs to remember how strictly she observed her newfound philosophy, but it was a serious motivator in her life. After completing her A-Level exams, she enrolled in Religious Studies in Arabic and soon traveled to India. "I went to temples and was totally inspired by India and came back to go to University. But as it turned out, it was a very dry academic subject and it wasn't alive enough for me, so after six months I quit and said I've got to go to South America!"

But she was sidetracked: her parents alerted her to a cottage for rent on Osea Island on the eastern coast of England. Virtually isolated due to tides, the island was a tiny (2 miles by .5 mile) bird sanctuary. Anne moved to the cottage and began a vegetable garden and, with the help of *Food for Free* by Richard Mabey, she collected foods from the wild. "The more I read about dandelion, rock sunflower, sea spinach, sea lettuce, the more I realized they were not only foods but also medicines. I completely fell in love with Mother Nature."

"The knowledge of flowers is a gift."

This quiet time with nature had a profound effect on Anne's perception of her life's purpose and inspired her future career as

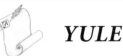

YULE

Yule is the winter solstice, the shortest day and longest night of the year, between the pagan holy days Samhain (Halloween) and Imbolc (St. Brigit's Day or Groundhog Day, February 2). *Yule* derives from Old Norse *Jól*, referring to a Germanic pagan feast. We still celebrate Yule Tide or Christmastide, vestiges of the ancient Anglo-Saxon calendar, which consisted of two "tides," each lasting sixty days: summer's Litha Tide, the months before and after summer solstice, and winter's Yule Tide.

Jól became *geol* in Old English, then *yoole*, and finally *Yule*. It gives us *jolly*, since the feasts of *Jól* were merry. (But not for the boar: each *Jól*, a boar was ritually slaughtered, a tradition evident in our Christmas ham.) Old French borrowed *Jól* to form *jolif* and *joli*, "pretty"; it originally meant "festive."

The word *Jól* is the root of "wheel," or *hjol*. The Wheel of the Year was sacred to ancient people who depended on the stars to predict the weather, the future, and what their lives would *entail* (a reference to divining).

an herbal healer. "I had a really strong sense that it was through Nature that we could heal ourselves not only on a physical level but also on an emotional level and a mental level. I felt so in harmony by eating so well and living a lot outside, I felt physically well but I also felt emotionally blissed out. It was probably the happiest time of my life."

Eventually, however, Anne "settled down and got a sensible job," and then traveled through the Andes mountains of Columbia. She returned to England and enrolled in the National Institute of Medical Herbalists, and in 1981 she qualified as a western herbalist with the NIMH. She set up her own practice and clinic with her husband in the Cotswolds, Gloustershire, but something was missing. "I found it hard to practice *just* as a western herbalist, so I studied massage and incorporated massage into my practice. Then I studied aromatherapy, then homeopathy, then counseling. Still it wasn't enough, somehow."

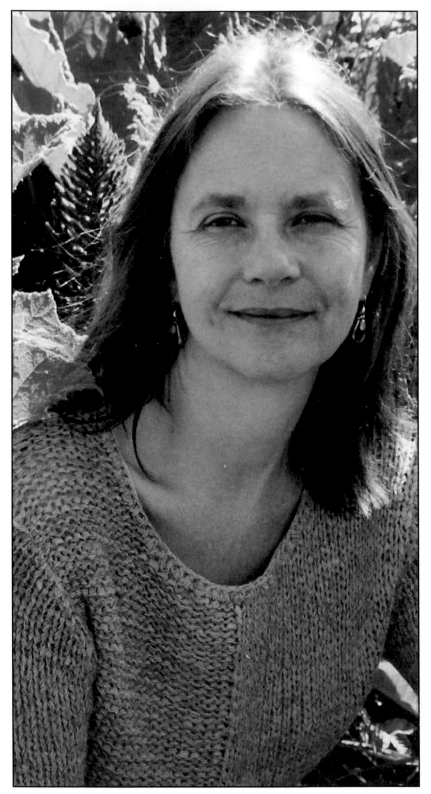

Finally she discovered Ayurvedic teacher Dr. Vasant Lad. "[Lad's method] is a marriage of my passion for Indian philosophy, which had never gone away, and herbal medicine. I had done some courses in Ayurveda but felt it was really complicated. With Lad's enormous depth of wisdom and knowledge, it made complete sense to me."

Anne incorporated this ancient method of healing and living into her practice for the next twenty years. "In my practice, it's a real mish-mash of the two. I use Ayurvedic and western herbs. If people come to me who know about Ayurveda, that's great because we can do Ayu-speak, as I call it. I can say, I think your dosha is imbalanced or your pitta is high, and we need to do cooling down or we need to do this . . . and it makes sense. Most people love it.

"I still feel that, even after twenty years of incorporating this into my practice, I'm always learning. I'm the kind of person that has a great need for more knowledge. I'm constantly studying more and there's so much more to learn. I find it really inspiring."

Herbs

Among Anne's favorite healing herbs are rose, holy basil, ashwagandha, rosemary, chamomile, and echinacea. She offers between 150 and 200 different herbs in her dispensary, and she's written numerous books about healing plants, including *The Complete Floral Healer* and *Dispensing with Tradition*. She dispenses herbal medicines in the form of tinctures, creams, lotions, and capsules, though she prefers clients take herbs as powders.

"The knowledge of flowers is a gift," she says. "We really need to be with the plants, actually growing them and being with them. You can get too involved taking herbs in capsules and pills. I think spending as much time in nature and with the plants is absolutely essential. Get to know what the plant looks like, feels like, and you'll never forget what the plant is about. The thing that's inspired me right from the beginning is being with them. So don't get too involved with all the pills and potions on the shelves. Just spend time with the plants."

Photo credit: Anne McIntyre

ANNE'S SPIRAL WOMEN'S GARDEN

From birth to paradise.

Anne has created a unique garden at her home, called Artemis House. It is designed in three circles: the first is the first thirty years of life, the second is the next thirty, and it ends around age ninety. "As you complete the spiral, each circle gets smaller because life gets faster, doesn't it?" says Anne. "Because the older you get, the quicker the years go 'round. Childhood feels like a long time."

The garden starts with the Birth Canal, with arches of raspberries, followed by the Children's Garden with nursery rhyme herbs. Then there's a Mary Garden for virginity, because medieval monasteries had secluded meditative spaces dedicated to the Virgin Mary with lavender, marigold, lilies, and chamomile. Then a Moon Garden edged with silver artemisias and red herbs for the moon and bleeding.

Next is a Male Energy Garden with a pottery Apollo, Artemis's twin brother. Anne planted phallic-shaped red-hot pokers, poppies full of seeds, and long courgettes (zucchinis). Then there's a Falling in Love Garden, with a secluded arbor and love potion herbs.

Next come two arches crossed for union, and the bed is rose-shaped. This Marriage Garden is adorned with hanging

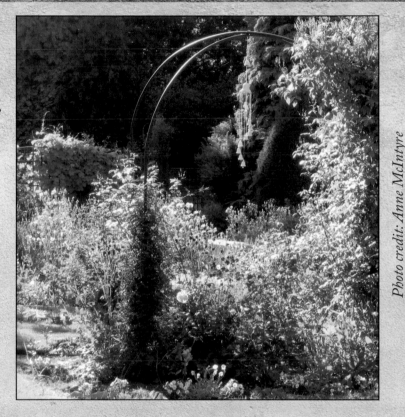

Photo credit: Anne McIntyre

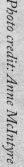

Photo credit: Anne McIntyre

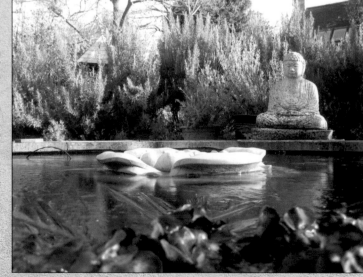

silver bells and herbs associated with courage and happiness like myrtle, rose, and jasmine. The last garden in this circle is a Fertility Garden with herbs for breastfeeding.

The dark side of the moon is a Menopause Garden edged with red sage, and then the Midlife Crisis Garden with a statue of a frantic woman surrounded by chaotic daisies. These gardens contain St. John's wort, borage, lemon balm, ashwagandha, and schisandra. A Wise Crone Garden sports the hallucinogenic herbs henbane and datura.

Finally, in the Garden of the Spirit, lavender, hyssop, holy basil, and gotu kola grow near a colorful pond with water lilies. A lotus-shaped fountain represents Eternal Life and Bliss. The last herb rosemary, an evergreen, represents eternal life, memory, loyalty, love, and, ultimately, immortality.

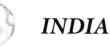

Bordered to the north by the 23,600-foot-high Himalaya mountain range and to the southwest by the 15,000-foot-deep Arabian Sea, India is a striking peninsula of ancient traditions and deep-seated respect for the value and efficacy of healing plants. The second most populous country in the world (after China), the majority of India's colorful and vibrant culture uses alternative medicine for healing. Nearly four-fifths[1] of India's billion population relies on Ayurveda, Siddha, Unani (a traditional and formal Persian medicine system based on Hippocrates and Galen and developed by Muslim scientist Hakim Ibn Sina, or Avicenna), and homeopathic medicines,[2] sometimes in combination with allopathic medicine. Recent scrutiny of the herbs used in rural India, in particular, has caused concern in allopathic circles since many of today's popular herbs are not the same as those listed in ancient texts or supported by empiric, traditional healing knowledge.[3]

In India, both women and men dress brightly, cows are sacred, and Hinduism is the main religion (along with Jainism, Buddhism, and Sikhism). Hinduism, a way of life termed *Sanatana-Dharma*, makes the awareness and understanding of life, death, and eternity its primary goal and it truly functions less as a religion and more as a spiritual pursuit, having no prophets or dogmatic leaders. It acknowledges reincarnation, the law of karma, and the sanctity of individual souls as common and equal to all souls.

For centuries, plants have held a sacred and central place in the medical systems of India, with hymns extolling their virtues in the ancient Rig Veda, the Indian scriptures written between 1700 and 1100 BCE. Hymn XCVII Praise of Herbs honors herbs as divine natural healers and celebrates them as generously curing all illnesses from humans. At times, the hymn addresses the plants themselves, saying, "Plants, by this name I speak to you, Mothers, to you the Goddesses," and also:

"Do ye who have a thousand powers free this my patients from disease."

"The healing virtues of the Plains stream forth like cattle from the stall,—
Plants that shall win me store of wealth, and save thy vital breath, O man.
Reliever is your mother's name, and hence Restorers are ye called. Rivers are ye with wings that fly: keep far whatever brings disease."

"Let fruitful plants, and fruitless, those that blossom, and the blossomless,
Urged onward by Brhaspati, release us from our pain and grief;
Release me from the curse's plague and woe that comes from Varuna…"

"All Plants that hear this speech, and those that have departed far away,
Come all assembled and confer your healing power upon this Herb."[4]

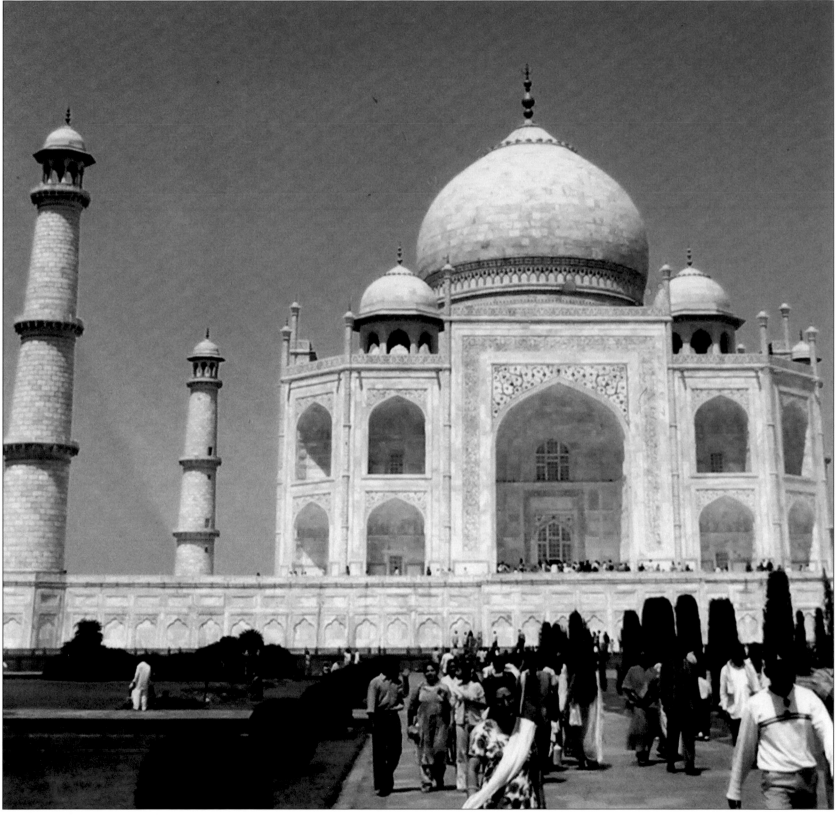

Taj Mahal, India

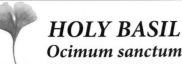

GINGER
Zingiber officinale

This favorite among spices, ginger is a circulatory stimulant that warms the blood and is diaphoretic, bringing sweat to reduce high fevers. Old Europe's wives relied on this exotic rhizome on cold days in a cup of hot tea, and they brewed it with elderberry or mint to relieve morning and motion sickness. Today, women still use ginger for cramps and nausea associated with premenstrual syndrome or pregnancy.

Externally, a poultice of shredded boiled ginger or a compress of strong ginger tea eases rheumatism and arthritis, as the stimulating juice is rubefacient and warming.

Called "pepper root," ginger stimulates digestive function. Allegedly, both Confucius and the Moghul Emperor Akbar included ginger with every meal, and the lusty cuisines of India and Asia use ginger for its enlivening citrus flavor and peppery, pungent heat. Ayurveda reveres ginger as the Great Medicament for treating colds, bronchial ailments, and stomach complaints, and it is used topically on children's chests for pulmonary relief.

After returning from China in 1292, Venetian explorer Marco Polo dictated experiences from his journeys, finally published as *Travels* in 1477. He mentions the thriving ports of Kayal, Comorin, Quilon, Thana, Somnath, and Cambay and notes that ginger, turmeric, and cardamom were major exports. "There is a great abundance of pepper and also of ginger, besides cinnamon in plenty and other spices, turbit and coconuts … Goods … that go to Aden are carried thence to Alexandria" (Lunde, 37–40).

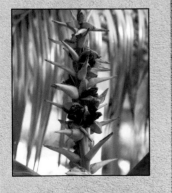

Ginger is not mentioned in the Bible, but the Qur'an bejewels ginger with high status and beautiful imagery, describing a flowing fountain called Salsabil, spouting a sustaining beverage of ginger and camphor for the righteous.

HOLY BASIL
Ocimum sanctum

It is said that no family courtyard in India is complete without a live tulsi plant planted there. Tulsi, *Ocimum sanctum* (also known as *Ocimum tenuiflorum*, Holy Basil, and Tulasi) is a revered herb native to India that has flourished for thousands of years. Praised in the *Padmapurana*, a five-thousand-year-old sacred hymn of Ayurveda, Tulsi confers health, longevity, and happiness upon those who worship and grow it. The plant is a favorite of the god Vishnu, "the Preserver," and was used in Egyptian mummification and Greek mourning rituals for centuries before it gained a more positive role as a plant for life, rather than death.

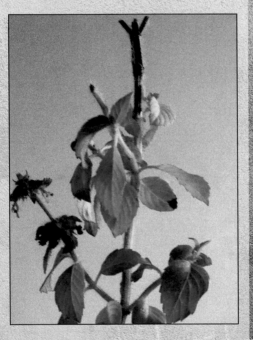

India's devout grow three main varieties of holy basil: Krishna (of greatest medicinal value), Rama, and Vana, a wild basil native to India. Krishna tulsi is commonly used for worship, where a single plant or an entire grove may be grown in containers or sacred gardens. Anne McIntyre lists the plant among her favorites. "Tulsi tastes amazing," she says. "I love the fact that it's dedicated to Vishnu in India. It gives the flavor of the spiritual life in India. It is very calming and uplifting, gives clarity, and creates resilience to physical stress on the body from the environment."

It is said that Tulsi, an Indian goddess, reincarnated herself as the sacred basil as her devotion to Lord Vishnu; in this form, she offered herself for worship on his behalf.

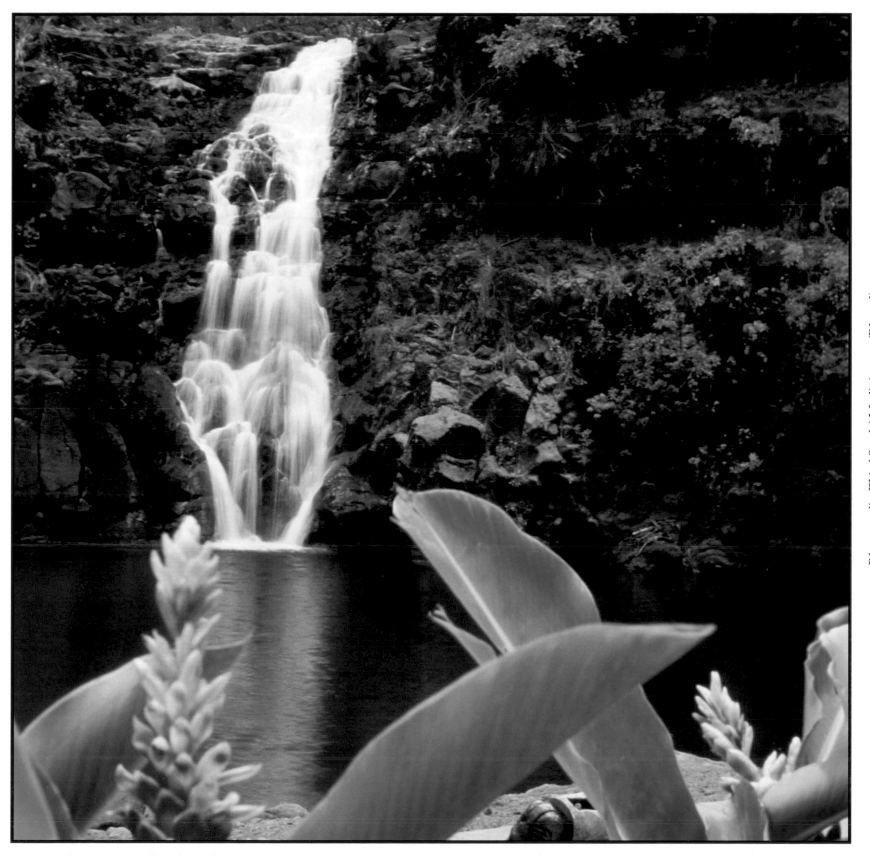

Chapter 7
EASTERN ORIENTAL MEDICINE

As one branch of Eastern medicine, Traditional Chinese Medicine (TCM) is a vast science that spans many cultures and thousands of years. It can include everything from acupuncture to bloodletting, massage, botanical prescriptions, and dietary guidance, and it generally includes teachings designed to point the patient toward a mystical though rational understanding of the illness. Early in its formation as a healing practice, TCM practitioners believed magic, astrology, and curses from ancestors were valid influences on a person's health, though since roughly the second century AD, practitioners have focused more scientifically on developing diagnoses and treatment based on a system of meridians of energy located throughout the body. Also, since about the same time, herbal remedies have become standard in physician-treated illnesses.

Ancient Chinese medical systems evolved in different but complementary directions. Both the philosophies of Yin/Yang (opposites) and the Five Elements (or Five Phases) have been accepted as standard methods of diagnosis and treatment in China for more than two thousand years.

The origins of the Yin/Yang Theory can be traced to the Shang dynasty of approximately 1600 BCE. Chinese medical practitioners explored the diagnosis of illness based on dualities of symptoms and body/mind characteristics. The symbolism of yin and yang refers to a person's general symptomatic picture: for instance, yin, being dark, passive and inherently feminine, presented with the following complaints: cold; moist tongue; pale lips; excess saliva; desire for warmth and warm food; thin and clear expectoration; plentiful urine; and a slow or deep pulse. Its opposite is yang, being hot, light and inherently masculine. Yang patients presented with symptoms including restlessness; red complexion; dry skin/nails/hair/lips; hard or leathery tongue/skin/lips; scant urine; constipation; warm

to the touch; and rapid pulse. Generally, yin is shady while yang is light, or yin is water while yang is fire. Attributing these images to the human body makes symptoms easy to group into categories for treatment.

Grouping symptoms and even diseases by oppositional category allowed practitioners to remedy the disease with its opposite, calling for cooling medicines that would alleviate hot conditions and bring the body back into balance (which is similar to the central tenet of India's Ayurveda). Over time, the yin/yang philosophy would group most patients under one of eight categories: cold, hot, deficiency (or emptiness), excess (or fullness), internal, external, and yin or yang.

Another traditional Chinese medical philosophy involves the Five Elements or Five Phases, which recall the Western images of fire, metal, water, and earth. In Chinese practice, great care has gone into this complex system to ensure that every illness, body part, constitution, food flavor, and symptom fits into one of the following categories: wood, fire, earth, metal, and water (some experts insert wind instead of wood). However, the system is generally called not the Five Elements but the Five Phases or even the Five Seasons, indicating that there is a natural flow or movement from one quality to the next, often in a sequential order and coming as a result of the previous quality. It is this dynamic and fluid concept of the body and its health that makes this type of Chinese Medicine appealing as people change and transition through diets, life stages, and age.

The Five Elements also includes the yin/yang system previously mentioned. In this philosophy, the organs of the body are identified by whether they are yin: heart, liver, spleen, lung, and kidney, or yang: stomach, gallbladder, small intestine, large intestine, bladder, and the so-called triple burner, an area of the abdomen that

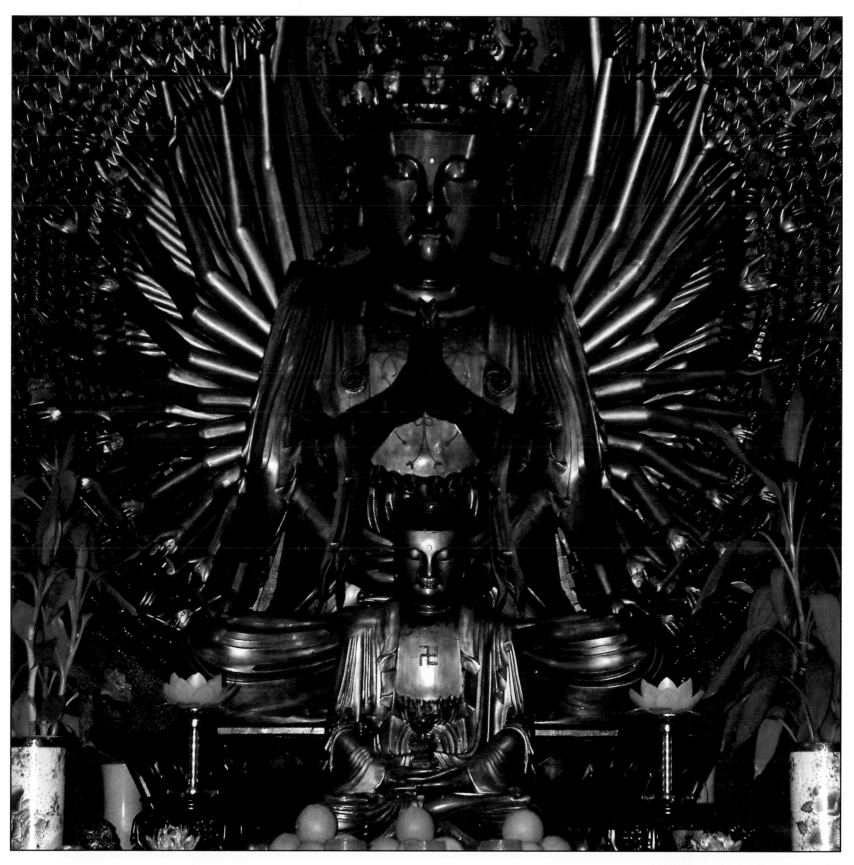

produces heat or the "fire of the life force." This organ (which has no equivalent in Western medicine) may be what is responsible for the fire of digestion and for anger, and it echoes yoga's hot Kundalini energy, which lies "like a serpent" at the base of the spine.

The healing philosophy of wood, water, fire, earth, and metal has become so ingrained in Chinese culture that it influences many parts of society, including not only health care, but also the military, music, and rituals such as the tea ceremony, which uses the Five Elements to determine how the ceremony is organized, which flowers are included, and how many people attend. Moreover, Chinese cuisine is organized into strict categories that reflect the Five Elements; the Five Flavors are acrid, sour, sweet, bitter, and salty.

Diagnostics was an early and flourishing skill taught to ancient Chinese practitioners. Typical methods for diagnosis included reading the pulse, examining the tongue, touching the skin, and examining the urine and feces. Once diagnosed, patients were prescribed remedies that traditionally included a majority of plant ingredients with corollary animal parts (from animals such as the snake, turtle, bear, rhinoceros, manta ray, tiger, and sea horse) as well as mineral ingredients. Ancient remedies also included the use of human parts such as fingernails, dandruff and earwax (see "Folk Medicine," chapter 4), but today's Chinese medicine, in an effort to modernize with Western medicine, tends to dismiss these.

Traditional Chinese philosophies in medicine have influenced a wide range of other Eastern methods, including Taoism, a philosophical and religious tradition that emphasizes health through harmony with a particular emphasis on herbal therapy and a connection to nature, according to Taoist master Chang Yi Hsiang (see later in this chapter). Considered a primary Taoist art, herbal therapy uses traditional Chinese philosophies (including yin/yang), diet and cooking, and meditation, often with direct one-on-one contact with plants.

Finally, for the herbalist interested in learning more about Chinese medicine, there is moxibustion: this is a practice within acupuncture (the insertion of needles into the skin to activate certain points of energy) that includes the burning of dried mugwort leaves close to the skin. The herb *Artimesia vulgare*, or common mugwort, is a bitter herb renowned in Western herbal medicine for its effect on digestion and, in ancient Celtic medicine, for its magical properties. In acupuncture, "moxa" is appreciated for its warming qualities and is used to treat cold and deficient conditions, as well as specific instances of breech babies before childbirth.

Tibetan Medicine

Dr. Phuntsog Wangmo is called Lhajen Wangmo, which denotes her status as a doctor. In ancient times, Tibetan healers were honored with the title Lhaje, meaning "King of the King," a title reflecting the greatness associated with the healer's skill and his or her sacrifice for the benefit of others. The Tibetan culture began more than 4,000 years ago in Shang Shung, the first kingdom of Tibet. The medicine of Tibet became fully formed approximately 2,500 years ago and is one of the oldest continuously practiced healing modalities on Earth. Just as the Tibetan healing system was influenced by its neighbors China, Persia, India, and even Greece, so did it incorporate the religions of time and locale—embracing Buddhism to form a unique practice of Tibetan Buddhism, which is central to its healing practice. Today, more than six million Tibetans (and many of the 7.5 million Chinese who live in the Tibetan provinces of Kham and Amdo) rely on Tibetan medicine.

Knowledge in Tibetan culture is generally classified into five major fields: art, craft, linguistics/poetry, medicine, and *inner knowledge*, considered the most important. Traditional Tibetan medicine is often practiced in conjunction with other therapies, such as Kunye (Tibetan massage), nutrition and prevention, acupuncture, moxibustion, astrology, and vinisection (bloodletting). Three humors are considered the basis of diagnosis and healing: wind, bile, and phlegm, each with its own temperature and pulse indications. All illness is the result of three states of being, or "poisons of the mind": ignorance, attachment, and aversion. These states of mind can infect the body, which is made up of three principles of function:

rLung is that which moves in the body. Consider it moving or kinetic energy, that which flows within the body, such as blood, energy, and even thoughts.

mKhris-pa is that which is heat, and includes thermoregulation, metabolism, liver function, and even the intellect or passion.

Bad-kan is that which is cold. In the body, this includes digestion (opposite Western herbalist's idea of digestive heat), the skeletal system, joints, and mental health. In the eighth century, four written texts called the Medical Tantras were brought to Tibet; these texts specified 84,000 diseases and 2,000 herbs and mineral mixtures as remedies. This literature, along with a strong Buddhist underpinning, has been the basis of Tibetan healing for centuries.

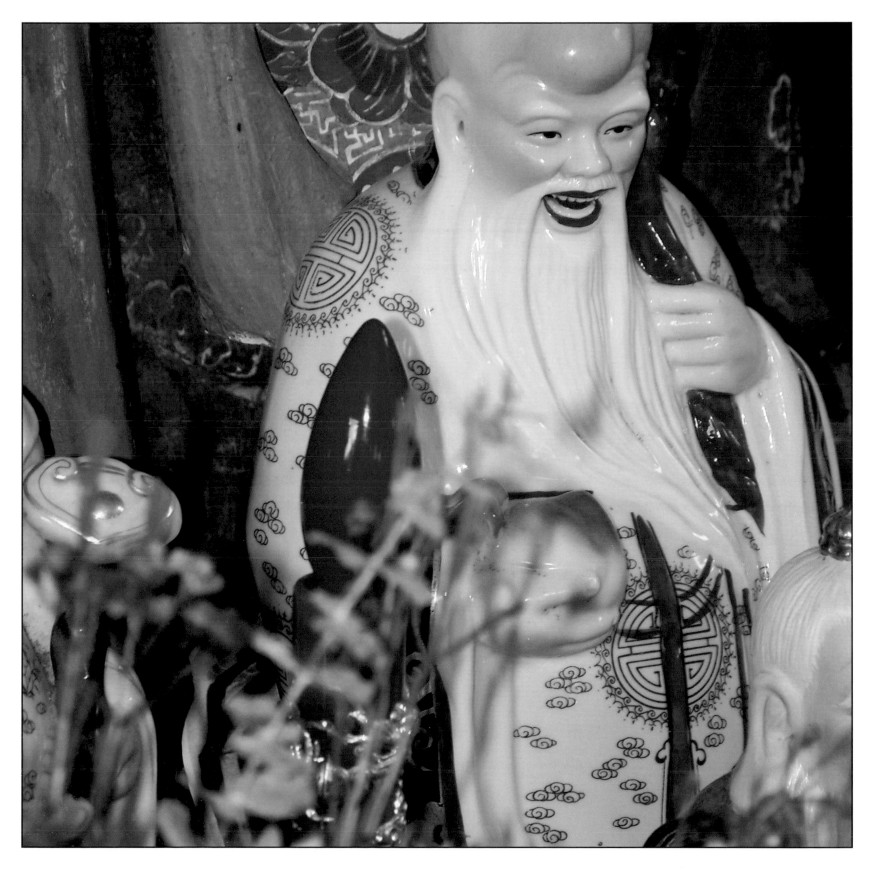

Dr. Chang Yi Hsiang

Outside the red-and-white painted Taihsuan Temple in Honolulu, the sky is a brilliant blue and the neighborhood is quiet. I slip off my shoes and enter a seating area filled with tempting books and a kitchen blooming with teapots and flowers. A lovely woman with dark, glossy hair smiles to me and indicates a cream-colored orchid growing in a pot. "It looks perfect, like plastic," she says. "I grew that from a tiny seed. It took twelve years! You have to appreciate her, because she's a queen, right?"

This woman may very well be a queen, too. She is cheerful and graceful, and with every step she exudes a lightness that makes me want to stand up straight and pull my tummy in. She is Chinese Taoist master Dr. Chang Yi Hsiang, or Lillian as she is fondly known, and she founded this temple and the World Medicine Institute in Honolulu to teach an intensive course of study in acupuncture, Chinese herbal medicine, and Taoist philosophy. Her Queen orchid has lived a dozen years in a temple, classroom, library, laboratory, and clinic with one of the world's most revered Taoist healers.

In the great room stands a floor-to-ceiling altar ornamented with Buddhist statues, fresh flowers, cups of tea, bowls of fruit, offerings, fresh flower leis, incense cones, and massive soccer ball–sized persimmons picked that morning from Dr. Chang's lush volcanic-soil gardens. The persimmons must ripen after being picked and they cannot be taken to the mainland, so I must decline when Dr. Chang offers me one. "It's too bad you're leaving today," she says, smiling. "You must come back and take a course with me."

I wouldn't be the only one: Dr. Chang is world-renowned and teaches thousands of students annually in conjunction with the University of Hawai'i. "For sixteen years," she says, "I had one thousand students a year. I don't do that anymore. I let go, got smaller," grateful to reduce her teaching load. "It's busy enough. We still have lots to do, lots to treat, lots to teach. I had one hundred patients a day. Same thing, I don't do that anymore, I cut down a lot, maybe 80 percent."

She is no ordinary acupuncturist. Beginning her Taoist training at age six in China, Lillian Chang learned the Six Secret Taoist Teachings from Master Chang En Pu. Her studies included Qi gong, herbal formulas, processing methods (including making the immortality pill of *Tsin Dan*), acupuncture, meditation, charm language writing, magic language with complicated Tiger form, palmistry, feng shui, astrology, Chinese brush calligraphy, painting, nutrition, Taoist chanting, *I Ching*, Lao Tse's *Tao Te Ching*, and other skills required of a devoted Taoist master.

A lifelong healer, Dr. Chang is the sixty-fourth generation Taoist lineage holder of a two-thousand-year-old tradition, counting from the Han Dynasty, or seventy-two generations counting her first recorded ancestor. She earned a medical degree in Traditional Chinese Medicine specializing in treating children with disabilities, and a PhD in Chinese Philosophy and Integrated Medicine in both China and the United States. She makes it clear that Taoist healing traditions emphasize natural healing, spirituality, and respect. "We appreciate the green earth, and what changes in Heaven there are for us, and how to adapt to these changes, how to make the best, healthiest happiest harmonious life." She travels the world every six months, visiting the Orient, Europe, the Middle East, the US mainland, Australia, New Zealand, and Canada teaching her primary core course in Taoist plant philosophy.

"For many, many years I never got sick once. I never caught a cold once. That's because I do it with plants. They're the ones who take my pain, take my fever, take all my sickness. So I appreciate the plants. I use plants for nutrition and for food, for healing and for rituals, as a guideline to live in harmony."

Dr. Chang takes her students into the wild to identify fresh herbs, especially the thousands of Hawai'ian and Chinese plants she grows herself on Oahu, where the twelfth State Legislature of Hawai'i designated her a Living Treasure of Hawai'i. "I take students to identify plants," she says, "not to [remove] them but to make a friend with them, to connect. You don't necessarily have to go get them, to cut them and boil them, in order to heal. Actually," she says, her eyes twinkling, "you just connect with them. The special Taoist appreciation of nature is your connection to nature and seeing the life source of support."

She mentions, for example, the herb Wedelia, a ground cover in the *Asteraceae* family with the unfortunate reputation as an invasive

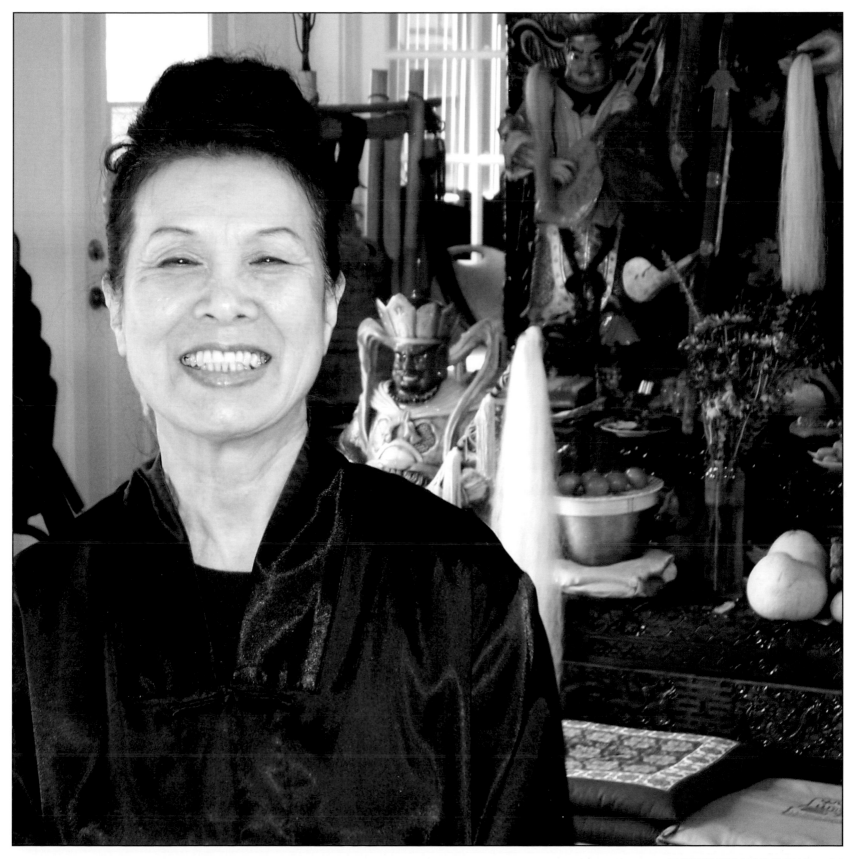

weed in Florida. "It has great qualities for people who are injured badly, even with a car accident, sports injury, broken bones, or torn tendons. These are difficult things to heal. So you reconnect with Wedelia. The Chinese call it *mo chi sa*. It's amazing—by the river the leaves grow really big and travel like a dragon around the pond and riverside. They have beautiful forms like [those seen] in Qi gong and tai chi. The place, the form, it's very humble," she says. "Wedelia stays very low. People step on them, but they never complain, they will just take it, go to the side and become stronger. It's not like a human being. If you step on somebody, they fight back. They're violent! The Wedelia is so useful as a groundcover and for beauty. It takes all the dirt, the dust, the things you don't want, and it takes it so nicely, never asking for a reward. It never claims you have to pay it back. For me in Taoism, I grew up learning to appreciate plants. This is what Tao is about."

An avid bonsai cultivator, Dr. Chang raises many bonsais, including banyans. She tells the story of one bonsai dropping down a long tendril, like a whisker, as if traveling. The tendril grew and stretched down more than a thousand feet until it reached her pond. "They are not aggressive," she says of the tendril-dropping trees, "they will not take anything. They just need to get water. It was just a thin connection like a wire. It's amazing how they know where to go. They don't make trouble."

By far Dr. Chang's greatest lesson is to always appreciate. While she harvests plants to prepare medicine and prescriptions, she finds the fresh, living herb more valuable. Some plants are used physically in her dispensary, such as in the free organic freshly picked herbal teas she offers patients. She says some plants like to be trimmed, but others are so rare, people need to enjoy them without touching them. "Don't even bother to go nearby, just appreciate them. They love your voice, they love your footsteps. I do Qi gong *with* them so they are part of our morning meditation, *mudras*, and Qi gong. They do it with me.

"We are very concerned about protecting the earth," she says of the Institute, "to help preserve life on earth. It's part of our responsibility and duty to not damage them." Her students plant trees in local areas needing botanical protection.

"You don't necessarily have to go get [plants],
to cut them and boil them, in order to heal.
Actually, you just connect with them."

Because she is Taoist and strives for immortality, Dr. Chang would not reveal how long she has been working and studying, and she certainly would not tell me her age. "But I can tell you that for many, many years I never got sick once. I never caught a cold once. That's because I do it with plants. They're the ones who take my pain, my fever, all my sickness. So I appreciate the plants. I use plants for nutrition and for food, healing and rituals, as a guideline to live in harmony." Her students observe plants through their many cycles, a philosophy that contributes to the ancient Taoist philosophy of immortality. "You can see that's why we don't have age, because the plants grow again and again. They rejuvenate."

Thus the Taoist search for the secrets to immortality: if humans can understand and express the plant's ability to live—as it were—forever, then so might we.

LEAVES

At the World Medicine Institute, Dr. Chang instructs her students in the ancient lessons of acupuncture and the meridians of the body, pathways of energy that flow through the extremities: hands, feet, elbows, ankles, and knees. These energies reach out to the Universe as leaves for nourishment. She trains her students to observe a patient's "leaves" in the course of diagnosis.

The word *leaf* can refer to the botanical part of a tree or shrub, of course, and also to the page of a book. The original Proto-Indo-European language may have used *leup*, meaning "to peel or break off"; Lithuanians used *luobas*, Old High German *loub*, Gothic and Old Norse *lauf*. Old English turned this into *leaf*, especially pertaining to thin sheets of metal.

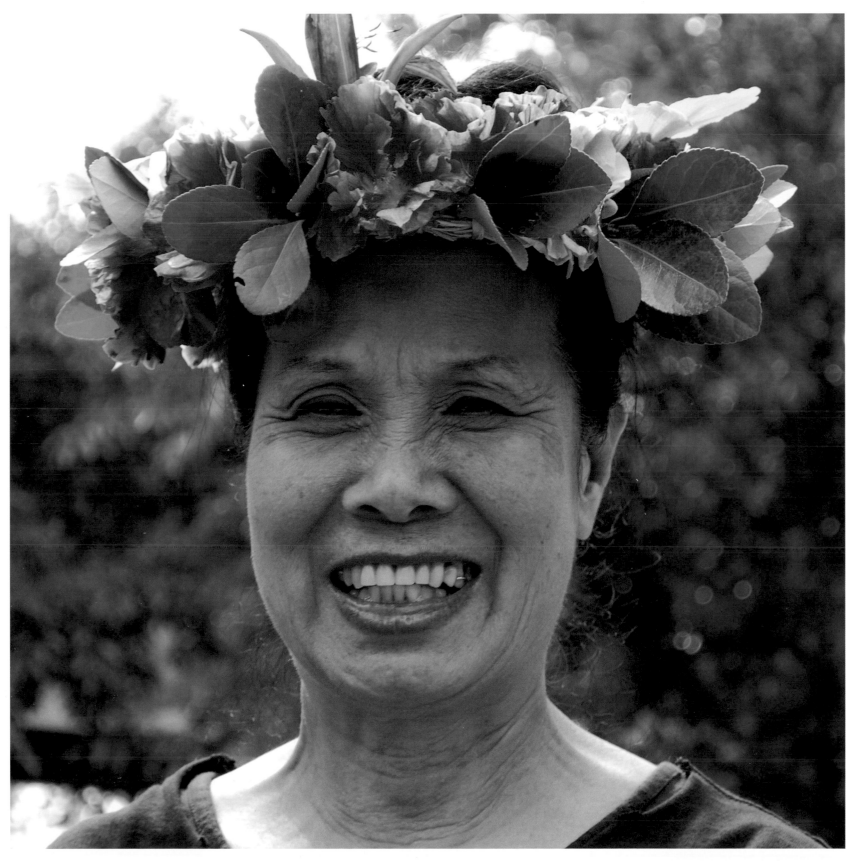

Photo credit: Lillian Chang

China is an enormous country with a population of approximately 1.3 billion people, mostly Han Chinese, but home to fifty-five ethnic minorities. Each minority, separated by high arid mountain plateaus, dry deserts, bamboo forests, mountains, grasslands, jungles, and wetlands, maintains its own customs and language. Despite their great geographic distances and myriad languages, Chinese generally honor three primary religions: Confucianism, Taoism, and Buddhism. During China's Cultural Revolution, the Communist Party outlawed religion, though today it is largely tolerated.

Taoism, as Dr. Chang practices it, centers on the pursuit of immortality and reverence for nature. One of its main concepts is an ordered universe, which can be expressed through a variety of art forms. Yin and Yang illustrate the concept of opposites, such as female and male and other "dualities" that also form the basis of Christianity. Qi is the energy that flows through life, and many Taoists work to harness or manifest Qi in their daily practices, through acupressure, Qi gong, martial arts, feng shui, divination, or I Ching.

Midway between Beijing and Hong Kong on the eastern Coast of China, Shanghai is home to the Huqingyu Tang Chinese Medicine Museum. The Museum, an old apothecary established during the Qing Dynasty (1644–1911), exhibits the history of traditional Chinese healing and—remarkably—still serves as a pharmacy, clinic, dispensary, and restaurant.

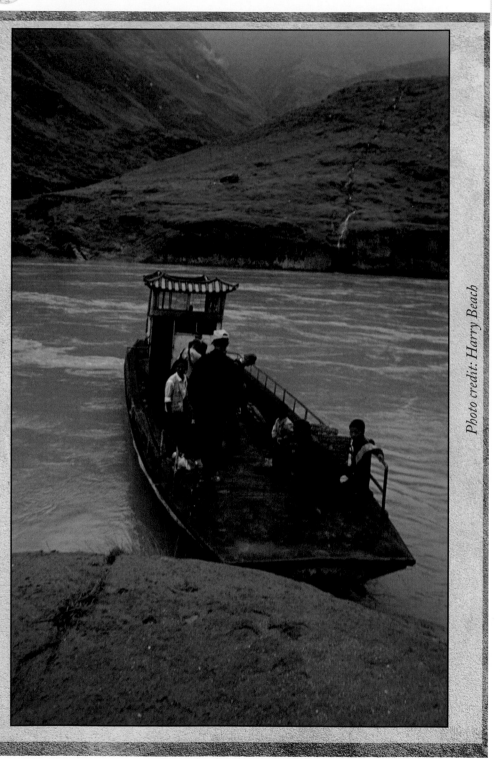

Photo credit: Harry Beach

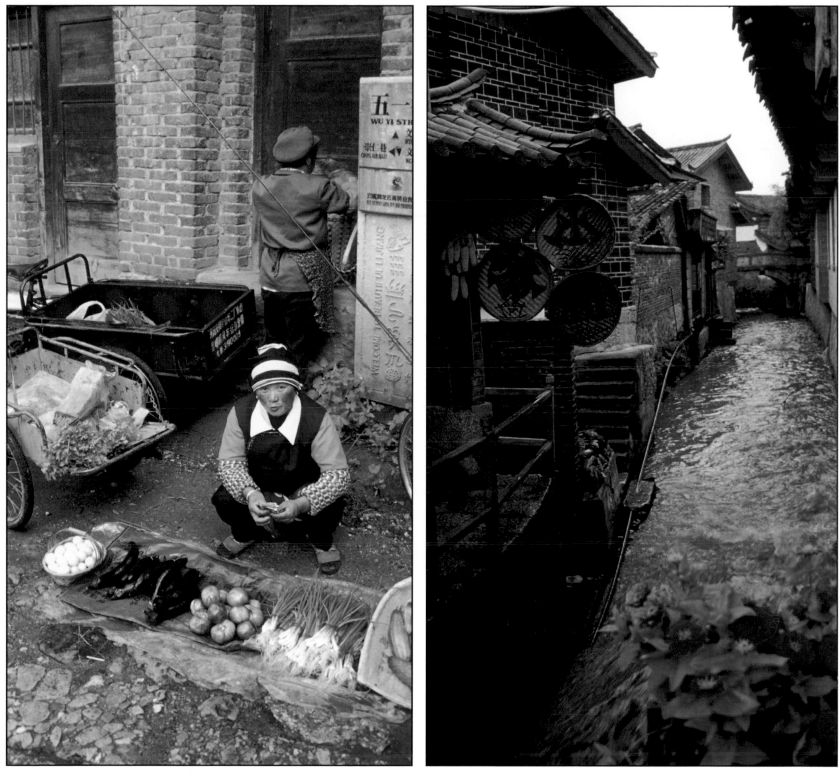

A woman sells vegetables in Lijiang, China

HIBISCUS
Hibiscus rosa-sinensis

Hibiscus rosa-sinensis (of the *Malvaceae* family) is a popular garden plant often grown in greenhouses. Named by the Greeks for mallow, the flower is also called rose-mallow because its blossoms resemble the folds of a rose, though it lacks thorns.

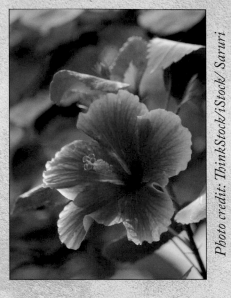

Photo credit: ThinkStock/iStock/ Saruri

In western herbal and Ayurvedic tradition, Hibiscus is considered cooling and is used in heat illness or "hot diseases." Ayurveda uses hibiscus as an emmenagogue to stimulate menstrual flow and as a contraceptive, uses being studied in India today.

Dr. Chang uses hibiscus leaves to "enhance the kidney areas, the hair, the bone marrow, all your joints, and sexuality, to make the next generation of children healthier."

In Polynesia, red hibiscus is given to "young mothers suffering from postpartum relapse sickness," and the flowers are boiled and applied to wounds. In the Cook Islands and the Philippines, the flowers were used to induce abortion, but in Hawai'i, mothers chewed the base of the flower as nourishment and to stimulate breast milk production.

Today, Hawai'ians cherish the beach hibiscus, a related small tree with a yellow blossom and lightweight wood prized for outrigger floats and tool handles. Pregnant women once consumed the slimy stem sap to lubricate reproductive passageways before labor. Surprisingly, the flowers are used as a dye in Jamaica to paint and condition shoes, and the lovely flower is called *shoe-black*.

MUGWORT
Artemisia vulgaris

Mugwort is an ancient herb revered across cultures as a medicine. High in liver and digestive stimulants, the leaves contain high levels of thujone and bitter principles, making them useful for treating worms. Dr. Chang teaches a variety of ways to use mugwort:

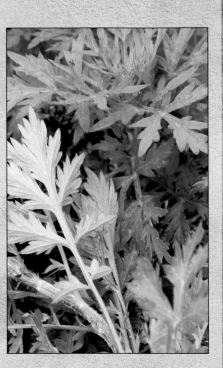

To make *moxa* powder for acupuncture, hang the long, silvery mugwort stalks on doors and windows to dry. "When we do an acupuncture treatment, it is like a ceremony because of the nice smell," she says.

Use fresh mugwort leaves in salad. "You cannot only have lettuce, tomato, cucumber, beets. Add a little mugwort herb. Of course you can have basil, mint, lemon grass. There's a balance in nature." She describes the Chinese springtime custom *e ay tah*, which uses bitter mugwort to cure viruses and infections. "Mugwort creates a fire, enhances the yang for inner strength, replaces what's damaged."

Soak leftover leaves in water for use as bonsai fertilizer and to make shampoo. Or dry the leaves for tea or to stuff pillows and blankets. "Make use of the useless things, that's what Taoists do," Chang says. "When people trim a plant, they throw it away. But you can soak your foot with ginger root peels and your body just loves them. After you finish the soak, don't throw them away: dry them and use them more. The whole plant is so useful."

Dr. Phuntsog Wangmo

Tibetan medicine: where mysterious meets modern, where ancient rituals at the top of the world simmer in pots of fragrant tea and baskets of hand-rinsed roots. It may seem a forgotten relic at the doorstep to the past, but Tibetan medicine is as vital today as ever, thanks in part to the efforts of Dr. Phuntsog Wangmo, who travels and teaches the art of authentic Tibetan healing. Long a mystery to Westerners unfamiliar with obscure Buddhist philosophy and domineering Chinese politics, ancient Tibetan practices are being revived and preserved as Dr. Wangmo shares her knowledge for the western worldwide. Now the director of the Shang Shung Institute's Traditional Tibetan Medicine Program in Massachusetts—the only school for traditional Tibetan medicine in the western hemisphere—Phuntsog is happy to be spreading the word.

"I liked to study Tibetan Medicine," Dr. Wangmo told me in her gentle voice, describing her entry into medicine as a girl. Keen to emulate her older brother, who was a doctor, Phuntsog yearned to be a doctor, too, and take a patient's pulse, analyze the urine and diagnose illness. Her uncle agreed that Phuntsog had an inclination toward medicine, and since Tibetan parents choose their children's occupations—matching the occupation to the child's character—it was a natural fit that Phuntsog would study medicine. Her aunt helped with her studies and her brother, who graduated when she entered school and has been a professor at Tibet Medical University for twenty years, tutored her.

> *"[A doctor] should have a warm heart, be humble, and be honest."*

Phuntsog attended Lhasa University School of Traditional Medicine and graduated in 1988, serving a two-year residency after completing the five-year training program. She studied with Khenpo (Master) Troru Tsenam for four years and Khenpo Gyaltsen, two of Tibet's leading doctors credited with the revival of Tibetan Medicine within Tibet under Chinese authority.

After earning her medical degree and becoming a *Lhajeh* (doctor), Phuntsog served as a doctor in eastern Tibet and collaborated on the development of A.S.I.A., a nonprofit organization serving the educational and medical needs of Tibetan people. Within the structure of this organization, soft-spoken Phuntsog created hospitals and training centers in the remote Sichuan Province and Chamdo Prefecture, and she coordinated the development of Gamthog Hospital.

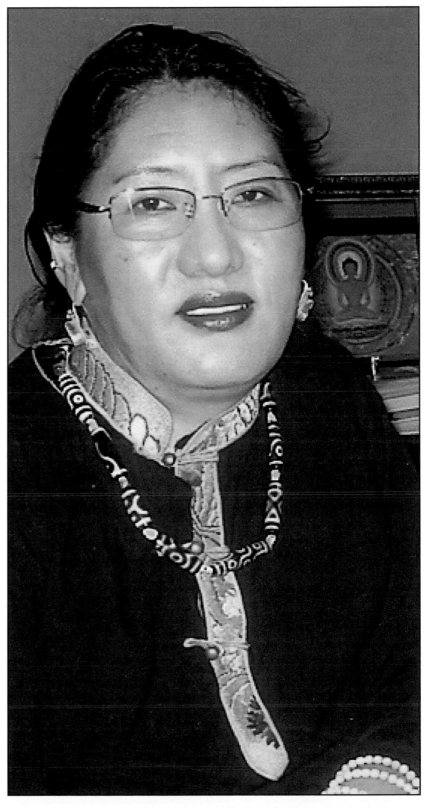

Photo credit: Phuntsog Wangmo

Eventually, Phuntsog served on the faculty of the Shang Shung Institute in Naples, Italy, where she presented seminars and spoke at conferences on Tibetan medicine. Later, she traveled to the United States, where interest in Tibetan healing increased in the 1970s along with other alternative healing arts, and she helped launch the Shang Shung Institute of the West. She returns to Tibet for two or three months each year to provide healing to the rural, nomadic peoples of eastern Tibet.

Tibetan Healing

Traditional Tibetan medicine includes a large variety of plants, but especially the common healing and culinary herbs, such as cardamom, nutmeg, garlic, and ginger. With the mantra "daily life, daily fruit," she advocates the use of very simple herbs that are easy to find and use. Of the potent medicinal herbs listed above, she notes that many cultures accept these as foods.

Tibetan cultures analyze plant characteristics and locale to determine proper use, much like European healers used the Doctrine of Signatures (a plant's color or shape) to guide them. "For example," she says, "the south-faced mountain herbs are good for the cool natured diseases. The north-faced mountain herbs are good for heat natured diseases. Since the Tibetan altitude is over 3,500 meters (10,000 feet), many herbs only grow at this altitude in the Himalayan region. These herbs are hard to find in other countries." Phuntsog was happy to discover familiar Tibetan herbs growing in such faraway places as the United States. "Angelica!" she says. "I can even find it in Massachusetts." She says Tibetans also include in their healing regimen herbs that grow elsewhere, such as dandelion and pomegranate.

> *"We have a long history of Tibetan medicine, it is a very deep knowledge. It is still very alive and much practiced."*

Tibetan medicine faces many of the problems besetting herbalists everywhere, namely: the commercialism of valuable plants is making those plants scarce. It hasn't been a big problem for long, she told me, "but now certain herbs are not growing anymore. They are difficult to find. From ancient times until just fifty years ago, traditional Tibetan medicine doctors would pick very carefully,

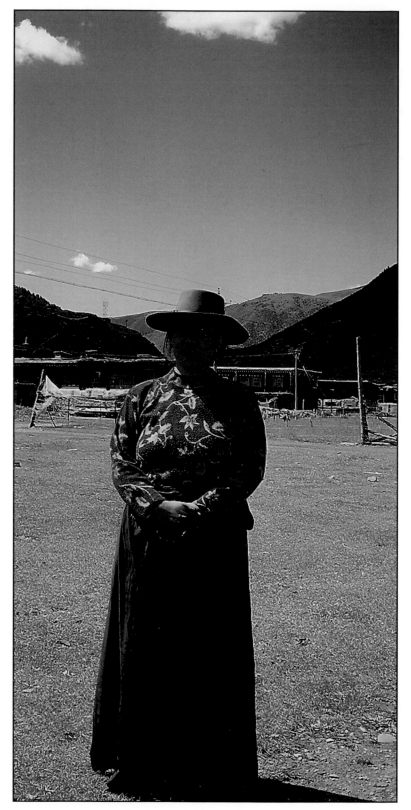

Phuntsog in Tibet

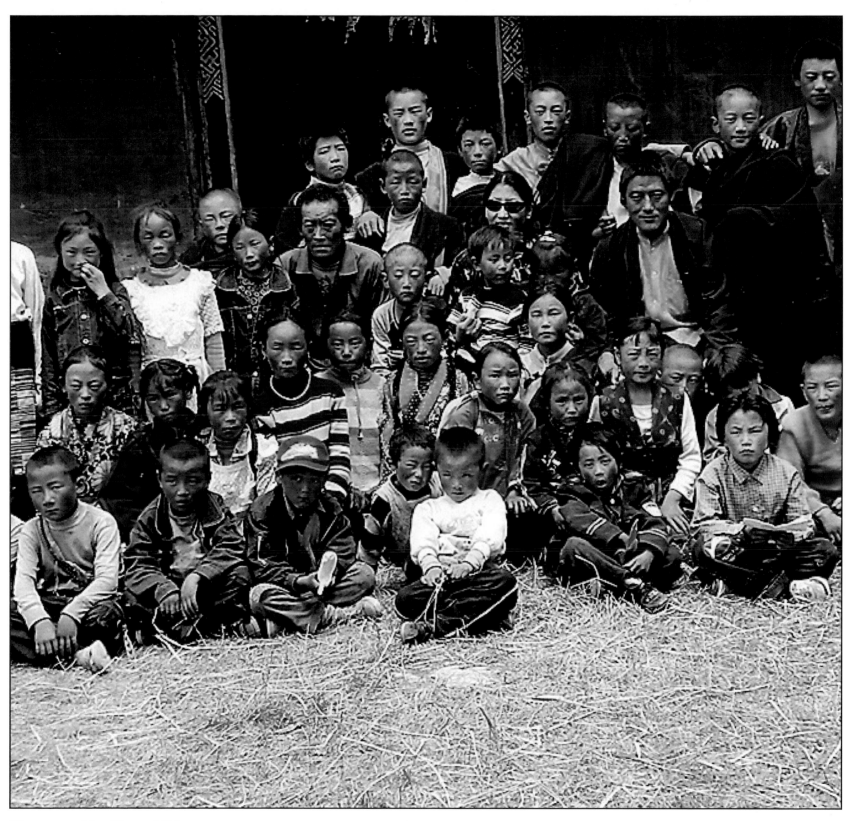

Phuntsog with village children

avoiding pulling from the roots. If they picked on this side of the mountain one day, the next time they would pick from the other side of the mountain. We tried to preserve and protect the plants. The locals would take their daily herbs"—only what they needed, and no more. "But," she says, "today there is big interest in the Industry, which is taking a thousand pounds a day [of medicinal herbs]. They need a huge quantity of herbs to put in the Machine. For this reason, many people pick the herbs in a careless way."

She also notes that certain technique is being lost, which is a challenge as she tries to teach the authentic ancient methods of Tibetan healing. "In the Western countries," she says, "many people don't know about Tibetan medicine. To introduce people takes time, and there is no [legal or official] standard for Tibetan medicine, and it is not licensed yet. This is hard for us at the moment." The Shang Shung Institute is creating a standard for practicing Tibetan medicine in western countries, especially in the United States, but this process will take time. "We still have qualified teachers and Tibetan medicine is very alive and much practiced. We have a long history of Tibetan medicine, it is a very deep knowledge."

Medical Philosophy

A great deal of Tibetan medical practice is actually based on the culture's religious tenets. "Our Tibetan culture is based on Buddhism," Phuntsog explains, so the philosophies inherent in the religion are integral to the way Tibetan healers are taught to live and work, and the standards for noble living are as much a part of the medical system as they are the religion. These religious concepts are taught to medical students not only from their families, but also from within the framework of the Tibetan medical system itself.

"[Doctors] get the teachings not only from school, but also from our parents: you should have a warm heart, be humble, and be honest. I always heard these teachings from my family, but I also learned them from the texts in medical school." The books taught her "*how* we should do, what is the purpose of learning medicine, what is our duty, and *what* we should do. I learned in medical school that you should try to think, 'I am the servant, so I should serve when I can.' I try to have good intentions. I always try to apply this information and knowledge to the daily practice. I think this has helped a lot because when you try to be honest or kind, other people are kind. I am confident we should keep this commitment. It doesn't matter

COMPASSION

Passion, etymologically, originated in the ancient Proto-Indo-European word *pei*, "to hurt or injure." Latin changed this to *pati*, "to suffer or endure," and Late Latin used *passio* and *passionem*. Old French coined *passion*, and in 1175 CE this applied specifically to Christ's suffering on the cross. One hundred fifty years later, English blended Latin's *com* "together" and *pati* "to suffer" to create *compassion*.

In 1579, *sympathy* entered English literature, meaning to commiserate with or to express a like feeling. This extended into folk healing, where sympathetic cures were believed to have supernatural powers. For instance, it was widely believed that if someone were injured with a knife, the healer should slather ointment not on the injured flesh but on the knife. Attributed to Paracelsus, the idea of a sympathetic ointment that would cure from a distance was taken seriously for hundreds of years before becoming superstition.

In 1668, *pathos*, "that which arouses pity or sorrow," entered English. Today sympathy means "pity," passion is used in the sense of sexual arousal or a vibrant feeling of life's purpose, and compassion means less to "suffer with" than it does to feel empathy and concern.

where you grew up or what you do," Phuntsog says, "it's important to *try* to be helpful, even if you cannot help other beings. Do not harm them and always have good intentions."

She tells her students that while it is important to study medical textbooks, "it is also very important to be humble, honest, and compassionate. It is not that easy," she admits, "but it is important because it is our best way for helping others."

"What I try to do here is a pure Tibetan medicine. I think that when we teach, it is important to teach it pure—the real knowledge. It is the real way we learned in Tibet—there are no shortcuts."

Saving the Heritage

Dr. Wangmo says her greatest challenge lies in preserving the ancient traditions of Tibet's healing practice. She strives to uphold the ancient ways as accurately as possible. "What I try to do here is a pure Tibetan medicine," she says. "I think that when we teach, it is important to teach it pure—the real knowledge. It is the real way we learned in Tibet—there are no shortcuts. And I do not put my own ideas in. I think when I am teaching, it is best to teach the correct thing." When students become doctors, they will apply this knowledge for their patients and they can do what they think is best on a case-by-case basis, she says. "I try to work with students honestly. It is my responsibility to introduce Tibetan medicine to western countries in a pure way, and I am doing that."

Phuntsog is happy to see more people learning Tibetan medicine because she believes this healing system benefits all sentient beings. "There are hardly any side effects because we use 100 percent herbs. We cannot say there are no side effects—sometimes when you eat food it makes you die," she notes. "But Tibetan medicine is a very simple method to apply, and it can also be quite a joyful process. Tibetan medicine is very good and can benefit all beings. That is my main motivation. That, and to protect Tibetan medicine by teaching it in a pure way."

TIBET

The mountainous "roof of the world" has a complicated history. Its borders and population have been the source of conflict for China, Britain, India, and possibly Russia, and, since 1956, Tibet has been under the forced administration of the People's Republic of China. In 1933, the thirteenth Dalai Lama died. In 1935, the fourteenth Dalai Lama was born (reincarnation is a central tenet of Buddhism) and, unlike his predecessors, was tutored in Western politics, geography, and philosophy. When China invaded Tibet in 1949, he was forced into exile in Dharmasala, India, where he remains the spiritual and political leader of the Tibetan people.

He has called for talks with China's government, offering to accept Chinese sovereignty though insisting on retaining Tibetan cultural and religious autonomy. The country is a political and spiritual entity, though due to early Persian influence, Tibet is home to an Islamic population.

Tibetan women face many of the same political hurdles Chinese women face, especially with health care and individual rights regarding pregnancy and birth. In 1982, China imposed mandatory abortions or monetary fines against women who become pregnant without the government's permission, and in 1995 China implemented a "Mother and Child Health Law" forcing abortions and sterilization for women who suffer "he-

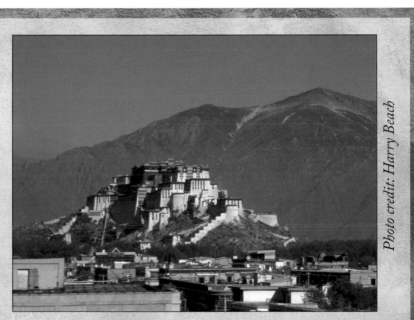

Photo credit: Harry Beach

Potala, Llasa, Tibet

reditary diseases," as defined by the government. According to the Government of Tibet in Exile, Tibetan women are not educated about other contraception methods, and they lack rights about conception and family planning.

Tibetans live comparatively sparse lives at altitudes above ten thousand feet. Many families are nomadic herders. Since

China's occupation, Tibetans must present ration cards to obtain their monthly allotment of dietary staples at government stores. Their favorite drink is butter tea, made from black tea (imported in bricks from China) with fresh or fermented yak's milk churned in bamboo butter tea churns. Salt (never sugar) or soda is added to the tea, and it is drunk hot. Many Tibetans drink forty cups or bowls of this beverage daily. Tea, *Tsampa* (roasted barley flour) and fatty meats form the typical Tibetan diet.

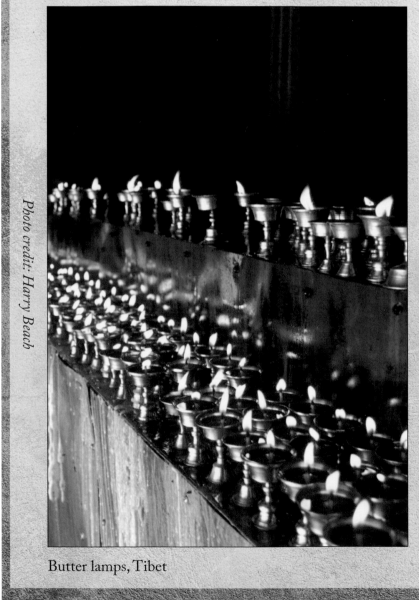

Photo credit: Harry Beach

Butter lamps, Tibet

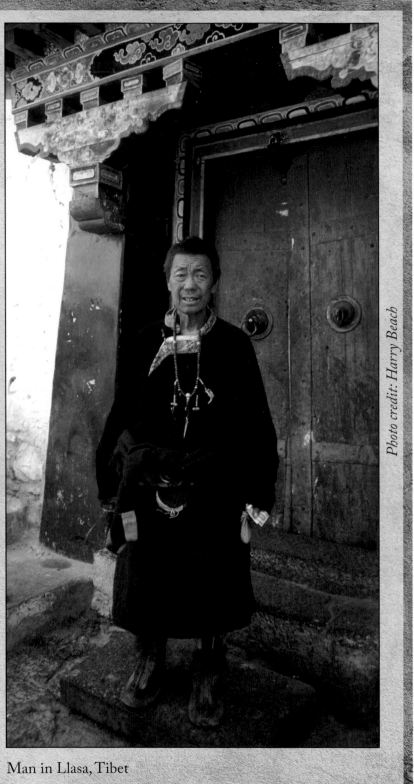

Photo credit: Harry Beach

Man in Llasa, Tibet

TEA
Camellia (Thea) sinensis

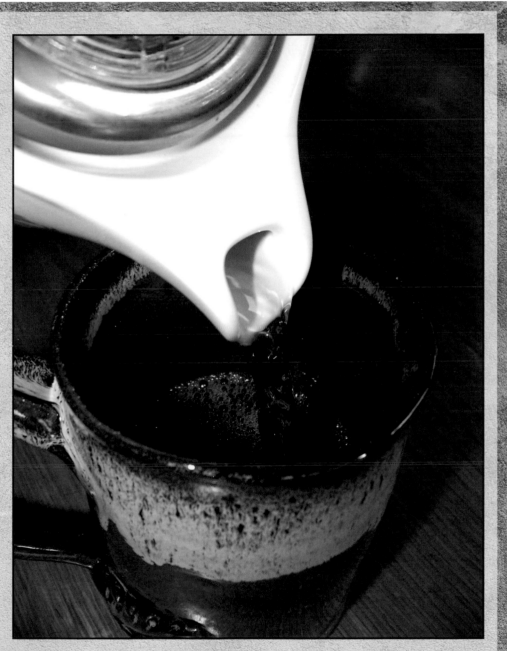

Discovered more than three thousand years ago in Ancient China, the beloved tea plant was named *Thea*, Greek for goddess. Later, the plant was placed botanically in the Camellia genus, but its alkaloid theophylline retained the heavenly moniker.

Native to southeastern China (*sinensis* is Latin for Chinese), tea is grown most notably in India, where most Darjeeling is cultivated. From the shrub's fermented leaves, a variety of energizing brews are made, including white tea (once reserved for kings), green tea, pu'erh, oolong, and black tea—the basis for Chai and all "breakfast" teas. The small, light green leaves are hand-harvested, mostly by women, and withered (spread on a rack to dry), rolled, sorted, oxidized, and fired.

Fresh leaves contain up to 4 percent caffeine, giving a six-ounce cup of tea between 30 and 60 milligrams of caffeine. (Other plants that contain caffeine include coffee, cacao, guarana, maté, and kola.) Unsweetened tea is bitter and astringent, thanks to its high tannin content, which stimulates digestion (see chapter 10, "Tannins").

The extraordinary history of tea includes the expansion of the Dutch East India Company and dangerous transports along the ancient Silk Road. Tea leaves were compressed in rectangular bricks, stamped with trademark symbols, and shipped to the American colonies before the Boston Tea Party. Tea is still shipped this way to Tibet, where butter tea is a favorite soup-like beverage.

The alkaloid theophylline is a white, odorless crystalline powder first isolated in 1885 and registered in the United States Pharmacopoeia and the National Formulary since 1916. Used as a smooth muscle relaxant, diuretic, and pulmonary vessel dilator, the alkaloid is useful in asthma and to lower venous pressure during heart failure. Recent research suggests that drinking a cup of tea daily, especially for women, helps eliminate free radicals from the body and provides antioxidants.

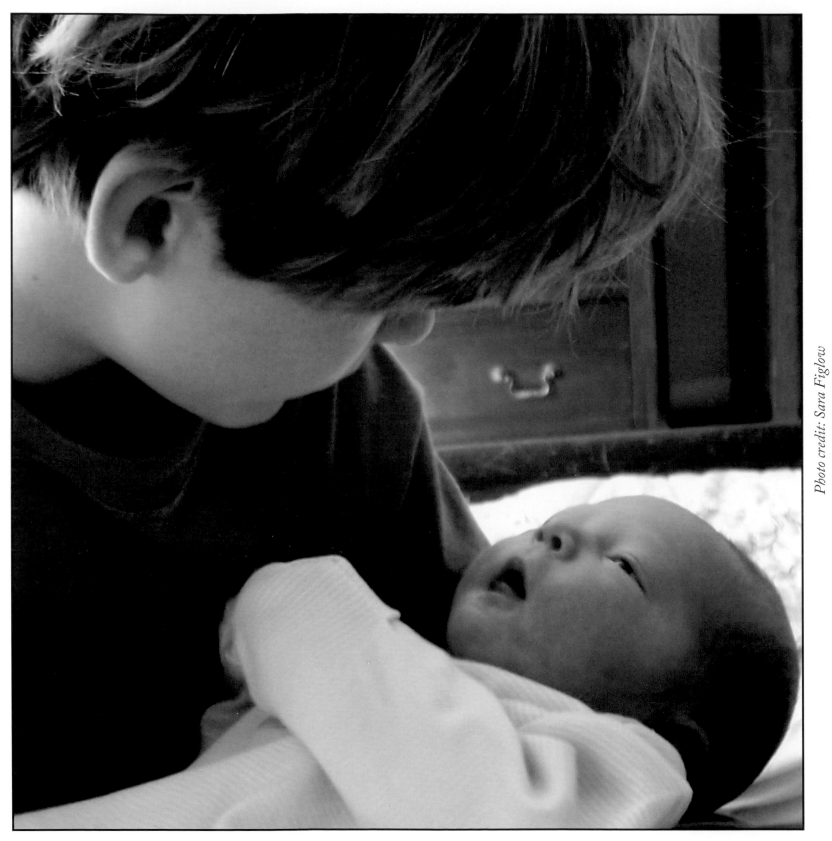

A brother is born

Photo credit: Sara Figlow

Chapter 8
MIDWIFERY

The practice of delivering babies has been a controversial profession for centuries, earning the attention of lay-practitioners, midwives, physicians, attorneys, and governments.

In 1716, long before America earned its independence, New York City required its midwives to be licensed. For the next century and a half, women enjoyed the role of primary caregiver during childbirth with little intervention from men or doctors. But in 1888, male physicians determined midwifery could be a lucrative practice: there was money to be made in the delivery of infants. They argued that obstetrics and gynecology should be removed from women (whether licensed or not), and they formed the American College of Obstetricians and Gynecologists (ACOG) as the first formal opposition to the right of midwives to perform birth services.

Male doctors quickly introduced controversial surgeries and drugs to what was formerly a natural event. In 1847 Dr. James Young Simpson of Edinburgh used chloroform for the first time to ease a woman's pain during delivery (a compassionate act, but he was condemned by doctors and ministers for "interfering with God's will"). Equally controversial interventions such as the Cesarean section, the use of forceps, electronic fetal monitoring, and the epidural would follow.

In 1894, the first Cesarean section surgery was performed in Boston. Childbirth was, however, still considered normal—95 percent of births occurred at home because of rampant poverty and inadequate transportation, and because male doctors found little monetary incentive for serving low-income women.

But a 1910 bulletin by the Carnegie Foundation for the Advancement of Teaching changed that. Surprising both the medical establishment and midwives, the Flexner Report claimed the majority of US doctors lacked a college education and had received substandard training. It recommended most medical schools close and the remaining schools operate on the lecture model of Johns Hopkins with stringent graduation standards. This led to fewer women's admissions and to the Federal Children's Bureau's rigorous investigation of childbirth practices.

Now both physician and midwife practices came under direct government scrutiny, and the work of Dr. Joseph Bolivar DeLee ensured that the pendulum would swing decisively in favor of medical intervention rather than midwifery. According to a 1936 *Time* Magazine article, Dr. DeLee was a forward-thinking obstetrician dedicated to relieving his patients' pain. He was praised by Franklin Delano Roosevelt and became a "celebrity" baby deliverer. Dr. DeLee forbade "meddlesome midwifery" and was instrumental, pun intended, in popularizing the use of forceps during delivery.

In 1920 (the year women achieved suffrage), DeLee denounced the idea that childbirth was a normal function of nature, claiming it was instead pathological, requiring active intervention from the medical establishment. His methods included heavy sedation, forcible extraction, episiotomy, and postpartum drugging. Encouraged by the medical climate, Dr. James Taylor Gwathmey of Manhattan produced a celebrated combination of drugs: an injection of morphine and Epsom salts into the mother's muscles for anesthesia, and an enema of quinine, alcohol and ether in olive oil into her rectum (*Time*, 1936).

Though the American Board of Obstetricians and Gynecology formed in 1930 and drugs and interventions became routine, the White House found no advantages to the new procedures. In fact, its Conference on Child Health and Protection reported that, despite these interventions, maternal mortality did not decline between 1915 and 1930, and infant mortality and injuries actually increased by an astonishing 40–50 percent. Despite what should have been a revelatory finding, between 1935 and 1950 the number of mothers delivering in hospitals rose sharply: from 37 percent to 88 percent.

In the early 1950s, The Midwifery Section of the National Organization for Public Health Nursing emphasized childbirth as a normal family process. The American College of Nurse Midwives (ACNM) was formed, and La Leche League was founded.

Childbirth Today

Despite these organizations' attempts at fostering competent care for natural childbirth in or out of a hospital setting, in 1960 a full 97 percent of births were hospital births, and America was introduced to the birth control pill and continuous electronic fetal monitoring (EFM). Nearly twenty years later, in 1979 the US Food and Drug Administration revealed behavior and motor handicaps in children whose mothers had received Demerol, a previously popular narcotic pain reliever used during labor. This prompted the conservative ACNM to change its negative policy to support "alternative" and homebirth services, a surprise move that opened the door for the establishment of the Midwives Alliance of North America, though the American Academy of Family Physicians (AAFP) still vehemently opposed nurse-midwifery, insisting midwives should be subordinate to doctors and payment should be physician-directed.

In 1993, a study showed a high rate of Cesarean section following epidural anesthesia. The investigators closed the study saying it was unethical, but the danger of epidurals went unnoticed: today, in 9 out of every 10 births the mother is given an epidural (*JPE*, 2004) and though the Cesarean rate has fallen from its high of 25 percent in 1988, it still hovers around 20 percent. The use of forceps is just under 4 percent, and, according to the *British Medical Journal*, an astonishing 85 percent of women are routinely subjected to electronic fetal monitoring in hospitals compared to only 9.6 percent of planned homebirths (*BMJ*, 2005).

Today fewer than 6 percent of US births are attended principally by midwives, compared to 75 percent in European countries. The World Health Organization (WHO) recommends "the curricula for the education of all health professionals should reflect the role of the midwife as primary caregiver in maternity care." WHO says the preferred location for most births is outside the hospital (at home or in a birthing center) and out-of-hospital births should be the standard for midwifery education and training. But many rural areas lack midwife services due to inadequate access to obstetric facilities or physician backup.

The Costs

What does this mean, in financial terms, for women and their husbands who wish to give birth naturally, in a natural setting? In 2001, the average fee for a midwife-attended birth in the United States was only $1,500, compared to $4,200 for a physician-attended vaginal birth. Educating a direct-entry midwife costs between $300 and $15,000, compared to a whopping $150,000 to $200,000 for an obstetrician-gynecologist.

According to Dr. Frank A. Oski, director of pediatrics at the Johns Hopkins University School of Medicine in Baltimore, nearly $20 billion in health care costs could be saved each year by developing midwifery care, de-medicalizing childbirth, and encouraging breastfeeding. Oski estimates that using midwifery care for 75 percent of pregnancies in the United States would save $8.5 billion annually.

Families must consider factors in addition to financial: emotional well-being, comfort, distance from caregivers, religion, maternal and fetal health, privacy, and independence. Carolyn Weaver, a certified practicing midwife in Tennessee (where midwifery is neither regulated nor illegal), says families need more education. "People don't know what happens in a hospital birth. With an epidural, a woman commonly spikes a fever. But when this happens, hospital staff treat the newborn baby as a sick baby, they separate him or her from the mother, they give 'routine' antibiotics 'just to be safe,' and they interrupt the bonding process. Women don't realize this. They're not informed."

The midwifery model of care includes lengthy prenatal visits, nutrition education, out-of-hospital birth options, practitioners trained in normal (and emergency) birth, and continuity of care with the same caregiver prenatally, during labor and birth, and postpartum.

Weaver cites the overuse of EFM during labor. "EFMs are really for litigation purposes," she says. Studies published in the *New England Journal of Medicine* and the *Lancet* show that, in the absence of specific indications for its use, EFM has no demonstrated benefit in reducing childhood disabilities and may even be dangerous. Dr. Oski estimates health care cost savings of $675 million per year simply by eliminating the routine use of continuous EFM.

"Commercialism and consumerism are propelling forward the surgical, medical, intervening, demoralizing model of hospital births," Weaver says, "even for completely normal pregnancies. This is not just a women's issue. It's a family issue. A global issue. When women give birth in a safe environment with minimal drug and medical intervention, our communities reap the rewards."

RASPBERRY
Rubus ideaus

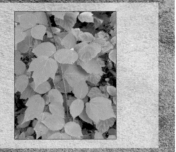

Children love raspberry fruits—those thimble-shaped, red sweet-tarts that grow on long, slender thorny branches—but herbalists prize the leaves. Raspberry leaves are soft green above but silver underneath and grow on bluish canes. The berries of the second-year canes are edible, but the first-year canes produce the calcium-rich leaves which, when brewed into an infusion with water, are cherished by midwives for toning the uterus and building strong bones. In western herbal medicine, raspberry leaves and roots are gentle astringents for dysentery and diarrhea.

TINCTURE

A tincture is a concentrated liquid extract of a medicinal plant that contains the "active" chemical ingredients minus the fiber: a pure medicine quickly and easily digested.

The hypothetical Proto-Indo-European language used *teng* (with a long A) "to soak." Latin coined *tingere* for something soaked or wetted, and Old French used *teindre* "to dye." Color played a large role in religious ceremonies and in establishing territorial boundaries and kingships, so dyeing clothing and other fabrics was top priority for women from the British Isles to the Mediterranean, Persia, and Arabia. From *tingere* Old French coined *teint* in the twelfth century, and *teindre*, "to dye or soak with color."

To remove color required a new word, a cognate of Latin *dis* "remove" and Old French *teindre* "to dye." *Desteindre* was borrowed by Middle English for *disteynen*, to discolor or remove stain. According to etymologist Douglas Harper, the word *stain* appeared around 1382, a merger of Old Norse *steina* "to paint" and Middle English *disteynen*.

By 1400, Latin used *tinctura* as "the act of tingeing with color or dye," and Greek used *tengein* "to moisten." In 1409, Anglo-French used *teinter*, "to color or dye," and in 1471, *tinge* meant "to dye or color slightly."

In 1543, the meaning changed drastically, barely resembling the original meanings of dye, color, or moisten. The revolutionary Paracelsus (1493–1541) accused physicians of quackery and schemes that failed to address the underlying cause of illness and frequently killed patients. The first to do so in nearly 1,700 years, Paracelsus rejected Galen's theories of humors; he emphasized chemical laboratory medicine and advocated drugs made with strong minerals such as mercury and antimony.

By Paracelsus's death, "chymical" medicine was popular and apothecaries created complicated remedies. Tincture of opium, or Laudanum, was hailed as a safe remedy for mothers and children. *Laudanum* comes from Latin *laudere*, "praise," or *ladanum*, "a gum resin." The word came to mean any alcoholic tincture of opium blend. Now *tincture* meant the concentrated extract of plants, minerals, precious metals, animal parts, and other ingredients chosen by the apothecary; the word exited the world of plant dyes for coloring wool and entered the realm of pharmacy.

Tincture of opium enjoyed centuries of devastating and addiction-causing success, but eventually its reputation was "tainted" with the news that it was not the miracle drug once thought. The word *taint* brings us full circle to the word *tincture*, because it derives from Middle English *teynten* "to convict, prove guilty" (c. 1375) related to Old French *teint*, "to dye or color." By 1573, taint meant "corrupt or contaminated" and, by 1591, it meant "to tinge or imbue slightly" with corruption.

In 1616, at Shakespeare's death, *tincture* was employed as the verb "to soak herbs and material in liquid to produce a medicine." Roughly one hundred years after the death of Paracelsus, *tincture* is recorded as a noun in literature meaning a "solution of medicine in a mixture of alcohol."

The next century brings us *tint*, meaning "to color," and two hundred years after that we have *dunk*, presumably from Pennsylvania Dutch *dunke*, meaning "to dip," which we can trace all the way back to the Proto-Indo-European *teng*, "to soak."

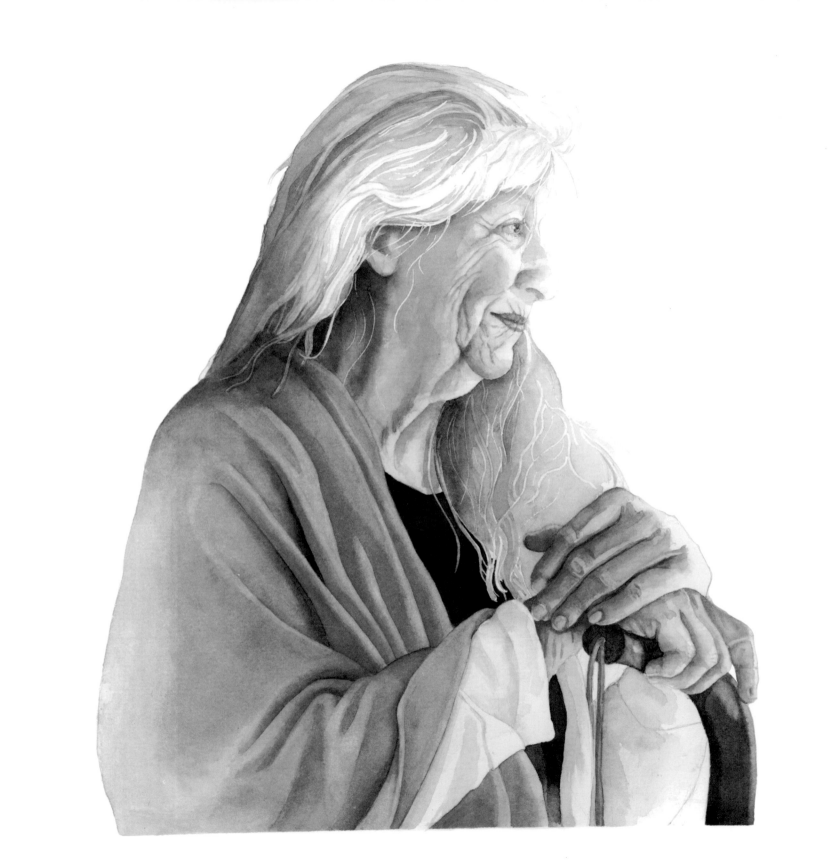

Marie-Henriette LeJeune-Ross

(1762–1860)

In the late eighteenth century, Nova Scotia was a remote and inhospitable region beset by the conflicts between France and England over the occupation of the northeastern edge of Canada. Roads were barely passable and hospitals did not exist. But in this climate of hardship, a young woman named Marie-Henriette became the unsung hero of pioneering, health, and freedom. She traveled dangerous paths to assist scores of women deliver healthy babies and she provided basic health care to rural families who had no access to medical professionals. Her heroism grew legendary with tales of tenacity and strength; some are true and some are beloved fable, but it seems clear she was a well-respected woman of her community.

Born and baptized in 1762 in Rochefort, France, Marie-Henriette immigrated with her family to Acadia, a region of Nova Scotia then owned by the French. But her family was quickly deported— twice—back to France during the English conflicts. Her parents gave up the idea of immigrating so Marie-Henriette was raised in France, where she married Frenchman Joseph Comeau. Soon, the pioneering young couple attempted what her parents had not been able to achieve, traveling in 1784 back to Nova Scotia. Sadly, soon after arriving in the new country, Joseph Comeau drowned, leaving Marie-Henriette a young widow.

Marie-Henriette was alone in a land consumed by political upheaval. Tensions between the United States, Canada, and France ran high. Marie-Henriette soon remarried, this time to Bernard LeJeune dit Briard. But tragedy struck again: her second husband drowned, leaving her a widow twice before she had turned twenty-six years old.

Finally, in 1792, Marie-Henriette married James Ross, her third husband in eight years. Ross was a Protestant Scottish soldier who took Marie to settle in Little Bras d'Or and then later around the East Margaree River, near Cape Breton Island. These communities thrived with Celts, Scots, and native Mi'kmaq people, and it was here that Marie-Henriette finally settled and raised her children. We know little of her family life, but legends tell of Granny Ross trekking through the northeastern forests to gather the healing herbs she used as the region's (perhaps only) midwife.

Herbs

Possibly learning from the native Mi'kmaq peoples, Marie-Henriette likely used common midwifery herbs such as raspberry leaves, partridgeberry, and bethroot (Purple Trillium, *Trillium erectus*), which she probably harvested herself, dried in her farmhouse, and carried with her across the region for new mothers. We can imagine that Marie used local evening primrose, violets, and St. John's wort to heal postpartum tears and tissues, and a strong tea of native cranberry to astringe tissues following birth. She may have collected wild boneset to relieve fevers in mother and baby, and she likely used chicory leaves and root, seaside mallow, and sheep lanolin as nursing salves for sore nipples.

In a story somewhere between fact and legend, Marie-Henriette is credited with saving many people from smallpox during an epidemic that swept the east coast. It appears Marie-Henriette had learned of Cotton Mather, notorious for the Salem witch trials and famous as a scientist-doctor who promoted the new "Turkish" practice of inoculating patients with a mild form of smallpox. Until then, inoculation was seldom used in America, though it was known in Africa and Britain, and Louis Pasteur's work toward clinical vaccination did not take hold until the late nineteenth century. Mather helped successfully inoculate three hundred people in an epidemic in 1721 and again in 1743. Nearly a hundred years later, Marie-Henriette is said to have successfully used these still-foreign techniques against smallpox in her own community.

When Granny Ross died in 1860 at age ninety-eight, she was already a legend in Nova Scotia. Many of today's residents of Little Bras d'Or and the East Margaree River are likely descendants of the babies Marie-Henriette helped welcome into the world.

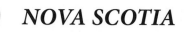

Nova Scotia was originally populated by the Mi'kmaq Nation before being taken over by the French and then the English. Triumphantly gained—and then forgotten and neglected by the English for nearly forty years—Nova Scotia's isolated Acadia region was hassled by both governments and expected to sign contradicting allegiances.

At Marie-Henriette LeJeune's birth, Europe's relationship with native nations was poor. The French and English usurped land, and many native people sided with French against English with attacks between the populations, while the fiercely independent settlers, who wanted little more than to be left alone, suffered in the middle.

Marie-Henriette's third husband, James Ross, was a Protestant Scottish soldier—an ethnic group that brought yet a fourth cultural dynamic to the region. Surely the couple would have been immersed in the region's highland culture alongside its French and English cultures when they moved to the Cape Breton region of Little Bras d'Or. The immigrants from Scotland brought their Gaelic language and heritage of bagpipes and fiddlers, traditions preserved today in Cape Breton; today, the area is known for salmon fishing and whale watching.

The native nations Métis and Inuit are recognized by the Canadian constitution as Aboriginal societies, and nearly one million people in Canada identified themselves as Aboriginal people in 2006.

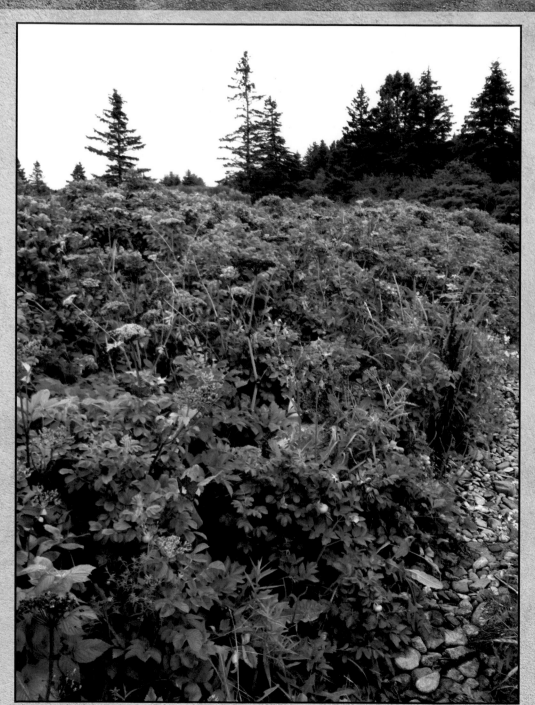

Because of its colorful history of Mi'kmaq, English, French, and Scottish residents, Nova Scotia abounds in rich healing traditions, including western herbal medicine, Native American sweat lodge and ceremony, and remnants of ancient Gaelic traditions.

Doña Enriqueta Contreras

Little Enriqueta Contreras was born into a family of seven children in the five-thousand-foot-high region of Rancho Tabla of the ancient Zapotec culture, a village known today as Benito Juarez, Oaxaca, Mexico. When Enriqueta was only seven years old—and her father had been dead four years—her mother made mysterious arrangements with a local childless couple, and Enriqueta was delivered, unceremoniously, to their doorstep. Abandoned by her family, she served this new couple as a daughter, but they suffered from alcoholism and thus neglected her. Instead of housing and feeding the child, they forced Enriqueta to work as a goatherd, sending her out into the open pastures distant from the village, without food, shelter, or protection.

Enriqueta lived in these wild goat lands for two full years. Had she been a weaker child, she would have died, but Enriqueta was nothing if not resilient. She tended the goats and followed them, observing what they ate, and in this way she fed herself from berries and herbs in the wild.

It was during this time that Enriqueta helped a nanny goat give birth, a formative act that led to her future calling nine years later, when she found herself with her family again and helped her sister during childbirth.

There seems to be something dangerous about Enriqueta today—something that causes unease in many typical physicians and government officials. It could be her demanding and fierce demeanor, because she stands firm with great resolve and can be intimidating. It could be her success, because she has flourished where lesser people have failed. It could also be that she has adopted a profession that threatens the establishment: she is a midwife. By following her calling, Doña Enriqueta (Grandmother, or Doni Queta, as she is fondly known) has suffered the pressures of a society that devalues women's desires to advance themselves professionally, and the consequences of this pursuit have been tangible: Enriqueta has lost blood, she has been attacked, she has even been fired upon. While caring for her youngest daughter, she "felt bullets whizzing by my head." This was in El Punto, when a faction of social services entered the town, divided the community, and literally did drivebys, taking pot shots at her.

When I met with Doña Queta, she and her translator, friend, and biographer Mary Margaret Navar were both wearing the bright colorful clothing and scarves of Doña's native Oaxaca. Doña's face was firm and unforgiving, and she looked about her with the ferocity of her Zapotec ancestors—until Mary Margaret slapped her on the knee and cracked a joke, and Doña permitted herself to smile. She gazed at me with a look that asked if I could possibly understand what she has gone through in her life, and she spoke passionately. "I have fallen," Enriqueta says, "but I lift myself. But thank God you see me, I'm here today, because I have to complete my mission in life to help people heal. My children were my goal, I wanted the best for them. I was mother and father to my children. Thank god my children love me, they respect me, they take care of me. Because I did the best that I could for them, for their best interest."

Enriqueta raised her children (after delivering three of them completely alone and without assistance) to be able to pursue their own dreams—a luxury Enriqueta had to fight for. "I didn't want them to repeat the same fate," she recalls.

> "They called me doctor, nurse, teacher. The people, the communities, have given me many titles. I am recognized by my own people. I don't have a piece of paper that validates my education. It's my own people that validate my life's work and what I have contributed to my own community."

After surviving years in the wilderness as a goatherd, reuniting with her family only to be forced to submit to an arranged marriage, then escaping bullets as well as government pressure to step down, Enriqueta has finally achieved success: she is a world-renowned midwife, herbalist, lecturer, and teacher who has the enviable record of facilitating more than two thousand births in sixty years without losing a single mother or baby during childbirth. It has been hard-won, but then again, Enriqueta is a Zapotec.

The Zapotec indigenous group of Mesoamerica is known as a fierce and formidable people, though they call themselves The People of the Clouds, since their homes grace the summits of the northern Sierra mountains, and their ancestors believed their rulers were direct descendants of divinity. Their communities nestle amid rich pine forests that housed their ancestors more than 2,500 years ago. Zapotec elders give advice on politics, family issues, and natural resource preservation, and Enriqueta advises on these issues as well as training the next generation to be healers and midwives.

With word spreading about her healing abilities and her natural grace during childbirth, Enriqueta was hired as the midwife for the village El Punto. The day of her arrival, the citizens unanimously

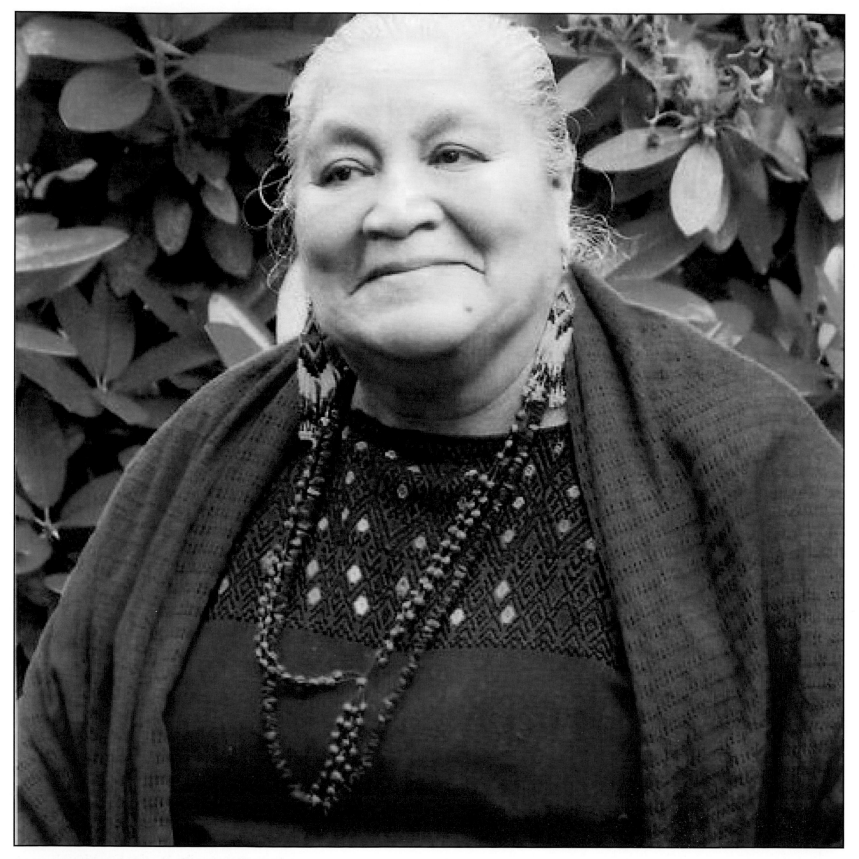

approved her position, collected building materials, and built her a new clinic and home. But by taking the position, she lost the support of her mother and brother, because she was now paid, which, to them, was taboo. The culture strongly disapproved of women working, but Enriqueta was determined, and she kept her position for eighteen years, traveling seven days a week between El Punta, Benito Juarez, and other villages.

Through unfortunate events (including jealousy and the bureaucracy of politics), Enriqueta was removed from her position in Benito Juarez for serving and healing people without "proper" government documentation. But her reputation was strong and she was immediately hired by the National Indigenous Institute. Here, she served as a health social worker, a translator for native dialects (including Zapotec), and as a representative to the Zapotec Indigenous Women's Forum in Guerrero.

This launched her more public role, and she became a much sought-after healer in Veracruz and Tuxtepec. Her midwife services brought her to remote Oaxaca villages, but she was forced to travel on foot because the government would not issue a vehicle nor provide transportation for her to tend women in need.

Just when Enriqueta was expanding her territory, an allopathic doctor at the Institute entered her herbal pharmacy, decried her indigenous methods and botanical remedies, and threw out all of her plants. She was mightily discouraged, but she didn't let him stop her. Naturally, Enriqueta mounted a loud protest, a move that could have resulted in her dismissal, but it eventually gained her an even better position at state headquarters. This greatly expanded her region of influence as she was able to assist dozens more villages and communities where women were giving birth without adequate medical prenatal and postnatal services.

In 1989, Enriqueta was invited to El Paso, Texas, to a midwifery convention by the agency *Maternidad La Luz*, and she enrolled in MANA (Midwives Alliance of North America). But at this peak of international camaraderie and professional advancement, she lost the support of many in Mexico, including her husband, who viewed women's "place" as in the home.

This brought Enriqueta to a crucial decision, one that, once made, demonstrated to her children just how dedicated and strong she was. She left her husband. "I left by my own means," she recalls. "I took a decision to separate from my husband in order to better my life and the lives of my children. My husband would absolutely not support my going. None of my family would."

I asked about the support of her colleagues. Weren't other women struggling to advance themselves professionally? Did they support her?

Mary Margaret (author of *The Life and Values of Doña Enriqueta Contreras—A Memoir*) helped answer. "No," she said. "Her colleagues had the same problem. Doña broke traditional rules by moving away."

Enriqueta, her face firm, nodded sadly while Mary Margaret translated. "In our community, for a woman to go out of her context from her home is completely forbidden. It's fatal to you. The traditions are so strict. But I did it, despite the fact I almost lost my

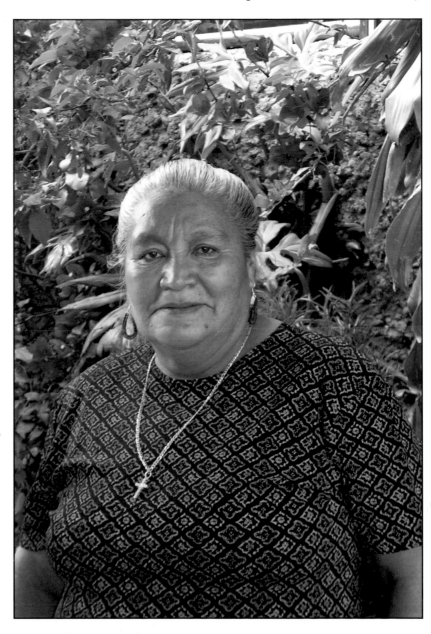

life a few times. So I thought the value of working toward putting my children through school and bettering their lives was more important than for me to sacrifice my life to stay in a traditional situation. So my children were more important to me than my husband or my communal context."

"Everything that we do, we have to do confidently."

Her great sacrifice was not lost on her children. Her youngest son, who now lives in the United States, remembers very clearly how much his mother suffered. When she decided to leave La Niveriea, her home village, to teach in Texas, rumors and accusations spread. But Enriqueta ignored them, insisting, "I'm pursuing this for my children."

Mary Margaret smiles. "She's an enormously dedicated mother."

And a skilled healer. Her impeccable record belies the fact that childbirth is always an intense and mysterious process, and she personally trains many up-and-coming midwives in Mexico and the southeastern United States. But her method of hands-on training is drawing criticism from academics who would prefer she focused more on book-learning. This has become a serious issue for her, as Enriqueta herself was empirically taught, having never attended a formal institution nor received a diploma or degree. Mary Margaret shakes her head. "Now there's a lot of pressure both in the United States and in Mexico to insist they go through nursing school and then specialize as a midwife practitioner, but she's against that. You don't have practical experience until you're *there*, and then what?"

The Sierras are beyond rural: when Enriqueta was growing up, they were isolated without adequate medical resources or emergency services. After years as a midwife and obtaining first aid training in Mexico City, Enriqueta earned the moniker The Doctor of the Sierras. "They called me doctor, nurse, teacher. The people, the communities, have given me many titles. I am recognized by my own people. I don't have a piece of paper that validates my education. It's my own people that validate my life's work and what I have contributed to my own community."

Mary Margaret nods. "They invite her to speak at rallies or conferences to defend this empirical position. You know she's very fierce, Zapotec people are very fierce, and she'll get up and have these arguments with the governor. Her colleagues will say, 'Doña Queta, you're going to get in trouble!' And she'll say, 'I don't care! For the years I have left? Let them throw me in prison.' But this

is an important issue. It's not easy to quell her. If she has a strong opinion, she'll let you know."

But Enriqueta laughs. "I continue my work. With a degree, without a degree, I know what I know. Am I going to stick my degree underneath the woman when it's time to birth the child? It's not going to help me!"

She shares the disturbing story of two professional midwives in Mexico who were educated without empirical, hands-on training. "The midwives had gone to see a mother, taking me with them, to give her an assessment about twenty days before the delivery. When I assessed her, I told her everything is okay, no problem. But to the midwives I said, 'Be careful! This lady . . . something is going to happen. Heads up! You will have problems.' But they didn't believe me. But in my gut, I knew that something was about to happen. So I warned them. It turned out the labor was coming, everything was going well, and the baby was born. In ten minutes, the mother died.

"What happened? What did they do since I wasn't there?" Enriqueta shakes her head, then informed me they already had this frightening experience under their belt when her own daughter hired them to be the midwives at her birth.

It is surprising to learn that her daughter chose a different midwife, but it is testament to the strength of the media and an unfortunate cultural stigma against traditionally trained and indigenous healers. Enriqueta, fierce and traditional, intimidated her daughter and probably seemed, as many mothers do to their children, somewhat "backward." Her daughter, convinced by the media that book-trained midwives were better, chose the two "professional" midwives mentioned earlier. Enriqueta stepped back, allowing the professionals to attend her daughter for hours. "But the baby would not come. So I knocked on the door and I could see immediately that my daughter was starting to lose her spirit. When I looked, the baby was stuck in one of the hips. So I grabbed my scarf, shifted the baby, put her legs on my shoulders, and the baby came out."

The midwives were horrified and embarrassed at their failure. "I could have never done that," one of them told her.

"So my daughter was going to die?" Enriqueta was livid, but because of her tenacity, she turned a potentially dire situation into a success. "I had to do something because we're talking about saving two lives. I let my daughter and her husband choose [their midwife] so they could appreciate what I do. Because I'm not always going to be here. One day I have to go and they have to stay, so how are they going to face life and make decisions? I tried to protect them a lot

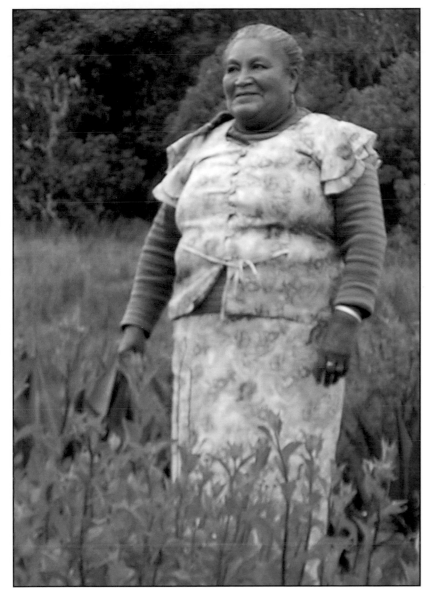

Photo credit: Doña Enriqueta

Enriqueta has encouraged Mary Margaret to become a midwife, but Mary refuses. "I don't do blood!" she laughs. "Being a midwife is not just a job, it's an enormous responsibility. You have two lives on the line, a mother and a baby. So be careful. *'Un ojo en el gato y el otro ojo en el otro gato.'* You have to have one eye on one cat and the other eye on the other cat. It's a very delicate profession."

Enriqueta leans in to Mary Margaret and whispers to her, a gleam in her eye. "No way!" Mary Margaret laughs. "See? She's still trying to talk me into it. It's been eleven years!"

"Breakdowns are breakthroughs. If there are no mistakes, how will you get better? You have to bump into a mistake in order to think and rethink and do better."

The Herbs of Midwifery

For Enriqueta, midwifery encompasses both herbalism and a strong sense of ritual. "I work from the perspective of both. You can't separate them. I bathe clients with flowers and plants. I cleanse them, give them massage. I use what is called *manpiada*, which is using the scarves to shift the baby around. So if the baby is breach, I put the scarf underneath the hips and manipulate so the baby shifts and is ready to go."

How many US obstetricians bathe their clients with floral water during labor? Most likely, the (male) doctor comes in at the very end of labor, often at the last minute of transition, to "deliver" the baby. But Enriqueta applies a hands-on loving approach. "If a mother is fearful, I'll get a sheet and fill it with flower petals, and wrap the woman in it. She'll breathe easier and come to a place of peace. There are so many techniques that I use in my practice. That's how it is."

Of all the plants and flowers dear to Enriqueta, those closest to her heart are roses. "*Todos las rosas.* All the roses, all of the colors of the roses. In my house, we may not have anything to eat but we have flowers. I cannot live without flowers in my house. I feel darkness when I walk into a house and there are no flowers. I choke."

When she was invited to the Lakota reservation at Rosebud, South Dakota, Doña Enriqueta experienced a community without flowers. "Just standing on the reservation, immediately the energy goes down," recalls Mary Margaret, who accompanied her. "It's

[when they were younger] because of what has happened to me, so in a way they have not learned that fierceness that I learned in life. But it was a good experience, so the husband and wife can realize life is not easy."

After the birth, the midwives thanked Enriqueta. They asked her forgiveness and admitted they had failed at their job. "I said, we all make mistakes. Our mistakes teach us to do better every day. Breakdowns are breakthroughs. If there are no mistakes, how will you get better? You have to bump into a mistake in order to think and rethink and do better."

very dark. The houses are dark and the only thing you can smell is cigarette smoke, alcohol. There's epidemic sexual abuse, domestic abuse, drug use. There's not one plant in sight, not even on the reservation. People don't plant things. It killed her. By the third day I had to ask the organizer to please take her off the reservation because it was affecting her. I could see her wilt."

"My life is nature," Enriqueta says. "That is a defect that I have."

"It would be a good thing if we all had this defect, right?" laughs Mary Margaret. "We wouldn't be in the situation that we're in."

Some of Enriqueta's favorite edible plants include mustard greens and watercress, and her favorite healing plants include arnica (*Arnica Montana*), elderberry (*Sambucus Canadensis*), called *saúco*, and raspberry (*Rubus idaeus*).

*"In my house we may not have anything to eat,
but we have flowers."*

The Nature of a Successful Healer

Her fierce Zapotecan heritage has been invaluable in preparing Enriqueta to be a powerful healer. When I asked her if you could simply be a gentle, peaceful, soft-spoken advocate, she recoiled. "No!" Then, laughing, "I sent that arrow straight! Otherwise, how can you be a shaman? You cannot fend off forces that are invisible to us, that are in other dimensions."

She stressed that it takes strength and confidence to be an effective healer, and that is the key attribute to anyone who wishes to enter healing professionally. "Before you even enter the camp, before you even walk in, you must have a huge discussion with yourself. You must evaluate yourself, and where your light is. You must have a light inside of you, and ask yourself: is it secure, are you confident in yourself as a healer? If you're not, and you give a recommendation and say, '*Maybe* it will help,' are you translating confidence or doubt? So before I even start, I evaluate students to see if they are confident. If they're not, the first rock they trip over they'll quit. So how will they convey trust to their patients and their clients? It's very important for them to analyze themselves and evaluate in terms of their spiritual life, their emotional life, and their physical life. 'If I have an illness, how am I going to deal with it? If I have an emotional imbalance, how am I going to deal with

BIRTH

The ancient Proto-Indo-European (PIE) word *bher* held two overlapping meanings: "to give birth" and "to carry a burden." This lead to Old High German's *beran* and Gothic's *bairan* "to carry," and finally to Old English's *beran*, "to bring or wear." PIE's *bher* gave Old Norse *byrdr*, which in 1230 AD became *birth*.

Later, birthroot (wake robin, *Trillium erectum*) became, through the gentle pronunciation of Appalachian mountain women, bethroot. Birthwort refers to *Aristolochia*.

it? If I don't believe in God . . . I want to be in childbirth, but I don't believe in the Great Spirit . . .' We already have a sickness there. That kind of evaluation is critical before you even touch a plant. Everything that we do, we have to do confidently. Because if you're not absolutely 100 percent confident of what you're doing, you're not going to have any results.

"This is an indigenous philosophy. If you don't love yourself, you may have fifty husbands, but that's not going to fill the void in your heart. You're not well in yourself. You're going to think that externally love is going to come to you, but love is born within ourselves."

I asked Doña if this was why white Westerners give their power away to doctors. "*Si!* Precisely, because they're allowing themselves to be manipulated. You give money, he writes a bunch of notes, gives you a prescription, but he doesn't even touch you, doesn't look at your heart, your soul, doesn't know where you are. He doesn't observe anything about your person. He sees you no different than that table, like a piece of wood. He thinks, 'Hey, I'm gonna get money for this session.' It's very important to not let ourselves be manipulated. Imagine, if I had allowed myself to be manipulated by my husband, his family, social pressures . . . do you think I would be here talking to you? What do you think? Honestly, I would be all submissive. 'Whatever that guy says, I'm gonna do . . .' Instead, I see how great the power and creativity of Mother Nature is.

"Everything is possible. Our work is very hard. As a shaman, I can sense human pain. And it hurts me, and I cry. I cry also in my

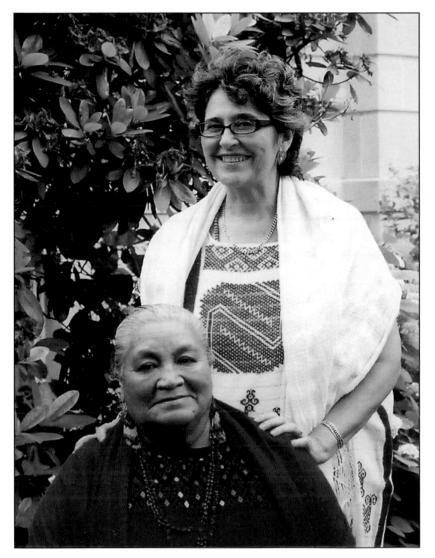

"A special sisterhood exists between Enriqueta and Mary Margaret Navar, an anthropologist and massage therapist who is also Doña Queta's translator and biographer. Navar memorialized the renowned midwife in her dual-language book *Zapotec Woman of the Clouds*. Such cherished friendships are important for women healers who need support throughout personal, professional, and political challenges."

own workshops, because I have feelings too. What is happening to someone else, I feel it. When I'm attending a birth, I'm birthing as well, because I remember the pain we have to share. My patients aren't a number to me nor a piece of paper."

CONCEIVE

The word *seed* has its origins in the Proto-Indo-European (PIE) *se*, "to sow," and it referred literally to the seeds of a plant for harvest. Proto-Germanic used *sædis*, Middle Dutch used *sæt* and Old Frisian *sed*. Biblically *seed* could refer to semen "planted" in a woman's womb. Another PIE word, *kap*, meant "to grasp," from which Latin coined *concipere*, "to take in and hold." By 1300 AD, this referred to taking a man's seed into the womb, and by 1340 it also meant taking an idea into the mind, as a concept. Today we use *conceive* as "create" with the implied understanding that the idea or baby will eventually be released into the world, though its original meaning was "to hold."

"That's why she has an impeccable record of two thousand births over sixty years," Mary Margaret says. "Because she's clairsentient, she's empathic."

"Step up!" says Doña Enriqueta, a call for all women ready to enter midwifery. "It's your turn. It's not a question of *whether* we can. It's, 'we *have* to!' A few weeks ago when I fell ill, I said to my students, 'You go! I can't, so you go! What is it I've taught you? It's not from a book. It doesn't have zeroes, numbers, ones, or tens. One remembers strong things that have happened [in their lives], you must go back and touch that.' I chose my path in life. I made my own path with no one's help. When I needed support from my family, nobody helped me. I couldn't count on anybody. I didn't want my children to repeat the same path that I had as a child where my parents abandoned me. I didn't want them to not be able to pursue their dreams, to repeat the same fate. It's not been easy for me in life. It's not the same to tell you about it, as it is to have lived it in flesh and blood."

Doña Enriqueta currently lives in Oaxaca, trains midwives, and lobbies the Mexican government for support for empirically trained midwives and healers. Her translator Mary Margaret Navar published *Zapotec Woman of the Clouds*, a vivid depiction of Zapotec heritage, Oaxacan life, and perseverance.

Where the earth heaves the giant mountain ranges Sierra Madre Oriental and Sierra Madre del Sur, this is the home of Oaxaca. The earliest Zapotecs lived here, at an average altitude of more than five thousand feet, and they believed their rulers descended divinely from the clouds. To this day, Zapotecs refer to themselves as The People of the Clouds, and they work to preserve their 2,500-year-old culture on this wild, rugged southern curve of the Yucatan Peninsula.

Zapoteca comes from the Nahuatl *tzapotecah*, meaning "the people of Sapote." This culture is credited with the development of one of the first writing systems of Mesoamerica, early cultivation of a variety of foods, including certain tomatoes and chili peppers, corn (*Zea mays*) as far back as six thousand to seven thousand years ago, pumpkins, squash, and cacao. Ancient Zapotec diets may even have included pineapples; avocados (first domesticated in the Chiapas-Guatemalan highlands); *maguey* (an agave from which *pulque* and tequila are produced); and *zapotes* or *sapotes*, the region's sweet, fleshy edible and medicinal fruit related to persimmons. In effect, they called themselves the People of the Sapote Fruit, illustrating the tremendous importance of this crop to their survival. Today, the region's largest export is shade-grown coffee.

Oaxaca, the fifth largest of Mexico's thirty-one states, was taken by Aztec tribes during Europe's dark ages and its capital Tenochtitlan was razed by Spanish forces in 1521. In 1858, Benito Juarez Garcia, a Zapotec Amerindian, became the first full-blooded indigenous national to serve as President of Mexico.

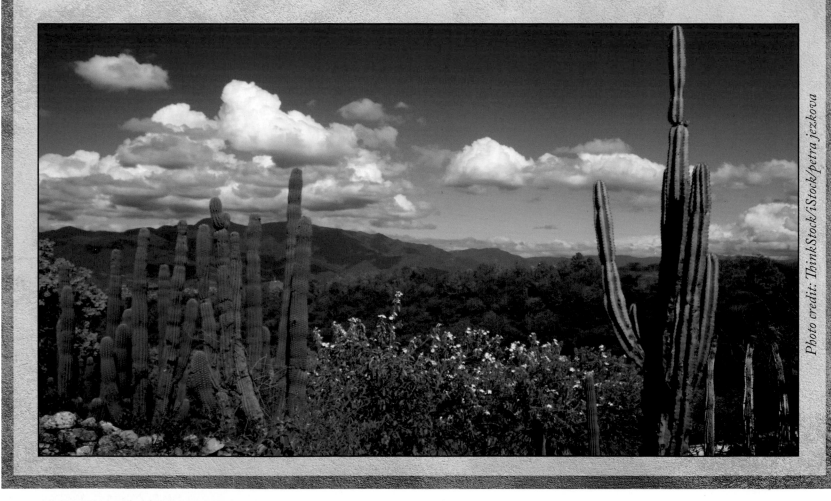

Photo credit: ThinkStock/iStock/petra jezkova

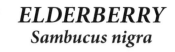

ELDERBERRY
Sambucus nigra

One of the world's more mythical plants—and certainly one of the most useful—the Elderberry (*Sambucus nigra* or *S. Canadensis*) graces many a trail, swamp, bog, and creek with its long, elliptical leaves and clusters of purple berries. Long used in Europe, the common or black elder earned its name from the Saxon Eller, meaning "kindler," since its hollow twigs were used to start fires. Scandinavians named the tree Hulde after their goddess of Love, a name that came to mean elves. This led to Elve and Hylde, and the Hylde-Moer or Hylde-Mutter was the Elder-mother, the magical Woman in the Tree. She protected the tree and avenged any wrong-doing, so that in time, few would cut the branches and even fewer built fires with its wood. Other common names include Bore Tree, Pipe Tree, and Sweet Elder, for its creamy perfumed flowers.

The tree was claimed by witches as well as their persecutors: witches and herbalists would plant elder by their doors, but many elder trees grow in the old churchyards of Europe.

Superstitions abounded: persecutors would snap off a piece of bark, dip it in oil, and float it in a glass of water where it would reveal any witch nearby by reflecting light in her direction.

Every part of the tree is useful as a medicine or a food. The rank-smelling leaves contain glycosides and the alkaloid *Sambucine*, making them a fine healing addition to topical oils and salves. The bark and root contain resin, viburnic acid, volatile oil, fat, wax, tannic acid, grape sugar, gum, starch, pectin, and salts; since the Doctrine of Signatures notes the stippling of the bark, it was used to treat pimples, acne, and skin eruptions. The hard white wood was fashioned into combs, pipes, and toys. The flavonoid-rich flowers are diaphoretic and anticatarrhal, making them useful to treat hay fever and sinusitis. The berries are expectorant and make a strong tincture or tea to treat colds, cough, and fever and to strengthen the immune system. Both flowers and berries are edible and delicious when prepared as fritters, pies, cobblers, and syrups.

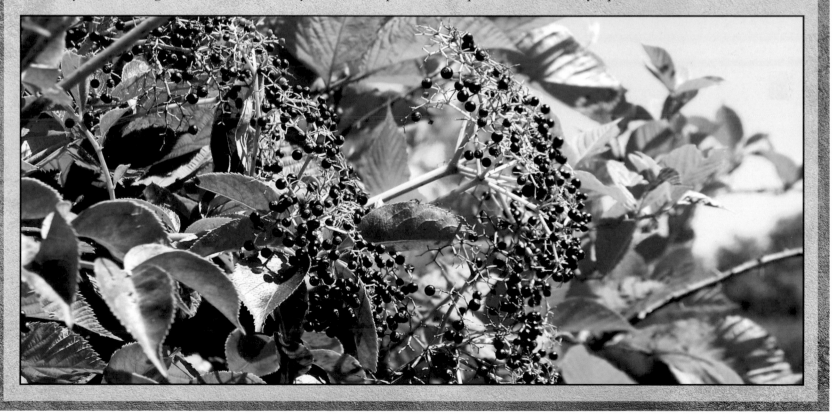

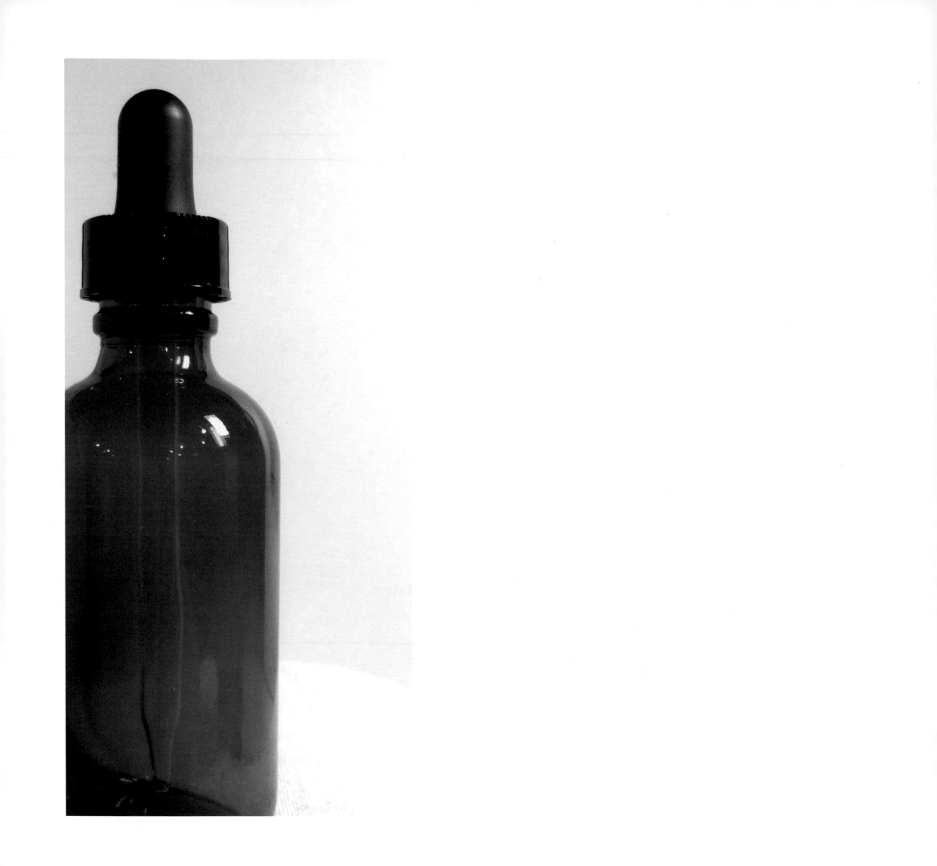

Chapter 9

ALLOPATHIC (MODERN) MEDICINE

Allopathic medicine in western countries is the conventional, or doctor prescribed, system of medicine. Allopathic is sometimes referred to as scientific, orthodox, or modern medicine. The word *allopathy* simply means "different from the suffering" or "other than the disease" and was coined by homeopathic healer Samuel Hahnemann in the nineteenth century, when he termed *allopathy* to distinguish modern medicine from his new "like-cures-like" system of healing, *homeopathy*, which used the cause of the symptom as the cure (*see* Homeopathy on page 171).

Allopathy is a mature branch of medicine and evolved for centuries into the sophisticated pursuit of healing that it is today. But early on, the debate between orthodox medicine and traditional therapies raged strong, beginning with the early advance of medical doctors into the arena of obstetrics and midwifery. It continued as herbalists argued with the English Crown that their methods were far safer than the barbers and surgeons of the day, while allopathic physicians bitterly called traditional healers quacks. And because of their limited knowledge of human anatomy and their insistence that they appear more effective than "simple" herbalists, allopathic practitioners through the early nineteenth century followed a useless framework based on Hippocrates's theories of the four elements (humors) and thus routinely engaged in surgery, lancing and bloodletting, cupping, purging, research on corpses, and the dangerous use of poisonous materials (hemlock, sulfur, and mercury) as curing agents.

Today, allopathy has dropped many of the more barbarous methods (except questionable practices such as irradiation, chemotherapy, and invasive surgery) and has outlawed many questionable and outright harmful practices that often caused greater risk to the patient than the disease itself, such as topical and/or internal applications of mercury. To its credit, allopathy has instituted high standards of hygiene, has developed invaluable questionnaires/intakes for patients, has improved record-keeping, and has an outstanding network of professionals writing in journals and teaching at universities. One downfall to orthodox medicine's spectacular achievements is that it has become a *system*, a bureaucracy in and of itself, and the enormous scale of this system has created related evils, namely treatment-influencing insurance companies, predatory lawsuits, a business atmosphere of middlemen, and—especially with the internet—misinformation.

Allopathy and "Integrative" Medicine

Many practitioners of modern medicine refer to themselves with the term *traditional*, and they call herbalism *alternative*. This implies that doctor-driven, surgical, and pharmaceutical methods are the norm; however, these are clearly new forms of healing compared to the ancient methods of botanic medicine, water therapy, shamanism, Eastern herbalism, folk healing, Gaelic pharmacy, and others that form the true backbone of tradition.

This isn't to say that these forms of healing are incompatible. Quite the contrary, it is very possible and even advisable to integrate them so that the patient receives the best care from a variety of knowledgeable and effective sources. Many of the healers profiled in this book advocate integrative medicine, believing that by being inclusive and working respectfully with practitioners of other systems, a healer truly serves a patient. Traditional therapists must work with standard doctors, they insist, and physicians and nurses must accept traditional practices. As no one therapy is perfect for all communities or to cure all diseases, the idea of integration in medicine is essential if we are to truly end suffering and promote health of body, mind, and spirit.

Together, modern medicine and traditional medicine can address a very wide range of disease. For instance, traditional medicine has a history of success with illnesses such as sleep disorders, anxiety, depression, mental illness, preventative care, midwifery, immune support, and wound healing—often succeeding where modern medicine fails.

On the other hand, allopathic medicine is poised to address trauma and emergencies, head injuries, allergies, communicable diseases, viruses, and vision, where traditional medicines are sometimes weaker. However, consequences of using allopathic medicines exist; for example, taking over-the-counter drugs to combat seasonal allergies can cause fatigue, stomach upset, and dependency even though the stuffy nose has been efficiently remedied.

Both systems—traditional and allopathic—provide strong treatment for cardiac distress, high blood pressure, hormone imbalance, and arthritis. Each person must weigh his or her own decisions against possible herb–drug interactions, side-effects, possible consequences, and the potential speed of recovery to determine how to proceed with traditional and/or allopathic care.

As Barbara Green recounts in *Green Pharmacy: The History of Evolution of Western Herbal Medicine*, the price of miracles is high. She notes that "miracle drugs" often demand a sacrifice, such as the touted Thalidomide drug of the 1960s that caused horrendous birth defects. Harmful adverse effects and allergic reactions were all-too-common consequences of many so-called miracle drugs,

and with the rocket-propulsion of women's rights and black rights in the 1960s and '70s in America came a new wave of "alternative" medicine and respect for traditional values.

Allopathic medicine uses one very important and incredible tool, however, that traditional methods rarely avail themselves of: technology. The use of magnification microscopes, invasive surgery, lasers, chemistry, X-ray technology, and of course advancements in hygiene control are second-to-none in learning about the human body and in finding new cures. This collaboration between technology and medicine has made for amazing recoveries and discoveries.

Obviously, no healing system is perfect and without mistakes. If a study were done on the fatal errors of herbal medicine, one would learn of mistakes with dosage, improper plant identification, and mistaken diagnosis. These mistakes, on both sides of the coin, teach a very powerful lesson: all healing systems must work together—generously, selflessly, and respectfully—to provide the safest possible environment for the alleviation of human suffering. And the emphasis of the importance of folk learning cannot be underestimated; using empiric knowledge (that which is gained by direct experience) is often vastly more valuable than copying words from a book. Only together—as integrative medicine—can we hope to achieve success that endures because it is safe, vital, open-minded, sustaining, and effective.

Trotula of Salerno

(12th Century)
A Female Physician

As a professor, as a physician, even as a woman, Trota is controversial simply because we know so little about her. Did she even exist? Did she write the famous and hugely popular women's medical and cosmetic texts that are attributed to her?

Commonly called Trota (a popular woman's name from the eleventh century through the thirteenth), Trocta, or Trotula di Ruggiero, this woman has long been hailed as the author of a group of works combined into one title, the *Trotula*—or, as researcher Monica H. Green calls it, *The Trotula Ensemble*. Originally penned in twelfth-century Salerno, Italy, three different medical texts were soon conflated into one large volume and, in 1544, they were heavily edited, rewritten, and reorganized by Renaissance editor Georg Kraut. For centuries, scholars have had only bits and pieces with which to study medieval women's medicine, until researcher Green translated a Latin-English edition in 2001. For the first time, we are able to extricate Trota's probable writings from the writings of others and to determine how a wide range of women's reproductive matters were handled in the medieval context.

Through her careful analysis, Green has determined that one of the *Trotula Ensemble's* three books (*Conditions of Women*) was likely written by a man, and that a third (*Women's Cosmetics*) was certainly written by a man; in fact, *Women's Cosmetics* originally contained a prologue by its author asserting that he was a male physician who obtained the recipes from women practicing the "art of cosmetics."[1] This leaves one book of the *Trotula Ensemble* that could have been written by Trota, and indeed it seems she was instrumental in the creation of this text. According to Green, the physician Trota and her medical knowledge was referenced in three other contemporary texts: 1) *Practical Medicine According to Trota*, which is now extant in only two manuscripts and displays an astonishing range of treatments for illnesses attributed to the physician Trota directly; 2) a compendium *On the Treatment of Illnesses* made in the second half of the twelfth century that includes excerpts from the writings of seven Salernitan medical writers, including Trota: "Trota is among them," asserts Green, "and the excerpts attributed to her here demonstrate her considerable expertise in the fields of gastrointestinal disorders and ophthalmology."[2]

And 3) an anecdote included in the text of *Treatments for Women* itself—the most professional of the Ensemble commonly called Trotula Major— refers to "Trotula" curing a young woman suffering a sharp bout of gas or "wind into the womb."[3] As Green notes, this third-person reference to Trota suggests she may not have been the author of *Treatments for Women*, yet it certainly confirms that she was a master medical figure,[4] that she did indeed exist, and that her knowledge was influential and primary in twelfth-century Southern Europe. Green speculates that Trota perhaps dictated her knowledge to a scribe who added to the text. Regardless of whether Trota wrote the entire *Trotula Ensemble*, it seems clear that many of her writings were included and in fact form the basis around which other physicians' works are structured. "Either way, it is in no way inappropriate to consider her the text's principal source"[5] with this primary text acting as a sort of magnet for the similar *Conditions of Women* and *Women's Cosmetics*, written by others and appended to the original text much later.

Though her life and accomplishments are incredibly vague, fascinating folklore abounds: that the woman called Trota chaired the School of Medicine at the famous University of Salerno; that she taught gynecology and obstetrics to both men and women; that she operated a clinic. In 1906, it was asserted that she married fellow physician Johannes Platearius (a family "dynasty" of physicians in Salerno at the time[6]) and had two sons, Johannes and Matthaeus, who both became doctors in Salerno,[7] though truly we know very little of her life whatsoever.

She may have been included in the *mulieres Salernitane*, the "Salernitan women" referenced by male medical writers of the twelfth century who lauded these women for their

WEED

Weed originates in Old Norse *vad*, meaning "cloth" or "texture," and was applied to plants for the cloth woven from their fibers. The ancient Proto-Indo-European *wedh* meant "weave," and these words form the basis Old English *uueod* and our *weed*.

STINGING NETTLE
Urtica Dioica

Stinging nettle has become one of western herbalism's most beloved herbs—and for good reason: it's extremely high in calcium, magnesium, trace minerals, protein, and chlorophyll; it's ideal for use during pregnancy, breast-feeding, menopause, and anemia. Growing in cool, rich woodlands, nettle contains formic acid, which is expelled through its tiny hairs when people or animals brush against it, resulting in a temporary, stinging rash. Practitioners of the Middle Ages used nettle as a hair rinse and tonic, following the Doctrine of Signatures.

Additionally, nettle juice was employed against itches and rashes, and the whole plant would be rubbed directly on the skin as a rubefacient for arthritis, rheumatism, and poor circulation (a process termed *urtication*).

Nettle fibers are woven into durable linen in Scotland and many third-world countries. Nettle makes a top-rate food: in addition to tea and steamed nettles with vinegar, Euell Gibbons recommends nettle purée and nettle pudding.

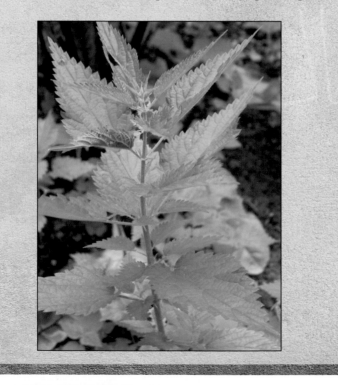

wonderful healings and treatments, though as Green notes "they are credited with no medical writings, nor are they referred to as teachers. The Salernitan women, to judge from all these references, are empirical practitioners: they know the properties of plants and are even credited on occasion with finding new uses for them, but they seem to participate not at all in the world of medical theory or medical books."[8]

It remains unclear if the Salernitan women were popular healers and midwives, or if they included a corps of respected and educated physicians, or even if they included Trota or any of her students. Likewise, it is unclear if these women were stripped of their titles by male historians or if they were simply celebrated as lay healers by either the general populace, by the university, or both. Later, Trota was affectionately called *Magistra Mulier Sapiens*, Wise Woman Teacher, and even centuries after her death, she was credited with great wisdom by historians and poets, including Geoffrey Chaucer in his *Canterbury Tales*.[9]

Based on the texts, we know Trota's medical expertise included the wide and prevalent use of herbs, though unlike her near-contemporary Hildegard von Bingham of Germany, Trota seldom used prayers, astrology, or incantations. She functioned less as a prophet and more as a hands-on physician and clinician and seldom refers to religious dogma at all. She dealt with the health problems of both men and women, treating swelling of the penis, hemorrhoids, intestinal problems, wandering womb, bladder and urinary problems, skin issues, cancer, incontinence, dysentery, gout, and more. Her dispensary included common herbs such as aloe, watercress, catmint, nutmeg, marsh mallow, wormwood, pennyroyal, camphor, wild rocket, elecampane, bistort, rue, sage, bilberry, nettle, mugwort, eggwhites, frankincense, mastic, and vinegar, as well as herbs and materials less than fashionable today such as worms, plaster of Paris, bacon, and fresh eels. What's more, her treatments unabashedly call for herbs and elements we consider quite noxious today, such as pitch, henbane, black nightshade, quicksilver (mercury), lead, arsenic, and powder of natron.[10]

The Texts

The lesser text *On Women's Cosmetics* (the one certainly written by a man) was less for academia and more for the housewife, with recipes and folk wisdom for healing common complaints such as

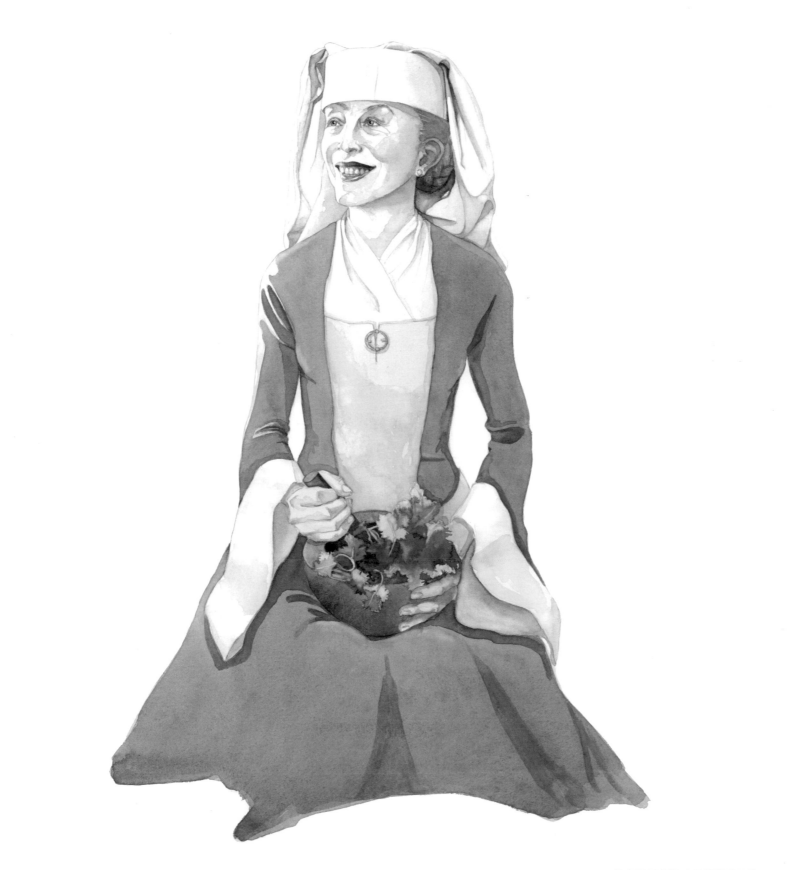

burns, headlice, wounds, and external dermal lesions including scabies, smallpox, eczema, psoriasis, and acne. Recipes abound for shiny hair, long black hair, thick black hair, and "various kinds of adornments."[11] It taught women to improve their beauty for their health's sake, in the context that a beautiful body must be a healthy body, and many references in the text are to Muslim women, or Saracens, whom Salernitan elite women wished to emulate.[12] Many of the herbs prescribed in this text are still used today for similar purposes: barley for nourishing skin and hair; dates and fennel for cleaning and whitening teeth; violet flower or leaf for burns.

The two major and more professional works, *On Treatments for Women* and *On Conditions of Women*, address a much wider range of illnesses specific to anatomy and medicine, especially menstruation and women's sexuality. These treatments, surprisingly, are pragmatic, yet they also address the desires and emotional well-being of women, a viewpoint generally not seen in twelfth-century writings on women's health where a straightforward mechanical view was deemed sufficient.[13] Indeed, a therapy is recommended for women who desire intercourse but must practice abstinence (such as nuns and widows), and it acknowledges both the emotional and physical pain that can accompany unfulfilled sexual desire. The therapy was likely seen as quite relevant since the general view maintained that regular sexual activity was necessary to maintain health and that abstinence could cause disease. This therapy instructed women in situations of forced abstinence that "sweet-smelling substances [should] be applied to the vagina" and that this therapy "constrains the lust and sedates the pain."[14] Trota's passage "On the Preservation of Celibate Women and Widows":

> "[141] There are some women to whom carnal intercourse is not permitted, sometimes because they are bound by a vow, sometimes because they are bound by religion, sometimes because they are widows, because to some women it is not permitted to take fruitful vows. These women, when they have desire to copulate and do not do so, incur grave illness.

For such women, therefore, let there be made this remedy. Take some cotton and musk or pennyroyal oil and anoint it and put it in the vagina. And if you do not have such an oil, take *trifera magna* [a blend of opium, cinnamon, cloves, etc.[15]] and dissolve it in a little warm wine, and with cotton or damp wool place it in the vagina. This both dissipates the desire and dulls the pain. . . ."[16]

Reading between the lines, women caught in the strict confines of forced abstinence might have seen a carefully worded acknowledgement that masturbation can be acceptable, healthy, and pleasurable.

Indeed, the harsh climate of Lombardi and Roman culture in twelfth-century Italy proved dangerous for new brides and widows alike, for a woman's ability to acquire and maintain property upon marriage or widowhood was tied to her sexual purity. It could be a life-changing event to be found, on the bridal bed, deflowered. To prevent this, in *Treatments for Women* Trota displays unapologetic concern for these women and bravely provides guidance for something heretofore unseen in medieval medical literature: straightforward deception. She recommends the use of "constrictives" for the vagina that would deceive a man into believing his bride to be a virgin. The text advised several options, many of which use astringent plant material, including a "douche" with pennyroyal; a douche with oak bark; a powder of natron or blackberry (natron is a sodium-soda ash deposit); and a fomentation with "oak apples, roses, sumac, great plantain, comfrey, Armenian bole, alum, and fuller's earth, of each one ounce." The most extreme of these prescriptions—and the one specifically called for on the wedding night—involves placing leeches in the vagina "so that blood comes out and is converted into a little clot. And thus the man will be deceived by the effusion of blood."[17] In his excitement, the young groom would be none the wiser—and many a bride's life would be eased thanks to Trota's straightforward counsel.

Sun-drenched Salerno, Italy, is a dream destination today, just as it was one thousand years ago when merchants, pilgrims, students, and the sick flocked through its city gates for selling, eating, schooling, and healing. The metropolis was modern and cutting edge even in the Middle Ages and, on top of its other attractions, Salerno boasted Europe's famous Garden of Minerva, with more than three hundred species of edible and medicinal plants. The spectacular garden operated as the "Hortus sanitatus" for the *Schola Medica Salernitana*, the world-renowned School of Salerno.

Near Salerno, the town of Velia had hosted a small school of medicine, but after the fall of the Roman Empire, the doctors migrated to Salerno; the School grew to become a collection of teachers and is now hailed as the first medical university in the world, offering studies in medicine, law, and philosophy. The school flourished from the eleventh century to the thirteenth century, and by 1811, it fell into decline and was closed by the Napoleonic government. In 1944, it was renamed Giovanni Cuomo University Institute of Education and, in 1968, it became a State university and is still in successful operation.[1]

As the most diverse educational institution in the world at that time, along with the universities of Paris and Bologna, the School of Salerno represented a kaleidoscope of cultures in its faculty and student body and was singular in its open acceptance of women professors and students. Today, this busy port city on the southwest coast of Italy boasts a waterside promenade, an ancient fortress, luxurious spas, and the Salerno Duomo Cathedral.

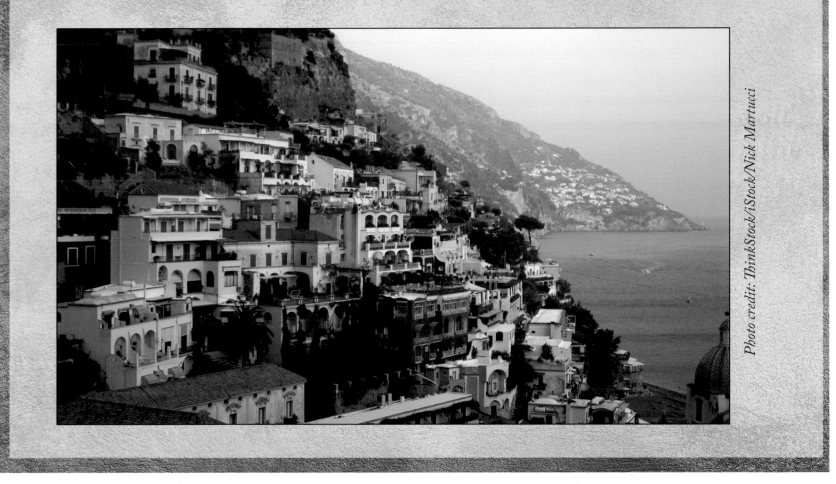

Photo credit: ThinkStock/iStock/Nick Martucci

Dr. Tieraona Low Dog

Dr. Tieraona Low Dog stands out in a crowd—she is a tall, powerful woman with long, sleek, black hair, strong features, a clear voice, and a warm smile. Wearing long skirts or leather jackets, with turquoise-and-silver jewelry and western boots, she appears to be the iconic desert Medicine Woman. She is this and much more—after a lifetime of learning the healing crafts from indigenous native peoples, Tieraona is a healer, a physician, and a highly sought-after speaker on phytochemicals and women's health.

There are, unfortunately, few tribal doctors who are also medical-system physicians. Most gravitate to either indigenous philosophies or medical degrees, but seldom both. Tieraona, however, sees no inherent division between the capability and intent of the indigenous herbalist and the physician. She represents a combination of interests and abilities, practicing both the indigenous and the allopathic healing systems as a world-class physician.

Tieraona sometimes takes to the lecture stage barefoot with a strong and unapologetic presence, teaching about women's health with a fireball-style and encyclopedic teaching approach. She is that rare breed of physician that successfully integrates the positive attributes of a clinical researcher with those of a compassionate healer—and a humorist.

Her interest in "folk" remedies began in her childhood, when her maternal and paternal grandmothers of the Dakotas and Oklahoma convinced her that the body could heal itself if given rest, good nutrition, and common sense remedies. "My grandmothers were both very practical," she says. "They taught me to use sage and salt water gargles, mint for tummy aches, thyme for a cold, and ginger and honey for a sore throat (sometimes with a touch of whiskey)."

As a teenager, Tieraona shopped at a local food cooperative and grew interested in bulk herbs. "Like lots of other folks thirty-five years ago," she says, "I got a copy of *Back to Eden* and starting making tinctures and liniments and salves. Interesting, I never considered that the remedies wouldn't work."

Tieraona spent a summer with southern Piute teachers and anthropologists in Arizona, learning Piute medicine. Later, she studied midwifery and massage therapy and became a respected herbalist in Las Cruces teaching the herbs of the Rio Grande in southern New Mexico. While she was a midwife and during her medical school residency, she birthed her own children at home, but admits she received negative feedback from her fellow doctors—even those in family medicine. Even for a normal function such as childbirth, she says, "They looked at women's health as a pathology."

She has since gone on to champion women's health as both natural and special. "I don't believe women are cycling men," she says. "Women are unique." She encourages women, including her own daughter, to hold true to their identities and be strong. "Women have surrendered their health to the medical system," which in turn treats women's bodies as somehow inferior or imperfect. "Is PMS really a *disorder* if 90 percent of women experience it? Be thoughtful about what's a disease," she teaches, "about what to treat pharmaceutically, and about what's normal."

Tieraona received her Doctor of Medicine diploma from the University of New Mexico School of Medicine, went on to study Tae Kwon Do for twenty years (earning a third-degree black belt), then delved into both Korean and Traditional Chinese Medicine.

Today, Dr. Low Dog can claim a long list of accomplishments relating to alternative health and healing: In 2000, she was appointed by President Bill Clinton to the White House Commission of Complementary and Alternative Medicine, and she serves on the Advisory Council for the National Institutes of Health National Center for Complementary and Alternative Medicine (NCCAM). She was elected Chair of the United States Pharmacopoeia Dietary Supplements and Botanicals Expert Committee. She ran a clinic in Albuquerque before joining the faculty of Tucson's Arizona Center for Integrative Medicine at the University of Arizona, where she serves as the Director of the Fellowship.

"I see myself as the gardener who loves to grow peppermint in her garden, the physician who gives peppermint oil to ease a woman's irritable bowel, and the scientist who researches the properties of menthol."

Dr. Low Dog works to bring the two "worlds" of medicine together. The word *integrative* is key to understanding her approach, as she combines historical knowledge with current science for a holistic approach to healing. "I am not interested in rejecting the past," she says, "nor am I interested in being stuck within it. I wish to take this rich tradition and continue to bring it forward—so

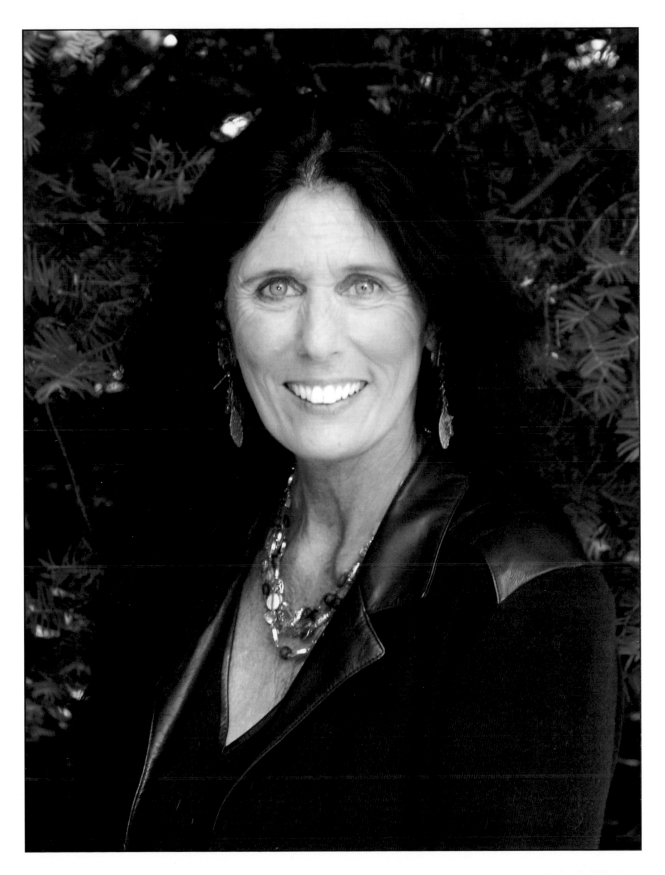

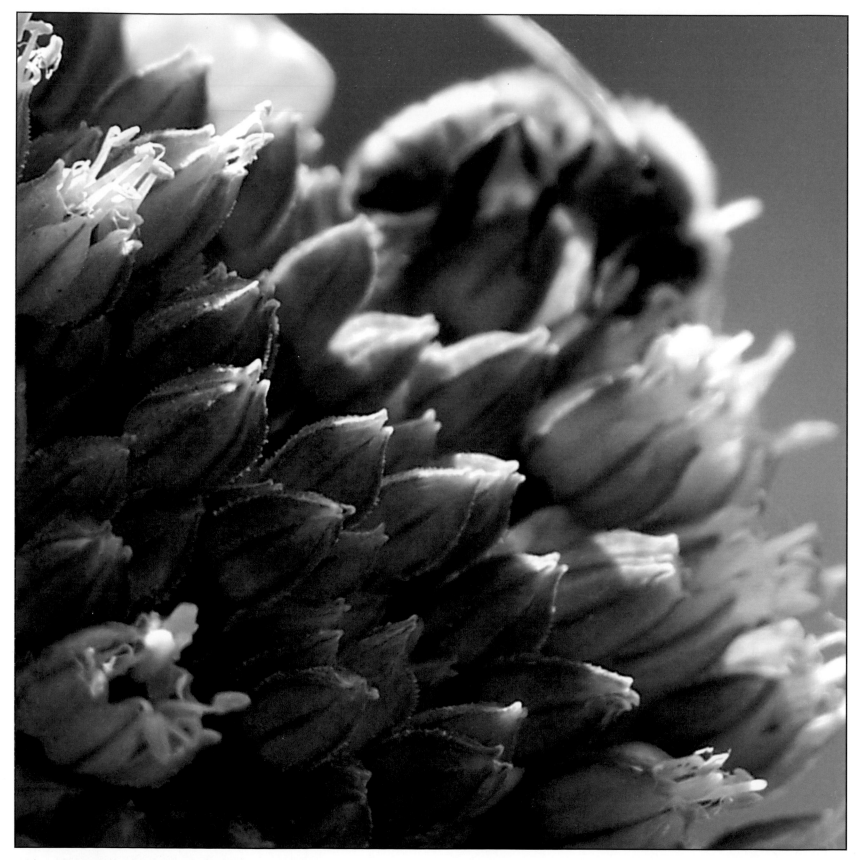

that herbal medicine can be used in a thoughtful, ecologically sound, scientifically rigorous, artful, and compassionate manner." She believes the one does not exclude the other, that it is in the best interest of both patient and science to bridge gaps between herbal medicine and allopathy. "I see myself as the gardener who loves to grow peppermint in her garden, the physician who gives peppermint oil to ease a woman's irritable bowel, and the scientist who researches the properties of menthol."

The Challenges

There were no formal training programs in herbal medicine in the early seventies in the United States when Tieraona was searching for guidance—no formal instruction in physiology, pathology, botany, green pharmacy, etc. She had to pick it up as she went along, which may have been a blessing in disguise. Though she laments it would have been convenient to learn the information in a more systematic fashion, she managed to piece together a broad range of traditions (indigenous US desert, Piute, Korean, Chinese, Western folk, and University allopathic) to build a strong foundation on plant interaction on human anatomy.

"The challenge," she says, "has been learning to walk with integrity and truth within both the scientific community and herb community. To be open to hearing all sides of the question, all voices in the conversation, and then retreat into the quiet and listen to my own voice."

She has since paved the way herself. Invited to speak at more than 350 scientific and medical conferences, Dr. Low Dog has more than forty publications to her credit. She serves on the editorial boards of *Menopause*, *Explore*, *Prevention Magazine*, and the *Kaiser Permanente Journal* and is the Integrative Medicine Doctor for KVOA Channel 4 TV in Tucson. She was *Time* Magazine's "2001 Innovator in Complementary and Alternative Medicine" and she was awarded the Martina de la Cruz Medal for indigenous medicines, Bioneer's Award for Outstanding Contribution to Medicine, the Burt Kallman Scientific Award, and National Public Radio's People's Pharmacy Award.

"The challenge has been learning to walk with integrity and truth within both the scientific community and herb community. To be open to hearing all sides of the question, all voices in the conversation, and then retreat into the quiet and listen to my own voice."

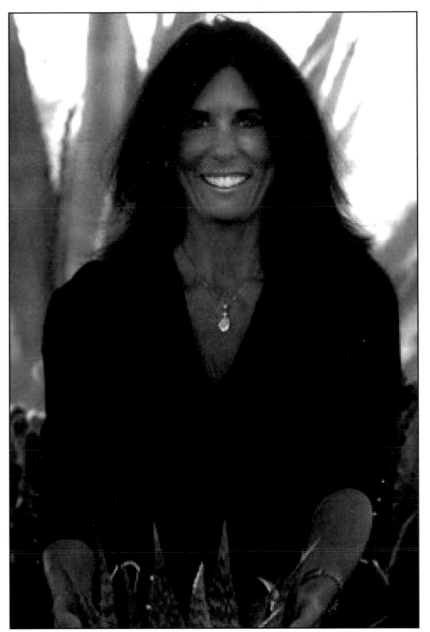

Photo credit: Tieraona Low Dog

"Science and Nature have provided the threads for the tapestry of my life," Dr. Low Dog says. "Learning about DNA, molecules, and the biochemistry of life has awed and inspired me—allowing me to expand my vision of the world, while Nature continues to provide a steady, gentle path for my soul to follow. The division between conventional and traditional medicine is as artificial as the division between science and nature. They can be woven together in a fashion that meets our physical, emotional, and spiritual needs. This is the foundation upon which integrative medicine is built."

By combining the strengths of herbalism (which some scientists see as "dubious") with the strengths of science (which some herbalists see as "artificial"), integrative medicine promotes better health. "Some conventional scientists and physicians will always think that herbal medicine is backwards and nothing but nonsense,"

Dr. Low Dog says. "Some herbalists will always reject anything that moves the field forward or reeks too much of science. I am not interested in working with either of these extremes. There is way too much to do. I will always be a student—constantly exploring, engaging, listening, learning. My work is to care for the sick, to help people feel better, to walk gently upon the earth, to do no harm. Herbal medicine is a part of that work."

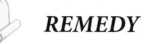

REMEDY

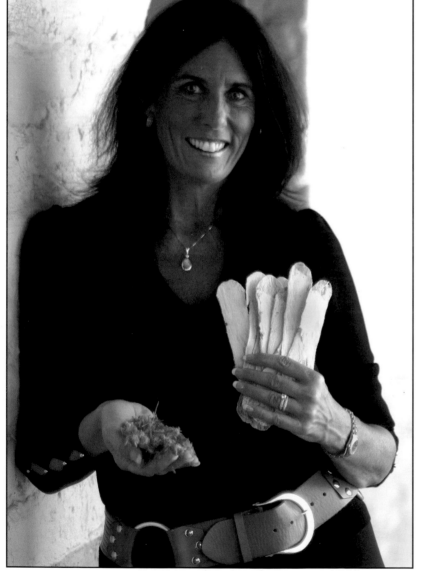

The Proto-Indo-European *med* meant "to measure," as in measuring amounts and placing limits upon, but also to ponder and think. To measure one's words or consider one's actions. Sanskrit *midiur* meant "to judge or estimate" and Welsh *meddwl* meant "mind, thinking." Both the Gothic *miton* and the Old English *metan* meant "to measure," and Latin coined *meditari* "to think, meditate, consider." By 1225, meditation meant "discourse on a subject" and *remedy* (*remedie*) in Anglo French combined *re* "again," with *mederi*, "to measure or consider." By 1646, *med* formed the French *médical* and Late Latin's *medicalis*, "of a physician," led to *medical*.

The dramatic paradise of the Sonoran Desert covers 120,000 square miles of Arizona (including Phoenix and Tucson, Arizona, on the Santa Cruz River), California, Baja and Sonora, Mexico. In 2001, the Sonoran Desert National Monument protected nearly a half million acres, and seventeen aboriginal cultures and two thousand plant species call this desert home.

Though it's the wettest desert in the world, water availability and quality are concerns; early desert cultures re-routed rivers to their homes and in the sixth century, the Hohokam built irrigation canals thirty feet wide and ten feet deep. They enclosed the trenches in plaster, bringing a safe supply of water from the Gila River to their villages.

The Santa Cruz River once flowed through the region, but its supply dwindled and the riverbed is now dry. As late as the nineteenth century, residents could purchase a gallon of water for a penny from traveling vendors who home-delivered drinking water in buckets and barrels. Today, Tucson receives its water from the Central Arizona Project Aqueduct, which pipes water from the Colorado River, three hundred miles away.

The Sonoran ecosystem provides for a rich variety of plants, including the Barrel Cactus (*Ferocactus wislizeni*) with its edible pulp; the Creosote Bush (*Larrea tridentala*), and the Saguaro Cactus (*Carnegiea gigantea*), which enjoys government protection since Saguaros grow only in this desert. Poppies and lupines sprout here as well as little-leaf Palo Verdes, desert ironwood, catsclaw, jojoba, and night blooming cereus.

Dr. Tieraona Low Dog is a self-proclaimed child of the desert. "I love the desert and our desert mountains," she says. "There is a vastness, an expansiveness that touches me deeply. I never feel so at home as I do when I am in the desert. And then the plants themselves . . . It's hard to go walking around in the desert or in the mountains and not want to learn the name of every creature that shares the world with us."

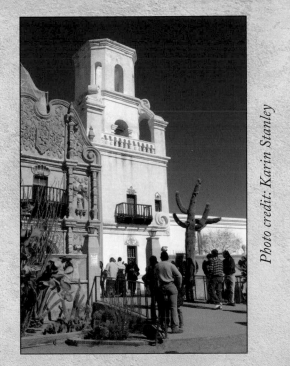

Photo credit: Karin Stanley

Mission, San Xavier del Back, in Tucson, Arizona

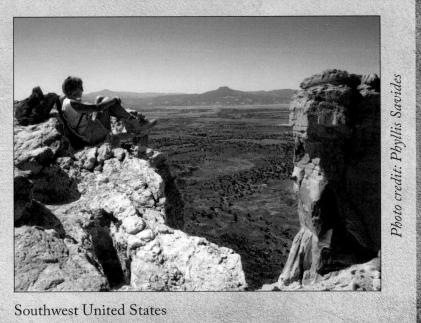

Photo credit: Phyllis Savides

Southwest United States

LEMON BALM
Melissa officinalis

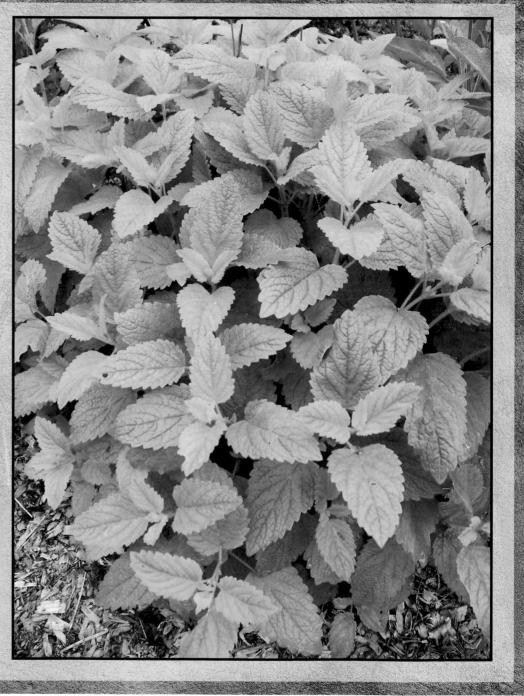

A medicinal powerhouse, *Melissa* (Greek for "bee") is affectionately called the Gladdening Herb since smelling its scent or drinking its infusion has a positive influence upon our emotions. It is rich in essential oils that reduce tension and relax the nervous system, at the same time heightening mental clarity. It is valued for promoting better memory and is a favorite of test-taking students.

Tieraona Low Dog recommends lemon balm for Attention Deficit Hyperactive Disorder because it "affects the limbic-hippocampal area of the brain. It is now believed that this plant can help 'filter out' excessive stimuli from the body. Melissa probably acts as a homeostatic modulator of nervous input from the inside and outside environment." Lemon balm can help a child determine subliminally what stimuli he or she needs and what can be ignored. Dr. Low Dog lauds its mild antidepressant effects as beneficial for children with social/behavioral difficulties.

Balm is also carminative, relieving spasms of the digestive tract and easing gas. It can be useful in lowering blood pressure and as a circulatory tonic. It has long been recognized as a powerful antiviral against herpes simplex and influenza.

CHASTE-TREE BERRY
Vitex agnus-castus

Chaste-tree berry, a member of the *Verbenaceae* family, is one of Dr. Low Dog's favorites. This beautiful, small tree with deeply serrated leaves and bright red berries acquired the name chaste-tree from the Greeks. They, along with English monks and pagan priestesses, used the dried berries to suppress sexual desires during ceremonies and in cloister: thus, the common names Monk's Pepper and Chaste Berry. The medically sophisticated Arabs similarly considered the berry and leaf calming.

But women today use the shrub for entirely different purposes: often to increase libido. How does this work? *Vitex* stimulates the pituitary gland, which increases leutenizing hormone and thus progesterone production. This inhibits the release of follicle-stimulating hormone and normalizes the estrogen cycle. Herbalists understand that, in some women, this increases libido because it fixes a disrupted hormonal structure and brings balance.

Etymologically, *Vitex* is an ancient word. Lithuanians used *gyvata* to mean "eternal life" and Old Persian coined *jivaka*, "alive." By substituting *b* for *v*, Greeks created *bios* for life, and later Latin used *vita* for "life" and *vitalis* for "belonging to life." Vitality was coined in 1592 and the sense of something being necessary or "vital" was first used in literature in 1619.

Herbalists today recommend *Vitex* for women suffering from dysmenorrhea or premenstrual syndrome and especially for menopausal women. Maintaining the health of the hormonal system is pivotal for women: indeed, Hippocrates used the word *hormone* to denote a "vital principle" from the Greek *hormone*, "that which sets in motion." Our hormones are meant to be in constant motion, continual flux and movement, as our reproductive system flows with the moon and is cyclical for repeated procreation. But dysmenorrhea or amenorrhea indicate improper cycling. *Vitex* is useful when menstrual cycles are fifteen days apart one month and then thirty-two days apart the next: this herb restores normal cycling for continuity, harmony, and a measure of sanity.

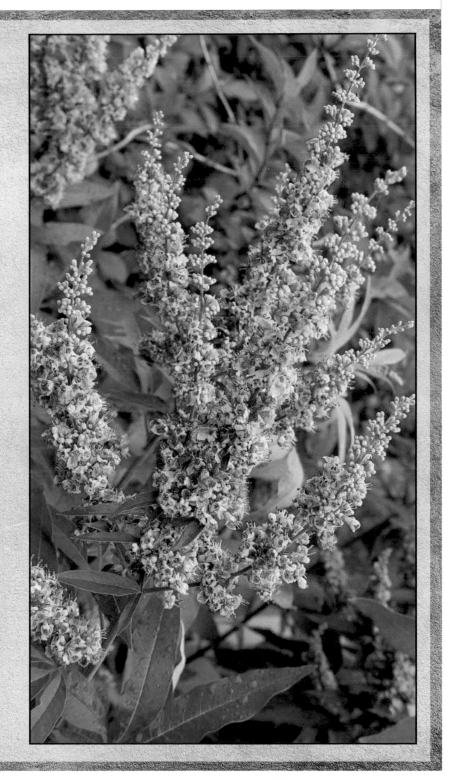

viral infection & chills

ORGANIC & WILD ORIGINAL
AWARD-WINNING ALL-NATURAL
WWW.VINEYARDHERBS.COM

Contains: Fre...
purpurea ro...
Willow bar...

Chapter 10
PHARMACOLOGY

Botany and chemistry are at the core of modern diagnostics and pharmacy; indeed, pharmacology is the basis of modern drug treatment. To the western allopathic practitioner, plants are chemical powerhouses containing resins, acids, alkaloids, sugars, tannins, volatile oils, triterpenoids, flavonoids, bitter components, glycosides, estrogenic and other hormonal substances, histamines, saponins, proteins, polypeptides, mucilage, and many other components not the least of which are our familiar vitamins and minerals.

The study of pharmacology is valuable to herbalists who wish to use not only spiritual, astrologic, or shamanic practices of healing, but also scientifically rigorous methods based on botany and science. The following are three of the most important and fascinating chemical components long valued by western herbal medicine: alkaloids, glycosides, and tannins.

Alkaloids

Defined simply, alkaloids are organic nitrogenous compounds found in many plants and some animals. They are famous because of their marked physiological effects *not only on the body, but also on the brain*. Most chemical compounds affect our bodies: they heal the skin, they trigger an enzyme, or they raise blood sugar level. Tannins, for instance, astringe tissue—but they don't affect the brain. Alkaloids, however, affect the body *and also* the mind, causing emotional, extra-sensory, and nervous system reactions—sometimes good, sometimes not.

For instance, nicotine is an alkaloid from the tobacco plant; nicotine relaxes muscle tissue and also calms the mind. Caffeine is an alkaloid from *Theobroma* and coffee that tenses the muscles, increases the heart rate, and speeds circulation. It also propels

the mind into over-alert hyperdrive, increases concentration, and keeps the mind awake. For these reasons, tobacco has been a valuable remedy for anxiety, and coffee a world-renowned aid for endurance. A single plant may possess two, three—even a dozen—different alkaloids in any part: the seeds, fruits, leaves, stems, roots, rhizomes, bark, and even in fungi. The word originated in the Arabic *al qualja*, meaning "ashes of plants," and most alkaloid names end in *–ine*: nicotine, caffeine, and berberine, for example.

Chemists ask the eternal question, Why do plants have alkaloids? An obvious answer might be for protection. A plant that produces a chemical that gives a predatory animal a severe stomach ache will discourage that animal from returning to eat more. But why would a plant cause an animal (or human) predator to have hallucinations? Or get the jitters? Or experience euphoria?

Most plants produce sweet fruits to entice pollinators, and they protect themselves with thorns or tall trunks for the advantage of height. But many plants rely on alkaloids, and there are a number of theories for why this may be so: 1) Alkaloids act as poisonous protection. Since most alkaloids taste extremely bitter, the cow/horse/human will not come back for seconds. 2) Because these are concentrated deposits of toxins that the plant cannot expel, it isolates them from its tissues to protect itself, much as an oyster wraps an irritating grain of sand within a pearl. 3) Or, perhaps these highly nitrogenous compounds serve as a nitrogen reserve.

Further food for thought: is protection a cause for the plant to produce these compounds, or is protection merely a result of alkaloids being produced for other reasons?

Michael Pollan, in his book *The Botany of Desire: A Plant's Eye View of the World*, believes that a plant produces a clue—a hint for us slow-brained animals—in its bitter taste. "As a general rule, sweet is good, bitter bad. Yet it turns out that it is some of the bitter, bad plants that contain the most powerful magic—that can answer our desire to alter the texture and even the contents of our consciousness" (Pollan, p. 114).

Alkaloids are those rare compounds that mystify our thoughts, muddle our feelings of success, scramble our tendency to fight. Alkaloids can also be extremely toxic and can kill animals and humans quickly, and they have been the means for murders (think Socrates, Nero, and Shakespeare's King Hamlet). Locusta of Gaul was an expert in achieving her desired, macabre results using alkaloid-rich plants such as yew, which contains taxanes. A certain amount of quinine is effective against malaria (tertian fever) while too much quinine-containing Monkshood can kill. A tincture of laudanum, with its high morphine and codeine content, can ease one into tranquility and lessen pain, but the dosage quickly becomes addictive and the patient's body debilitates thanks to the very drug used to heal it.

Glycosides

Have a sweet tooth? Much of our daily sugar intake comes from innocuous sources, foods we generally don't consider sweets. Corn, for example, is a starchy food high in fructose, one of the many 'oses that indicate naturally occurring sugars: dextrose, fructose, glucose, sucrose, and lactose are the official sugars recognized by the US Pharmacopeia and National Formulary (USP-NF).

One or more sugars can be created when a glycoside compound is "hydrolyzed" or acted upon by a particular enzyme often found within the same plant but in different tissues. Glucose occurs most frequently.

Glycosides have profound effects upon the body; cardioactive glycosides, for example, affect the heart muscle by increasing its tone (acting as a tonic), exciting it, and causing it to contract. This can be useful for those with low blood pressure, as the glycoside will empower the heart by strengthening the pumping action. This is why herbs such as strophanthus, squill, convallaria, and especially *Digitalis purpurea*, or Foxglove, have earned their place in the medicine halls of fame. *Digitalis* is one of the few plants still used in modern drug making—its dried leaf contains digitoxin, digoxin, and ouabain, among other powerful cardioactive glycosides.

Many plants contain glycosides, including black mustard, wintergreen, and the laxatives senna, aloe, rhubarb, and cascara sagrada. Traditionally used fresh or dried (but in their natural state) by herbalists, these plants can also be compounded in laboratories as official formulary drugs.

Tannins

Typically, plants contain enzymes and proteins. Enzymes break proteins down into smaller particles, such as amino acids. Plants also contain tannins—astringent or antiseptic compounds that bring enzyme action to a screeching halt. Tannins restrict enzymes so they can't break down proteins. This is harmful for human digestion—think of black tea, for example, because the tannins in *Camellia sinensis* bind with living tissues to hamper proper digestion. (To avoid this, simply add milk to the tea, which negates the process.) When tannins are applied to living tissues, the action is called astringent because the tissues are "astringed" or tightened.

But tannins aren't all bad—they can be helpful to living tissues in the right circumstances. For instance, tannins can form a protective barrier under which new tissues can grow. Pharmacologist Varro Tyler gives the example of a burn patient: the exposed tissues of the burn contain proteins, and when tannins are introduced to these proteins, a protective (and antiseptic) coat is formed under which new tissue can regenerate. Tannins can also be used as an antidote to toxic alkaloids, because the tannin will bind with the alkaloid to form an insoluble substance (a tannate), rendering those poisons ineffective.

The binding action of tannins is also useful for activities involving non-living tissue, such as "tanning" deerskin. When tannins bind with proteins to form a coat, they create a pliable yet tough skin that is inherently preserved. Some scientists believe tannins are a waste product of the plant, because tannins are often found in the leaves of deciduous trees and, by falling off, will rid the plant of excess toxic tannins.

Pucker up! Here are some of the many plants used medicinally for their tannins:
- Witch Hazel (*Hamamelis virginiana*) leaf and twig. Astringent, hemostatic.

- Oak (*Quercus spp.*) leaf, twig, acorn. The nutgall from Asia Minor is the result of an insect depositing its larvae in a mass on the oak tree's leaves. The gall contains a great deal of tannin. Known to Greeks since 450 BCE, the nutgall is a chief source of tannic acid.
- New Jersey Tea/Red Root (*Ceanothus)* leaves, root. This was a tea substitute for Colonists during the Revolutionary War. Considered potent blood-coagulators.
- American Cranesbill *(Geranium maculatum)* leaf, root. Styptic, hemostatic, vulnerary. Contains gallic acid, similar to roses. These tiny roots are a traditional remedy for diarrhea and internal bleeding. They are taken internally (as a douche or tincture) or externally (as a poultice or compress).
- Rose (*Rosa spp.*) petals. Harvested (especially from southern France and Morocco) for their tannic and gallic acid content. "Gallic" is from *Rosa gallica*, meaning "of Gaul," or France.
- Raspberry (*Rubus ideaus*) and Blackberry (*R. villosus*) root.
- Hemlock tree (*Tsuga canadensis* and other spp.) bark.
- India Tree/Kino (*Pterocarpus marsupium*) astringent red juice from trunk of tree. Collectors make an incision in the trunk to collect the juice, which is dried in shallow pans in the sun. Once dried, the drug is shipped from Bombay; the preparation shipped from Madras is known as Malabar Kino.

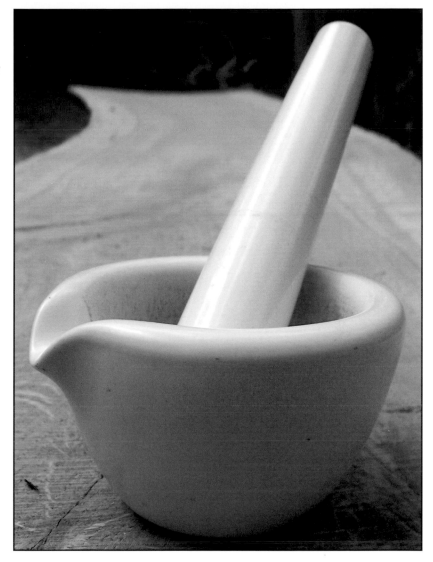

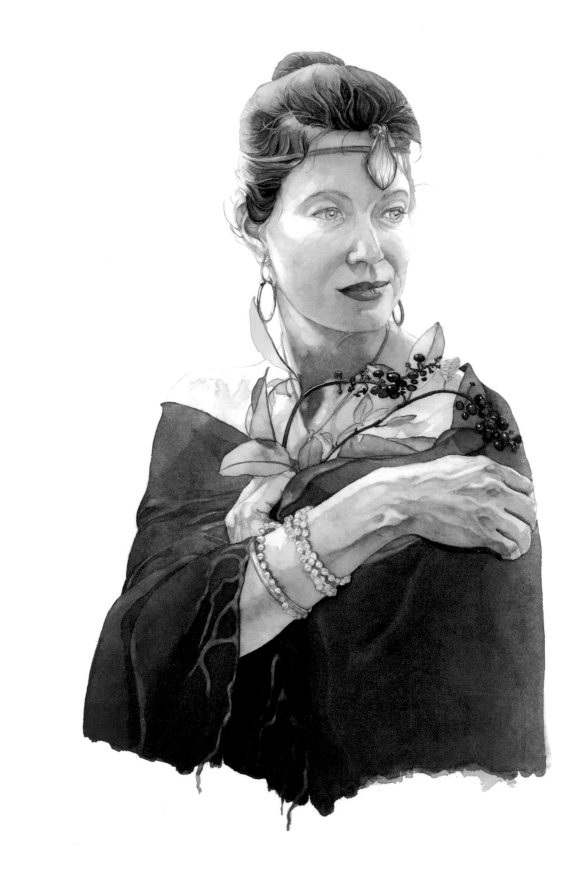

Locusta of Gaul

(? - 69 CE)

Though this book is generally a celebration of healers, I could not resist including the fascinating story of Locusta of Gaul, a first-century poisoner skilled in the chemistry and use of plants. We know of her frightening occupation today thanks to writings by Seutonius and Tacitus, historians who recorded the events roughly one hundred years after her death and, though she lived her life as a professional murderer—being paid to poison people—she nevertheless captures our attention for her guile and even her desperation.

Young and probably pretty, Locusta likely arrived alone and on foot to the loud city of Rome from Gaul, or southern France. Neither a girl nor an aged woman, she was a young woman anxious to keep her head on her shoulders in a time of bitter unrest between citizens and their governments.

Born in the first century CE and roughly a contemporary of Mary Prophetissa in Alexandria (see chapter 5), Locusta became a manufacturer of herbal and chemical poisons which she distributed (presumably for a substantial price) to the nobility of Rome. She is even said to have given consultations in poisoning and (at one point) offered training through a school specially set up for her by Emperor Nero.

Poisoning was a rich trade in first- and second-century Rome. It was not uncommon for family members to arrange to have loved ones "knocked off." Hadrian was rumored to have murdered his young wife Sabina; in 192 CE Marcia killed Commodus. So many people were downing poisoned wine or consuming toxic foods from their trusted friend's hands that historian Peter Macinnis says in his book *Poisons*,

> "By Ovid's time (he died in AD 17) everybody was hard at it, and the poet wrote of how men lived on plunder, much of it won by poisoning. Guest was not safe from host, he said, nor father-in-law from son-in-law. Even among brothers it was rare to find affection, while husbands longed for the deaths of their wives, who reciprocated, and murderous stepmothers brewed deadly concoctions, and 'sons inquired into their fathers' years before the time.'"

Locusta likely used a combination of plants, fungi, and minerals in her poisons, including strychnine, cyanide, arsenic, yew, mushrooms, and hemlock.

In this atmosphere of revenge and accelerated demands, Locusta's skill with poisonous plants was in great demand, and as news spread

---

POISON

Today, many a bartender asks, "What's your poison?" Historically, people have had liquid, semiliquid, and solid options.

The Proto-Indo-European *weis* meant "to melt or flow," especially for rotten fluids, from which Latin conjured *virus*, originally meaning the poison sap of plants, or a slimy liquid. In 1392, virus meant "venomous substance." Sanskrit's *visam* meant "poison, especially of a foul or malodorous fluid," and Latin used *viscum* to refer to any sticky substance.

The Yew Tree secreted a sap considered a venomous substance to be used on arrow-tips to kill deer or invaders. (Yew wood itself made longbows.) The Greeks used *toxikos*, "pertaining to arrows or archery," and Latin used *toxicus*, "poisoned." The Greeks created *toxon* (from Scythian) to refer to the bow itself. From this, Latin coined *taxus* to give the Yew tree its genus. (Arrowroot earned its name in 1697 because it absorbed toxin from poison-dart wounds.)

A less sticky and more liquid substance is drinkable, from Latin's *potare*, to drink. This gave *potionem*, and Old French's *puison* in the twelfth century meant "a drink." Later *puison* came to mean a potion or a poisonous drink.

Who were the poison bartenders of ancient yore? They were the pharmacists. Ancient Greeks termed anything that was a "drug, poison, philter, charm, or spell" a *pharmakon*, and those who prepared them were *pharmakeus*. Middle Latin used *pharmacia*, Old French *farmacie* and, by 1386, most drugs and poisons were considered medicines. The word *pharmacist* appeared in 1834.

---

of her ability (and willingness) to kill, Locusta became the queen of an odd and exceedingly dangerous profession. She grew famous for her ability to make a deliberate poisoning appear to be nothing more than a natural death—and perhaps scores of unsuspecting people met their demise at her skilled hands.

But even Locusta could not shake off justice. She was eventually discovered, accused, and sentenced to prison on poisoning charges, but her punishment was short. Agrippina, the last wife of sixty-four-year-old Emperor Claudius, summoned Locusta from prison to poison Claudius, to whom she had been married only five years. Locusta was successful: according to Pliny the Elder, the aged emperor famously died after consuming poisonous mushrooms in 54, and Agrippina's conniving seventeen-year-old son, Nero (and Claudius's son by adoption), gained the throne. Claudius's nearly fourteen-year-old son, Britannicus, was booted out of line, and Locusta was re-imprisoned.

But Nero showed no appreciation to his mother, Agrippina, and she grew frustrated with her lack of control over him; to her detriment, she began favoring Britannicus, which proved fatal for the boy. Jealous and ambitious, Nero secretly commanded Locusta to poison his step-brother whom he believed would steal his throne.

It was an awkward moment in history. A tribune named Julius Pollio escorted Locusta from the praetorian guard so she could prepare the poison for Nero. Historian Suetonius, Emperor Hadrian's secretary, records that she duly concocted a poison but it succeeded only in giving the boy abdominal cramps. Nero was so outraged that he imprisoned both Locusta and Julius Pollio. He ordered Locusta flogged but ultimately gave her a second chance, threatening execution if she failed.

Under dire circumstances, Locusta upped the strength of her poison and tested it on a baby goat (some sources say she tested it on a slave), but found it too weak. Again she strengthened the dose and tested it on a pig, which died instantly. Within hours, on February 12, year 55, Nero summoned his family, including Claudius's son, Britannicus, to a dinner party. The boy's wine was tasted and found satisfactory, but wines were served hot and he asked for it to be cooled. After cold water was poured into his cup to cool his wine, Britannicus began convulsing and fell to the floor. Frightened and concerned, Agrippina and Britannicus's mother (some say sister) Octavia moved to help him, but Nero kept them at a distance, claiming the boy suffered from epilepsy and demanding no one help him. The boy writhed in agony until Nero ordered him removed, and he died later that evening.

Nero soon pardoned Locusta and released her from prison. Because she enjoyed a growing reputation, continued her poisoning commissions, and is reported to have conducted a training school in Rome—receiving pupils sent by Nero himself—it is plausible that she and Nero became lovers, though there is no evidence. Nero is said to have granted Locusta lands and gifts and even hired her to poison his own mother Agrippina (which failed). The historians Tacitus and Suetonius record that Nero then arranged a shipwreck, intending to drown his mother, which also failed. Finally, the

APOTHECARY

Our ancient near-eastern and African ancestors used clay pitchers and pottery bowls to store perishable milk, oils, powders, and resins in their mud-floored cellars, far from the cooking area to avoid rancidity. Hard-won food, medicine, ritual resins, and incenses were among a community's most valuable goods, and with neither refrigeration nor locks, these items—and wine, precious metals, jewelry, and fabrics—had to be secured. Sanskrit used *apadha* ("concealment") and Greek combined *apo* (away) with *théké* (receptacle) to form *apothéké*, storehouse. Latin coined *apotheca*, storehouse, and Late Latin formed *apothecary*, storekeeper, to refer to the person responsible for maintaining supplies in the *apotheca*. He or she became the specialist who dispensed foods and medicine. By the seventeenth century, *apothecary* meant the person behind the counter; i.e., the druggist. In 1617, the idea of foods being separate from drugs cemented in the minds of the London elite, and the Apothecaries' Company of London separated from the Grocers Guild.

Moreover, *apotheosis*, meaning "to elevate a person as to the status of a god," reflects the high status of doctors and surgeons. It derives phonetically and historically from the same prefix and it's possible *apotheosis* and *apothecary* evolved concurrently since the safekeeping of a community's most valuable possessions was worthy of the highest title. Consider also that Ancient Persia's word for the High King's palace was the similar *apadana*.

In 1848, the Spanish word *bodega* arose, meaning wine shop, from the Greek *apotheke*. Many ancient medicines were dissolved in wine, as wine was plentiful, stable and strong. Bodega gave way, in 1953, to the Old Provincial words *botica* and *boutique*. Thus, the ancient apothecary's art of safekeeping foods, medicines, cosmetics, ritual ingredients, and beverages split into at least three types of shop: the apothecary for medicine, the bodega for wines, and the boutique for cosmetics.[1]

emperor ordered her execution but publicly disguised it as a suicide. Agrippina died in 59.

In 68, the Roman Senate captured Nero and, rather than face execution or imprisonment, he committed suicide. The new Emperor Galba quickly imprisoned Locusta and publicly executed her in January 69. But the swift sequence of death continued: Galba himself was murdered within the week.

ROME, ITALY

Rome has proudly claimed its share of notable residents, from Julius Caesar to the poet Virgil to the artist Raphael. That list can also include the famous physician Galen, but well before Galen was born in 129 CE, Rome was home to the notorious poisoner Locusta and to the Greek surgeon and writer Pedanius Dioscorides (circa 40–90 CE). Originally from Greece (*see* chapter 4), Dioscorides was a surgeon in Nero's Roman army, and since he and Nero's poisoner, Locusta, were contemporaries, it is possible they met. It is unknown, of course, but since she was employed by Nero as a poisoner and Dioscorides as a healer, it is plausible that they interacted in some capacity: did the two herbal experts share information about the dangers of Rome's plants? It is fascinating to think that Nero's favorite Locusta might have studied with Dioscorides or even contributed to his wildly popular herbal classic *De Materia Medica* before her death in 69 CE. It seems reasonable that, since Locusta "became one of the first to systematically investigate the use of poisons with state sponsorship,"[1] she may have been a resource for Dioscorides and his understanding of plant toxicology, including belladonna, aconite, hemlock, yew, and opium.

Over the centuries, Roman gardens developed not only as a source of food and herbal medicine but as popular ways to worship, relax, and advertise a family's status. Watered with cisterns, Roman gardens were useful for the production of medicines, cordials, perfumes, garlands, and of course food,[2] but they were also an important social marker: poorer residents had small gardens and monasteries and publicly owned entities had open gardens that likely grew rue, pepper, grapevine, cucumbers, mushrooms, figs, roses, violets, rosemary, acanthus, hart's-tongue fern, ivy, smilax, and parsley,[3] among others. Wealthy residents maintained expansive private gardens that were separated into distinct regions: tree-lined promenades, covered and tiled walkways, and flower-filled gardens where the owner and his or her guests could stroll, gossip, and conduct business.

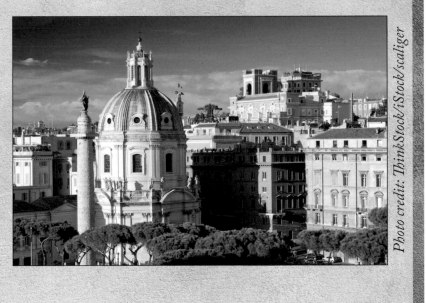

Photo credit: ThinkStock/iStock/scaliger

YEW
Taxus baccata

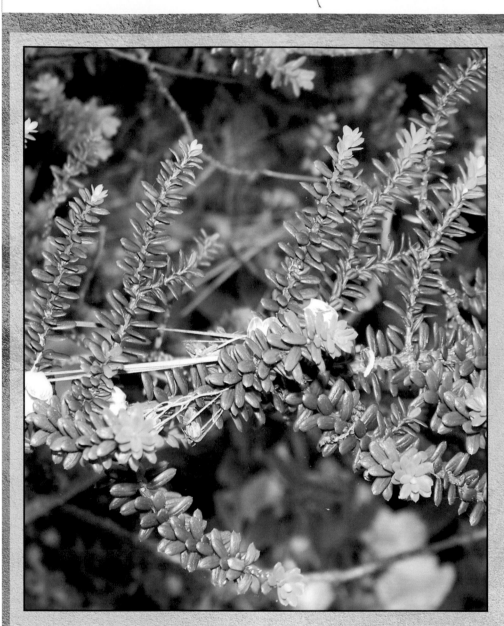

Living monuments that can survive more than 1,000 years, the great yew grows 40 to 50 feet high with reddish brown peeling bark on a wide trunk that grays as it ages. Several individual trees are believed to be more than 1,500 years old.

To the ancient Breton, the yew was sacred, as was holly and alder, and druids built temples and performed ceremonies in yew groves. Many ancient religions believed gods to be born from trees (consider the Egyptian myth of Osiris and Horus). Old Norse myths from the Eddaic literature suggest that the great Norse god Odin was born from a yew. Other literature says he was born of a woman named Bestla, a word Skaldic scholars believe derived from *bast*, meaning "yew." Odin legendarily sacrificed himself on the Yggdrasil tree to attain eternal and infinite knowledge; though the tree may be the ash, it's phonetically possible the tree was the yew. The fifth vowel in the Celtic Ogham tree alphabet is *idho*, with the Old English version originally spelled *iw* or *iow*.

The hard, impervious wood was used for personal protection, breastplates, and military longbows. Yews were felled by King Henry IV's royal decree beginning in 1350 to supply the English military and, by the 1600s, yews were virtually eliminated from England and Scotland.

In folklore, the yew oversees the separation of spirit from body, and in Breton legend, the tree sent roots into the open mouths of the corpses below to provide the soul a way out. The ancient Celts believed the soul of a person would be captured in trees. Certain of these trees were set apart for worship, although Sir James Frazer says this worship began as a way to honor (out of fear) one's dead relatives, not necessarily because of the sanctity of the tree itself. In Classical Greece and Rome, yew was sacred to the moon goddess of death, Hecate, and Shakespeare incorporated the magic of yew into *Hamlet* and *MacBeth*, where three of Hecate's witches brew yew to foretell the future.

Botanically, all parts of the tree are extremely toxic; its seeds and leaves secrete taxine, a dangerously strong cardiac depressant, and many cattle and horses die after grazing on yew clippings.

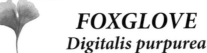

FOXGLOVE
Digitalis purpurea

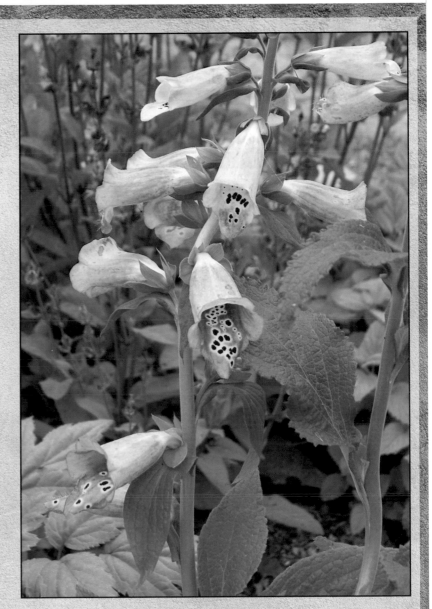

Originally called Folks' Glove, the flowers' spots were imagined by ancient Brits to be fairy footprints. The name morphed into *foxes glofa* (glove of the fox), and in Germany it was called Fingerhut for its resemblance to a thimble. German botanist/Lutheran minister Hieronymus Bock classified the plant as *Digitalis* (from Latin *digitus*, "finger") in 1539.

Culpeper referred to foxglove's "gentle cleansing nature" under the dominion of Venus, saying foxglove poultice was "familiarly and frequently used by the Italians to heal any fresh or green wound." He advised making a decoction with honey to cleanse and purge the body "both upwards and downwards, sometimes of tough phlegm and clammy humours, and to open obstructions of the liver and spleen."

Did Locusta experience clammy humours? We don't know, but it's likely she appreciated Culpeper's word *purge*. Purging—or vomiting—is the most visible indicator that something is happening inside the body. From ancient Galen to nineteenth century Samuel Thompson, a plant that could make one vomit, salivate, cry, defecate, urinate, bleed, or ooze out the blameful sickness was heroic. Locusta knew that if heroic herbs were used to excess, the patient would expire. She likely used poisonous mushrooms and foxglove leaves (also called Dead Man's Gloves or Witches' Gloves) in stews, porridges, and beverages for her clients' enemies.

Today, thanks to the village women of Shropshire, England, who shared their recipes with William Withering, physicians use foxglove to treat dropsy, epilepsy, and seizure disorders. Certain doses of *Digitalis* demonstrate a regulating effect on the pulse, but determining the quantity of drug in an ounce of dried foxglove is difficult, so amateur herbalists avoid the plant. *Digitalis purpurea* extract contains cardiac glycosides that increase cardiac contractility and control heart rate. It is prescribed for patients in atrial fibrillation and heart failure. Foxglove poisoning can produce bradycardia (lowered heart rate) or tachycardia (increased heart rate), extreme nausea, vomiting, and diarrhea. Non-fatal doses produce headache, delirium, hallucinations, xanthopsia (jaundiced or yellow vision), and reduced appetite leading to anorexia.

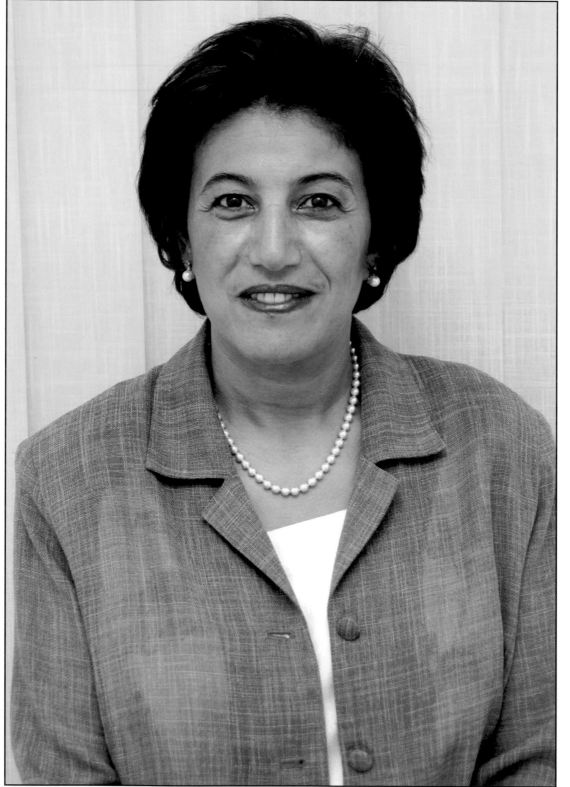

Photo credit: Zoubida Charrouf

Dr. Zoubida Charrouf

A chance drive past a group of women selling oil on the side of the road changed Dr. Zoubida Charrouf's life forever—and in the process saved a threatened tree and liberated thousands of women with financial independence. She didn't expect it. A woman with bright eyes and a smart, contemporary style, Zoubida had no idea her daily commute to University to study for her PhD would result in one of the world's most successful and celebrated women's business cooperatives—and that it would involve, of all things, argan oil.

Born in 1952 and raised in western Morocco in coastal Sfaafa, near Rabat, Zoubida grew up loving and appreciating plants. Her mother instilled in her a deep appreciation for medicinal plants and their many family uses and, as a young woman, Zoubida decided to pursue doctoral chemistry; for her dissertation, she surveyed people in her community to understand the many traditional virtues of medicinal plants and to obtain firsthand reports by Moroccan men and women who used native plants daily.

After an eye-opening journey to Lille, France, to study chemistry, Zoubida returned to Morocco in 1977 ready to devote her life to medicinal plants. She began using a variety of plants, and among her favorites are rosemary, the artemsias, *Nigella* (black cumin seed), chamomile, and—especially— the little-known oil from her country's own native desert tree, the argan. This scrubby, thorny tree so captured her imagination that, by 1985, Zoubida had completed her doctorate on it and, though she didn't realize it, she was on her way to becoming the country's chief expert.

> *"When I was young, my mother was treating us with plants. I read a lot about caring for plants and Morocco is very rich in medicinal plants."*

The Women's Cooperative

While researching the argan tree and commuting to her university classes, Dr. Charrouf noticed some of the women who had participated in her survey: they were standing hundreds of yards apart on the roadside selling oil pressed from the argan nut, and they were anything but professional. They suffered individually with no guidance, no standards, no collaboration with each other,

COOPERATE

Latin speakers used *opus* to refer to work, or *opera* to refer to effort toward work. Today, opus generally refers to a musical composition, as does opera. But the sense of work and labor is not lost: *operation* was first recorded in 1368 to signify work performance, and *operate* appeared in 1606 from Latin's *operari*, meaning "to have an effect," "to be active or cause something to happen" (Harper, 2008). Today, to *co-operate* means "to work together."

and they used low-quality practices such as packaging the oil in reused glass bottles. Dr. Charrouf also noted they took home very little money, and she realized that, since argan oil was valuable, they could increase their income if they had some business help.

Thus the brainchild cooperative was born: Dr. Charrouf approached the women with the offer to establish a cooperative in which the women would unite in their work, and within the year, in 1996, the first women's argan oil cooperative was formed. It proved highly successful and since then Dr. Charrouf has founded two more women's regional cooperatives, providing employment for the country's women and at the same time gaining utility from—and protecting—a threatened native tree. In 2003, she formed Targanine, a nongovernmental organization dedicated to bringing to fruition the work of the cooperatives and introducing argan oil products to the international market.

Assisted by the International Development Research Centre, Zoubida Charrouf helped free Moroccan women from their expected domestic restraints and was instrumental in helping them gain financial freedom. Her goals for the cooperatives were to produce argan oil, to preserve the tree in the Moroccan forests and deserts, and to be a catalyst for native women to realize their full potential. Her surprising career in Muslim Morocco has liberated and educated hundreds of women and simultaneously secured protection for one of the country's most valuable trees. She is widely credited with saving the Argan tree from eradication and in the process slowing the desertification that threatens Morocco's southwestern communities.

In addition, she has advanced the technical process of extracting argan oil from the nut. Traditionally, women had pressed the nuts between rocks or by hand, a painfully inadequate and time-consuming method; Zoubida and her husband developed new machinery to make the oil extraction easier. The new technology made the women's cooperatives much more efficient: one of her cooperatives produces certified organic edible argan oil meeting international health standards and enjoys $100,000 worth of business per year. But she doesn't stop with economics: Dr. Charrouf's cooperatives train women in business as well as literacy, marketing, and quality control—subjects never previously taught to women expected to work strictly in the house. "Benefiting our local communities by initiating these research cooperatives in argan oil has been the most beautiful part of my career," she says. In 2001, she was awarded the International Slow Food Award for Biodiversity.

She credits early discussions with pharmacist and doctor Jamal Bellakhdar for her desire to pursue the study of medicinal plants, and "many of Dr. Bellakhdar's books are my bedside books," she says, listing titles including *Maghreb, Artisans de la Terre,* and *La Pharmacopee Marocaine Traditionnelle.*

Not everything has been easy for this strong Moroccan woman. Gaining the support of her colleagues has been a challenge for her. "The most difficult part of my work with plants," she says, "is finding partners to carry out pharmacological tests." But she's not stopping: she has future plans to research leaf and wood pulp products to benefit Morocco's citizens, particularly its women.

MOROCCO

Renowned for its brilliant roses, lush annual rose festivals, rose water, and floral extracts, Morocco is a jewel on the northwest coast of the African continent, just south of Spain and the Strait of Gibraltar. To the east lie Algeria and Mauritania; to the southwest the sub-Saharan desert stretches to the Atlantic Ocean.

Moroccan architecture delights the senses with elaborate geometrical designs, archways, curves, and domes. Its structures are embellished with colorful tiles, patios, courtyards with fountains, and intricately carved stone recesses, reflecting the brown Sahara sands and the mounds of fragrant spices sold in *souks,* the specialty markets of Marrakech. Vendors hang fresh and dried botanicals in great strands and ribbons from the *souk* ceilings or lay them in stacks on long tables; spices may be displayed in the forms of solid cones or they may be stored in tall, cylindrical white or yellow woven baskets—all ready for sale to flavor the evening's *diner* (French is the country's unofficial second language). Sunni towns often contain a communal baking oven, a *hammam* (a steam bath for personal ablution rituals before prayer), a Koranic school, and a grocery. In the intimate setting of the neighborhood *hawma,* families can purchase vegetables, fruit, sugar, and spices; oil and coal can be purchased for home heating and cooking.

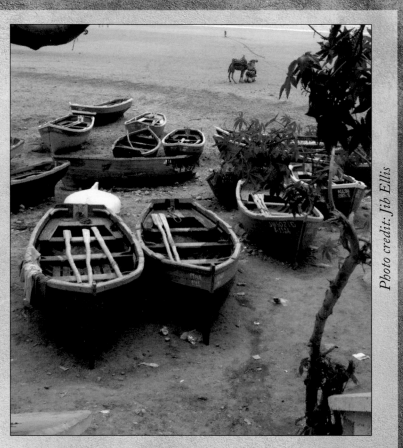

Photo credit: Jib Ellis

Morocco, Tahagazout Beach

Berber (Amazigh) women, especially those of the Atlas mountains, apply henna to their hands and feet and clothe themselves in brightly colored veils when they reach adulthood. Cosmopolitan women, such as those in Casablanca, Marrakech, Tangier, or in the capital, Rabat, may wear more western clothing, but because this is a Muslim country, strict dress codes are culturally and even legally enforced.

Women generally maintain the home life, often collecting water for their families. In 1957, personal status statutes prevented women from claiming their rights as adults, no matter their age. In 1972, the country's constitution granted women the right to vote and to be elected and, in 1994, seventy-seven women were elected to the Chamber of Representatives. In 2004, after King Mohammed VI succeeded his deceased father King Hassan II, women gained more rights: to seek divorce; to demand half her spouse's wealth upon divorce; to collect child support; the right to be alerted if her husband wishes to take a second or third wife (and the right to try to veto this attempt); and the right for women over eighteen to marry without parental consent. Many citizens seek greater reforms, more precise wording, and better training for the country's judicial and democratic systems.

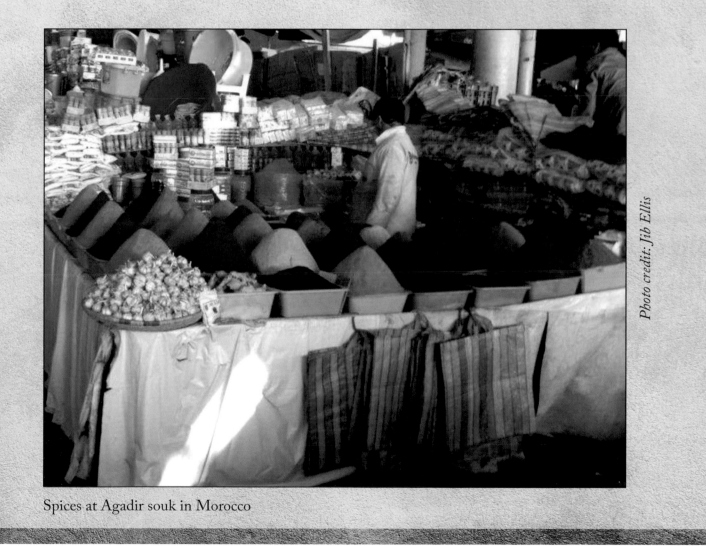

Photo credit: Jib Ellis

Spices at Agadir souk in Morocco

ARGAN TREE
Argania spinosa

The tree beloved by Dr. Zoubida Charrouf—and the mainstay of her women's cooperative's financial income—is the argan. A scraggly tree with a weather-beaten appearance, the thorny argan shelters many a hungry goat who love to climb the tree and eat its fruits. But argan collectors dislike sharing their precious crop with the goats since, in the past two decades, argan oil has become the world's most expensive oil at about $300 per liter.[1] Now overharvested by abundant goats, the argan tree is endangered and is protected by the United Nations Educational, Scientific, and Cultural Organization (UNESCO). Moroccan Berber families use the tree much as Italians use the olive: as food, fodder, timber, and fuel.

HYSSOP
Hyssopus officinalis

An ancient herb, vegetable, spice, flavoring, and medicine, hyssop (Hebrew: *ezov*) was hailed in the Old Testament of the Bible for cleansing and purification and as a purgative, though the word *hyssop* may have referred to caper, oregano, or herbs other than *Origanum syriacum*. Throughout ancient Greece and Europe, hyssop was a favorite anise-flavored expectorant from which syrups were made for cough, congestion, flatulence, pain, and inflammation. Pastes of the aromatic leaves can be made for fresh wounds and a tea of the leaves is fragrant and calming. The minty leaves give a fresh zing to salads and to Chartreuse liqueur.

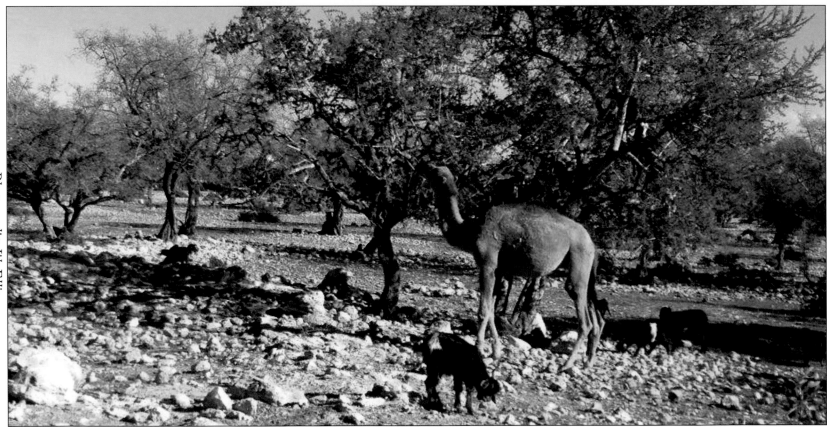

Camels and goats enjoy the argan trees

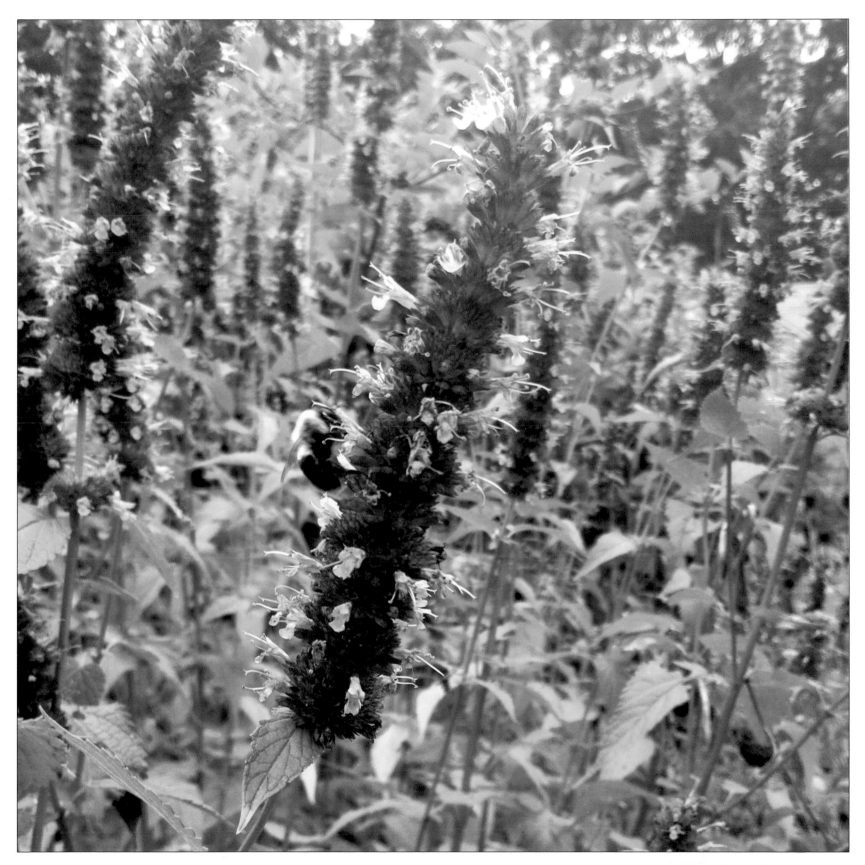

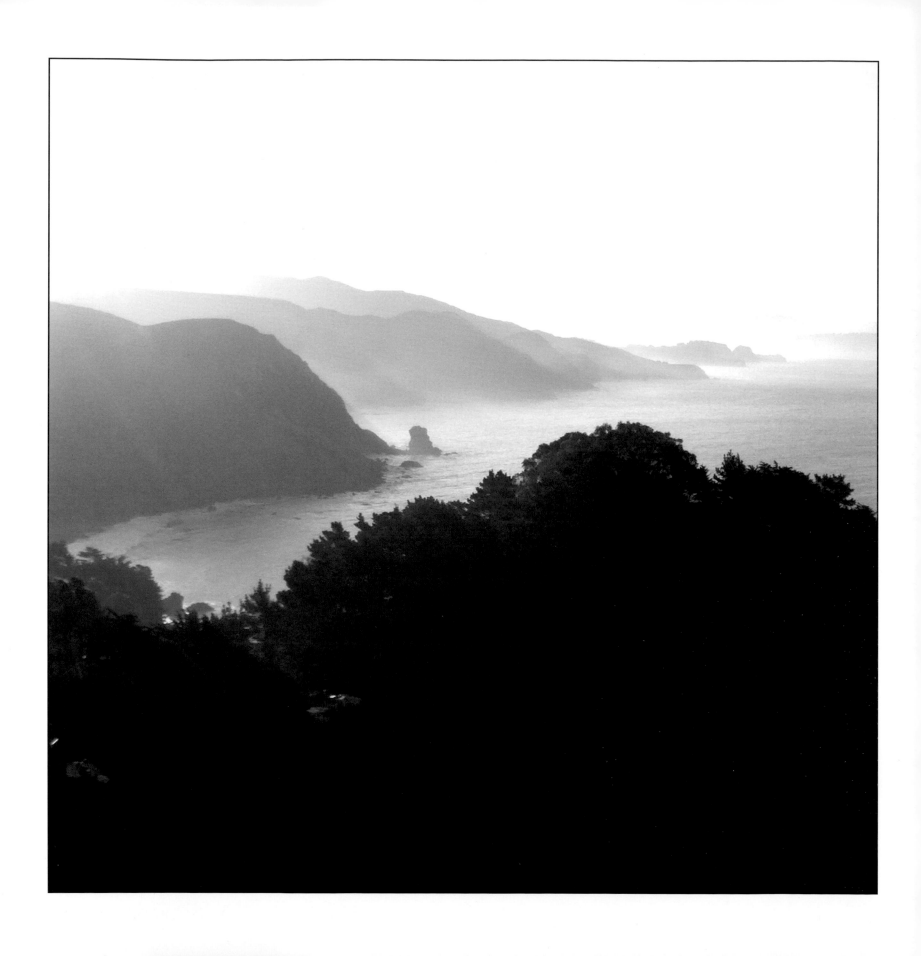

PART III:
SPIRIT TRADITIONS

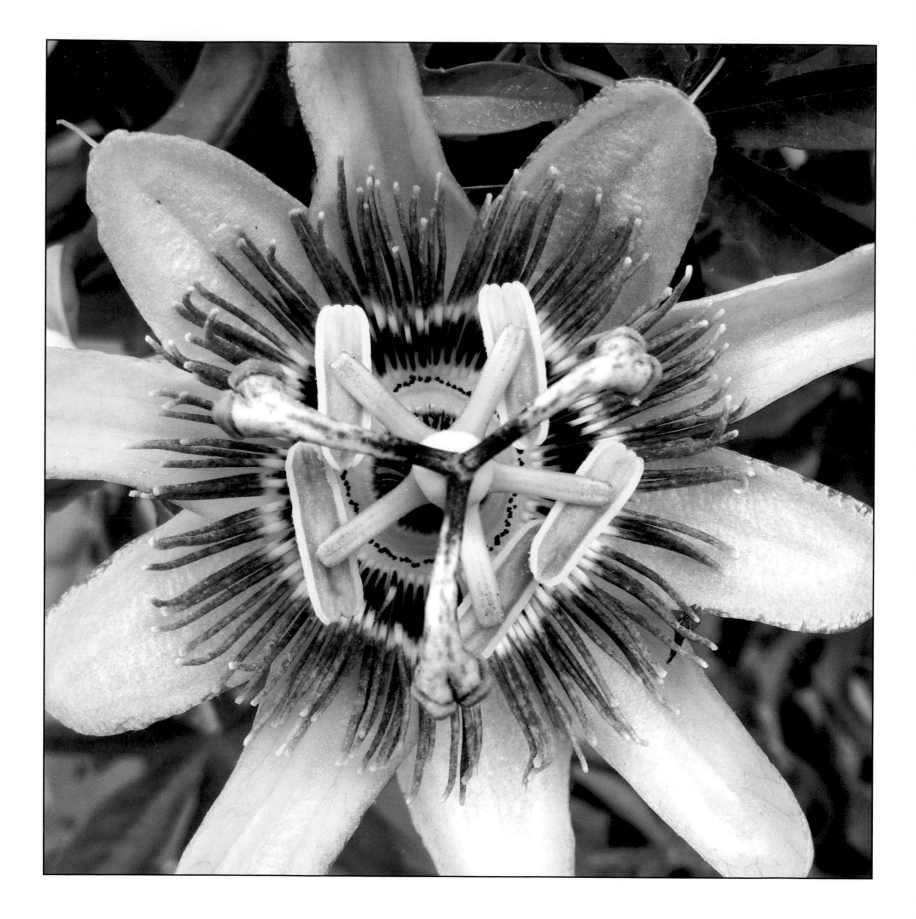

Chapter 11
FLOWER ESSENCE THERAPY

Flower Essences

Throughout history, flowers have been used for medicinal purposes: rituals, healings, prayers, blessings, benedictions, art therapy, and as pure ingested medicine. In 1930, English bacteriologist and pathologist Edward Bach conducted research into pure medicines from natural substances—from the essence, or spirit, of nature. He developed a system of liquid remedies based on emotional imbalances and their medical effects in people. His gentle system established itself quickly as an alternative to invasive and impersonal conventional medical practices and drugs.

Today, a flower essence is a liquid preparation of the "energy" of the plant—often the whole plant, not necessarily the flowers. The preparer often conducts a type of ritual in harvesting this energy, using glass or crystal bowls, pure spring water, and sunlight or moonlight. Generally, these essences soak throughout the day or overnight, imbibing the energy of the plant. Similarly, alchemists in the first and second centuries AD would collect the water caught on a plant's leaves, especially with plants considered magical such as ladies mantle, *Alchemilla vulgaris*. The morning dew that collected in the curved shape of the leaves was drunk as a healing tonic or applied to the skin or the eyes in the belief that the dew (already a magical substance) had absorbed some of the healing powers through its contact with the leaf. Modern flower essence collectors either lower flower stalks into the water for that same immersion or they place the bowl of water in direct proximity of the plant without physical contact.

Direct contact is not necessary, as this is an energetic medicine. Kate Gilday, flower essence therapist and director of Woodland Essence in New York State, calls these therapies "a vibrational healing modality that holds the essential nature of flowers in a liquid form."

Due to their inherent energetic nature, flower essences serve to balance our emotional and spiritual states rather than our physical bodies. Sometimes, a plant works with dual capacities, providing chemical medicine for an illness and also a flower essence for the emotional pains that accompany that illness. For example, Gilday noted at the 2007 International Herb Symposium that *Echinacea* flower essence is used for maintaining an integrated sense of self, especially when one is severely challenged; Echinacea is widely used in herbal medicine to address infection and immunity. Additionally, American Ginseng is used in herbal medicine for vitality, strength, and support when experiencing depletion, and its flower essence provides similar effects for the emotions.

Bach pioneered his work with English flowers, while others, such as Flower Essence Services of California, followed his lead to create essences from North American flowers. Clare G. Harvey, author of *The New Encyclopedia of Flower Essences*, uses orchids, water lilies, and other Thai and tropical flowers. Hibiscus calms the nervous system, helping a person relax mentally and physically. Kate Gilday's Woodland Essence creates essences from native plants of the Adirondacks, using red cedar to promote courage, mountain laurel for guidance during times of confusion, and sassafras for learning self-love. Ian White, the grandson of herbalist Inez White, profiled in this chapter, offers hard-to-find and little known flowers from the outback, such as Monga Waratah and Sydney Rose, through his signature company Australian Bush Flower Essences.

Part of the allure of flower essences is that they are gentle and safe enough to be used by children and sensitive adults; they are also "people's medicine" and can be made by anyone with minimal equipment and ingredients. Flower essence therapies are notably positive, encouraging, and specific to supporting a strong sense of self, which is central to all forms of healing.

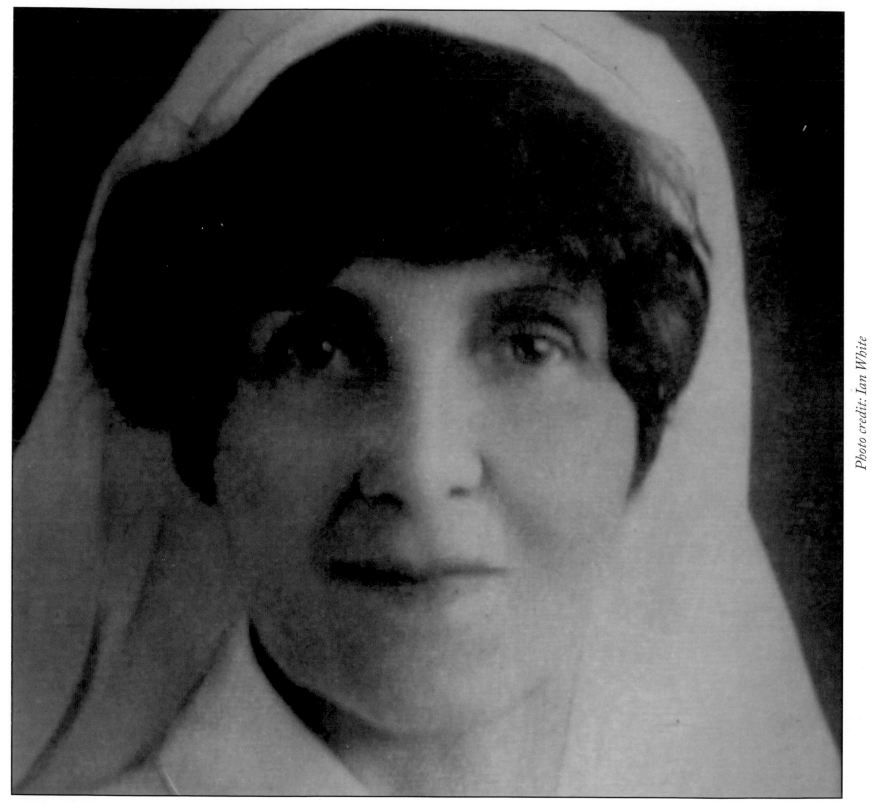

Photo credit: Ian White

Tulsi Le Brun

Inez White

(1896–1966)

In the 1850s, Australia experienced a gold rush similar to the California rush of 1848, and single men flocked to the "outback" seeking—and finding—sudden and startling wealth. News of this gold rush caught the attention of a young woman herbalist in England who left her homeland on an adventure to find her share of Australia's gold. Her dreams went unrealized, however, and she eventually left the demanding work in Australia to explore the mysterious healing plants of New Zealand. Here she gave birth to a daughter she named Tulsi Le Brun. The call of Australia was strong in young Tulsi's blood and, when she became a teenager, she convinced her mother to return to Australia with her. Together the adventurous women moved back to Australia and, at Tulsi's urging, they established an herbal practice and a home clinic.

Years later, in 1896, Tulsi gave birth to her own daughter, Inez; just like her mother and grandmother before her, Inez showed an early and powerful desire to learn botany and healing. Together Inez and Tulsi became among the first non-Maori people to seriously study the medicinal properties of Australia's wild plants.

In a family story told to me by Inez's grandson, sixth-generation herbalist Ian White, there was an external influence in Tulsi's and Inez's pursuit of botany: an English doctor, the illegitimate son of a British prince, was sent to the colonies with a large stipend so as not to embarrass his royal family. He met Tulsi and Inez and worked with them from a very strong British herbal tradition as well as with allopathic medicine. His work profoundly influenced (and probably empowered) both women, who determined to conduct extensive research on Australia's native plants extending two hundred kilometers north and south of Sydney. By now, the gold rush was more than sixty years in the past and Australia was blossoming into a vibrant and artistic country. Young Inez practiced medical botany in Sydney operating a clinic that specialized in treating children, and she ran a general herbal clinic.

Her grandson Ian, a flower essence practitioner and herbalist who wildcrafts plants in the bush, affectionately recalls spending time with Inez in the wilderness. Until he was ten years old, he lived next to her and near the wild national parks that bordered his family's property. As a young boy, Ian would pretend to be sick to avoid school, so his working parents would take him to his grandmother's house. "I would, of course, make spectacular recoveries as soon as my parents left for work," he told me, "and my grandmother loved it. I would help her make extracts and tinctures and go for walks in the bush with her as she pointed out plants." Ian recalls that Inez was very excited one day to discover a Sydney Rose, which she had believed to be extinct.

At Inez's elbow, Ian discovered the amazing diversity of healing bush plants of east Australia. She taught him about *Telopea mongalensis*, which is valued in indigenous Australian medicine as the highest healing plant and called *Monga Waratah* (meaning "beautiful") by the Eora Aboriginal people, the indigenous people of the Sydney area. Ian was also gifted with the knowledge of Old Man Banksia, *Banksia serrata*, a striking plant with a strong action on the thyroid. This plant was named by Carolus Linnaeus the Younger, son of botanist Linnaeus, to honor Sir Joseph Banks who had accompanied Captain James Cook on his first expedition to Australia.

Just as her grandmother and her mother Tulsi had taught her, Inez taught her grandson about the Daggar Hakea (*Hakea teretifolia*) with its sweet cinnamon scent that would perfume the air in summer's hot weather, as well as the Grass Tree (*Xanthorrhoea*) with its huge spear, commonly called Blackboy.

"Inez was a leading herbalist in Sydney," Ian says of his grandmother, but her career was not easily accepted by her husband, who was a product of his post-colonial society. "My

PIONEER

A pioneer is the first to attempt or succeed at something new. The word takes its roots from Latin's *pes* and *pedo*, relating to the foot, later *peon* and Old French's *paonier* "foot soldier" in the eleventh century. Middle French smoothed this to *pionnier*, and Douglas Harper records that in 1523 this meant a "foot soldier who prepares the way for the army."

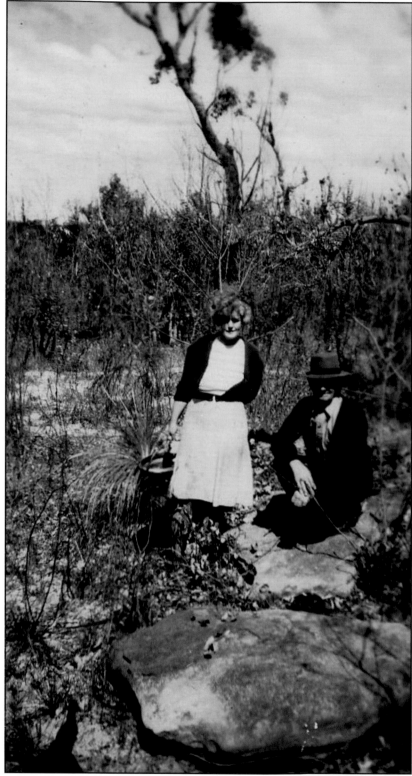

Inez White in the Australian outback

grandfather had his own career in the clothing manufacturing industry, and he was embarrassed of my grandmother's work when she spoke of it at dinner parties. A lot of women didn't work then, and he thought it was belittling of him that his wife had her own career. My grandmother was a strong woman," Ian says, "and she always persisted in that. But it was a challenge at the time." Neither was Inez content to sit primly in the stylish lifestyle typical of Europe's society women: instead, she could often be found trudging through the rugged outback searching for plants with a shovel in hand.

*"One of the tragedies is when the family tradition
has passed on."—Ian White*

Inez White researched the native plants of Australia all her life, even when her body became riddled with cancer. She kept this information secret from her family and managed to keep the illness at bay for ten years after Ian was born. She treated herself, somewhat successfully, with *Phytolacca* and sorrel, both non-native plants, as well as native plants, but an unfortunate turn of events on a trip to Europe proved to be too much. As she was traveling, Inez was separated from her luggage, which contained her valuable herbs, and by the time her husband was able to send new herbal supplies to her, the stress of traveling and the cancer took its toll on her body. Inez went into a coma and was flown back to Sydney where she died in 1966 at age seventy.

Very little was written down of her herbal research, her clinical practice, or the work of her mother Tulsi Le Brun, and virtually nothing survives about Tulsi's mother, the intrepid explorer who heeded the call to Australia's gold rush. The loss of Inez's research left an indelible mark on her grandson, who encourages herbalists to record their work. "Read as much as you can about the early texts," Ian advises. "In Australia, there is not a long written tradition of working with plants. There was the oral tradition of the Aborigines, but many of these people died of small pox and influenza when white settlers arrived 220 years ago," leaving colonists with scant information about Australia's botanical treasures. Sadly, little survives of Inez's pioneering work with native Australian plants or her work with children. "That's another time knowledge was lost," he says. "I'm very curious about how they did their experimentation and work, about how they worked with aborigines. One of the great tragedies is when the family tradition has passed on."

Incz and her mother, Tulsi, were pioneers in the field of Australian native plant research and children's healing when there were few herbalists, fewer women herbalists, and little appreciation for recording knowledge for future use. Ian White honors his grandmother's and great-grandmother's heritage by operating Australian Bush Flower Essences, supplying many of his sixty-four flower remedies from the blossoms originally shown to him by his grandmother Inez.

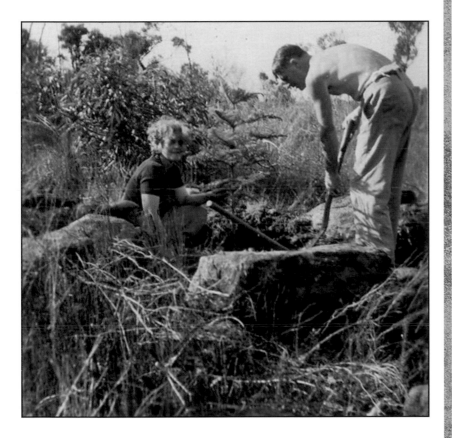

OLD MAN BANKSIA
Banksia serrata

Some people may not consider the gnarled, misshapen Saw Banksia tree to be lovely, though its large, creamy-colored flower spikes are certainly impressive. The tree, often called Old Man Banksia, can grow fifteen meters tall in the windswept arid lands of Australia, and the flowers provide an important food source for bees and small mammals.

Its bark is fire retardant, allowing it to survive the many bushfires of the open outback; it oozes a red sap when injured and, in many Banksia species, the fruits require burning to open. The large seed pods inspired local nineteenth-century folklore and stories, including the popular children's tales *Snugglepot and Cuddlepie* by May Gibbs.

Sixty of the seventy-six species of Banksia occur in Australia, and many Australian artists carve Banksia wood. The indigenous peoples of southwestern Australia sucked the nectar from the flowers and made sweet drinks from the flower cones, and they had used the tree for ages before the son of Linneaus named the plant after Sir Joseph Banks, who accompanied Captain Cook to Australia.

It may be the cheery gold of the flower or the persistence with which the tree survives fires that give it use as a modern flower essence remedy for renewing enthusiasm and promoting interest and enjoyment in life.

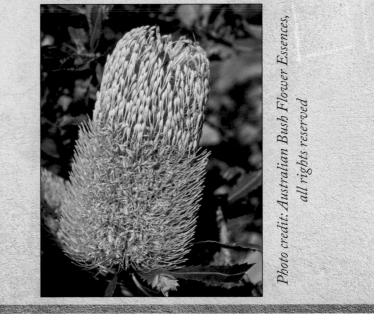

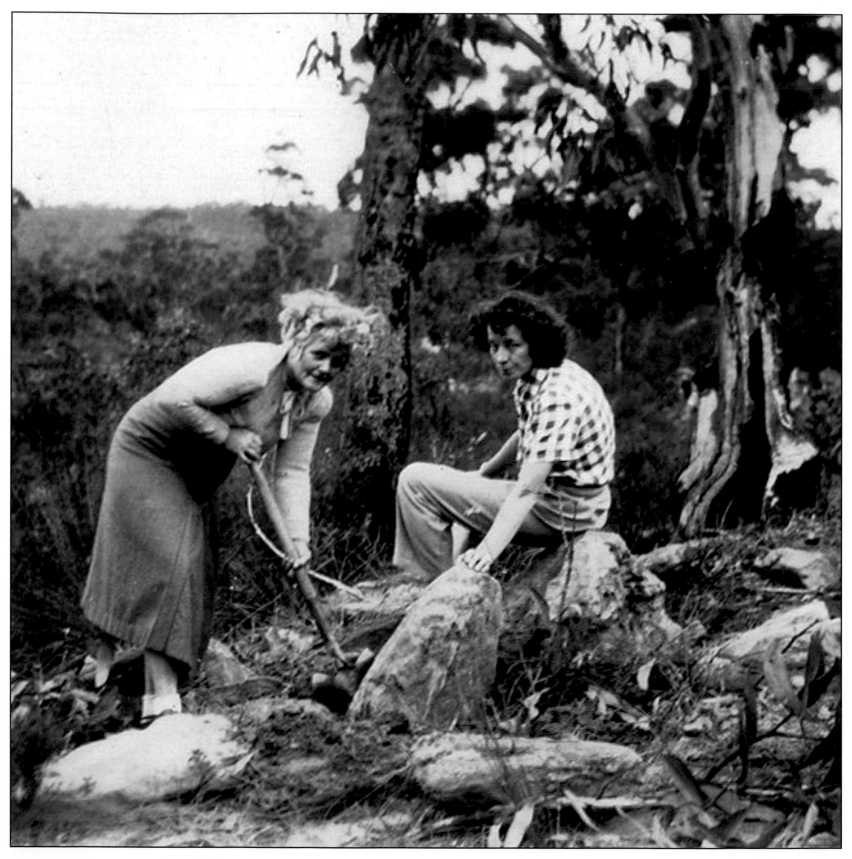

In about 1606, European sailors first discovered an unknown southern land, and they called it *terra australis incognita* and were immediately enchanted with it. Over the next 170 years, fifty-four more ships voyaged from Europe and the Dutch East India Company to explore this land now named New Holland.

In 1770, the ambitious Captain James Cook claimed the entire east coast for England's King George III, rechristening the area New South Wales. He and Carolus Linnaeus the Younger documented the wealth of plants they found to such an extent that Cook nicknamed their ship's harbor Botany Bay.

Life was slow and colonial, with frustrations between the Eora natives and the colonists. But in 1851, gold was discovered, changing the socioeconomic structure of the fledgling country forever. Gold fever (like it did three years earlier in California) attracted prospectors and, in 1852, a whopping 370,000 immigrants arrived in Australia, tripling the population by 1871 and introducing the nation's first railroad and telegraph service.

Today Australia is popular for commerce, education, and recreation. World-class Sydney, the "Gateway to Australia," is famous for opera, symphony, and theater—and alternative healing. The

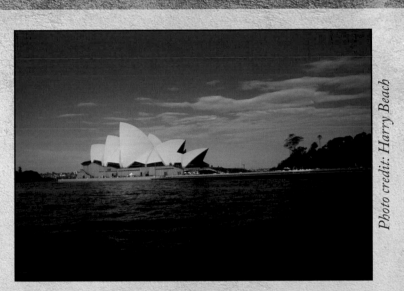

Photo credit: Harry Beach

Syndey Opera House, Australia

Australian Traditional-Medicine Society boasts nearly twelve thousand members, including massage therapists, herbalists, acupuncturists, homeopaths, naturopaths, and nutritionists.

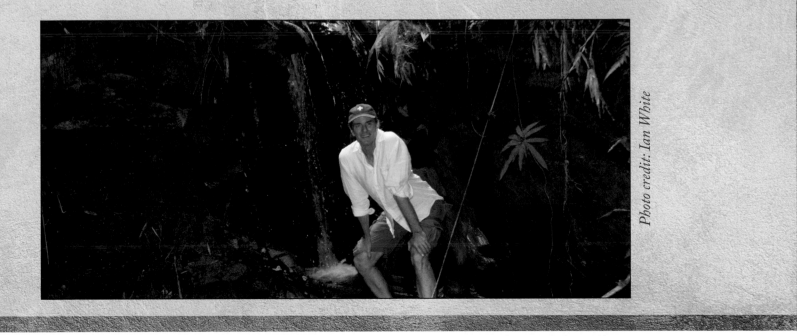

Photo credit: Ian White

Kate Gilday

You'll either find Kate Gilday in the Adirondack woods harvesting the medicinal mushroom chaga or at the podium of a women's conference leading songs and chants. Kate, who is renowned as a flower essence therapist and gentle intuitive healer, approaches the collection of botanical medicines the same way as the sharing of songs: with compassion, kindness, and a deep, flowing rhythm.

Kate trained as a nurse, attending evening courses at Boston College's nursing school and at Boston City Hospital in 1979, but she never finished her degree because her two young daughters were frequently diagnosed with ear infections. When their pediatricians continuously prescribed antibiotics for them, Kate grew alarmed. Determined to learn about natural healing, she visited bookstores but found little available until she discovered *Back to Eden* by Jethro Kloss. The only herb book on the shelf, its approach opened a new world for her and she began treating her children's common ailments—their colds, tummy aches, pinworms, and lice—with herbal teas and syrups. She was amazed to find these methods worked.

As the oldest of ten children, Kate and her siblings never went to doctors, which was fortunate, she realized, because she didn't have to revolutionize her healing mentality when she sought out more earth-friendly therapies. "My introduction to herbal healing was organic, slow and steady," Kate recalls, a process that mirrors her calm and steady personality. She opened The Herb Field near Boston to sell salves and oils and she lived for seven years in a little cottage with no electricity or running water; it was here she planted the herbs that would remain her healing standbys: echinacea, calendula, comfrey, mullein, plantain, and hawthorn.

"I am especially fond of the indigenous plants, the plants that were here even before we Europeans arrived on the scene. Of course, most of these are the at-risk forest plants now." Kate's husband, Don, is a knowledgeable woodsman who introduced her to the trees. "I was familiar with the forest plants," she says, "but I didn't *know* them. I'd always seen the woods. But Don taught me to see the individual trees and shrubs and plants that made up the forest."

Flower Essences

During her studies, Kate became enchanted with flower essences. "I took to those like a duck to water," she says. "I just loved the idea of flower essences, it made sense to me." She and Don woke up one March morning having experienced the same dream: they were to make flower essences from the plants of New England. This was pivotal because theirs would be the first essences made from the region, as Bach flower essences were made in England and FDS essences were made in California. "It's been seventeen years now and we're still learning. People relate to me because I started herbs as a mom, with a family, really slowly. And most of the information I share is experiential—it's not a rehash of other people's experiences. It's what I've seen and experienced. That's a big part of what people are looking for."

"I'm very happy to be a local herbalist, offering what we can from what we grow or gather, and to offer plants that are different."

Kate now works with many people with cancer and has completed Ayurvedic training. She still works with indigenous plants or those she can grow, but the plants she uses most are those that help severely depleted people, including calendula, Reishi mushrooms, sacred basil (Tulsi), ashwagandha, and hawthorn. She harvests birch bark for oils and crèmes (betulinic acid, she says, is useful for skin cancer) as well as chaga mushrooms, which grow on the upper branches of birch trees and are very valuable. "Chaga is used for gastrointestinal cancers to both prevent and support the person going through therapy," she says. "Chaga is also used for melanoma; it is being shown to have antioxidant values even more than açai berry." Kate and Don gather the chaga, dry it, chop it with axes, put it through a chipper/shredder, then grind it to a tea-leaf consistency—a labor-intensive process that produces a superior product. Kate also gathers evergreen branches to infuse for massage oils, and she harvests hawthorn berries.

"My biggest challenge is being able to meet legal requirements so we can offer our herbs without having to do all kinds of standardization," she says. "People are buying processed pharmaceuticals and have little access to fresh and conscientiously

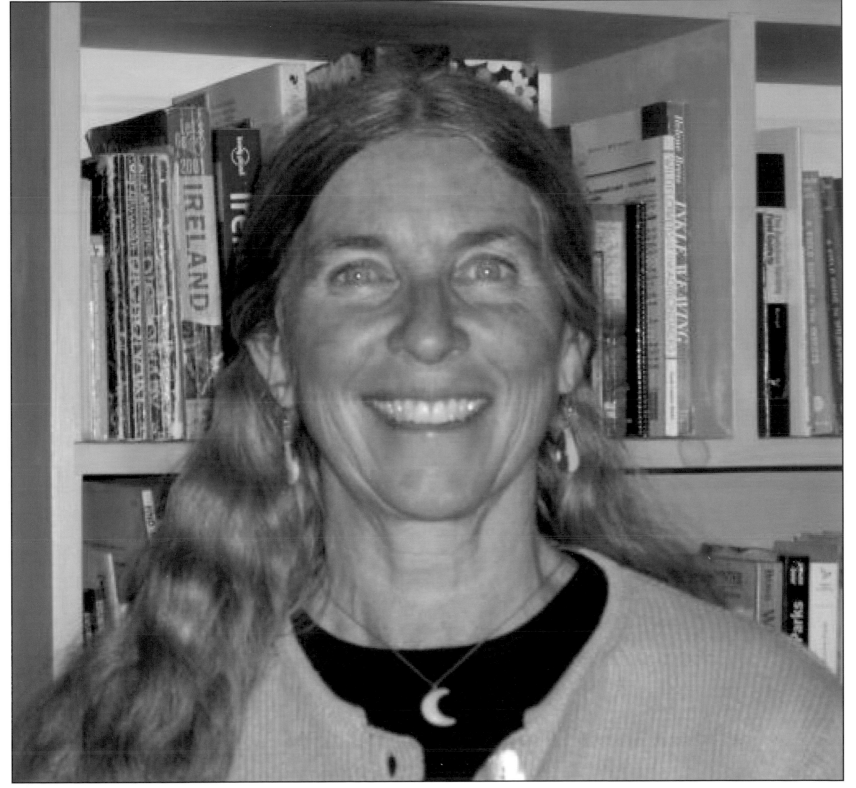

Photo credit: Kate Gilday

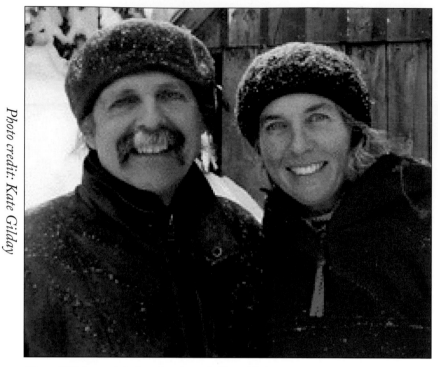

Kate Gilday with her husband, Don Babineau.

harvested plant medicinal." The FDA is trying to make it difficult for herbalists to produce their product, she says, and it's not just about cleanliness. "It's about having to prove that a plant is what you say it is. Only a huge business can afford to get a product out to people: chromatography tests, lab equipment. It's sad. We're getting more and more pulled away from the roots of what we love to do," Kate says. "I'm very happy to be a local herbalist, offering what we can from what we grow or gather, and to offer plants that are different."

Kate's company Woodland Essence offers flower essences, salves, crèmes, massage oils, handcrafted birch bark baskets, pine pollen sold by the ounce, and a formula of pine pollen, *American ginseng* and *Aralia nudicaulis* featured in herbalist Stephen Buhner's books. Kate crafts simple and compound extracts, an herbal gum rinse, a restorative herb blend with Ayurvedic herbs, and extracts of woodland mushrooms—the steady, calm, nurturing presence of a singer offering her melody for the forest.

Anointing the body or a special object has long been reverential. In the "Inscription of Ashurbanipal," in *Assyrian and Babylonian Literature*, Ashurbanipal hopes his descendents will "anoint [his inscription] with ointment and offer sacrifices and set it up along with the inscription." In *The Magical Texts*, the Babylonian writer complains "they have anointed me with an ointment of noisome herbs, they have taken me for a corpse," an ancient act of anointing the deceased. Margaret Starbird, in *The Woman with the Alabaster Jar*, makes the case that Mary of Bethany or Mary Magdalene famously performed the sacred rite of death and immortality when she broke the jar of spikenard perfume upon Jesus's head. The great kings of history were ritually anointed with oil cementing their god-given role as ruler.

The six-thousand-year-old hypothetical Proto-Indo-European (PIE) language used *ongw*, "to salve or anoint," giving us *unguent*. To anoint with oil was *anakti* (Sanskrit), *aucanem* (Armenian), *anctan* (Old Prussian "butter"), *ancho* and *anke* (Old High German and German words meaning "butter").

The PIE word for fat or butter was *selp* or *solpa* (from which we derive *soap*), and Greek used *elpos* for fat or oil. Sanskrit *sarpis* meant "melted butter."

Old English created *sealfian*, "to anoint (a wound) with salve," because they simmered healing herbs in butter and lard. In this context, the patriarchal king is forgotten and the word means "healing." *Sealf* meant healing ointment, a word derived from Germanic *salbo* and *salbe*, "oily substance." Old Saxon used *salba* and Middle Dutch used *salve*.

In Shakespeare's lifetime, servants presented food to the king on a platter so the king knew foods were free of poison. The tray was a salver, from the French *salve* (tray) and the Spanish *salva* (testing of food and drink). Both terms originated in Late Latin *salvare*, to save or render safe.

"God save the King!" This verbal cry might have originated as a greeting between two people, as common salutations typically include a wish for the other's health. ("God be with you" turned into "goodbye," "fare thee well" became "farewell," and "you are well come" became "welcome.") The Romans greeted one another with a *salu*tation (literally, a wish for safety). Italian's *salva* is a salute or a volley of firearms in one's honor.

In about 1440, English borrowed Latin's *unguere* "to anoint or smear with ointment" to create *ointment*, and herbalists' safe, healing ointments are *salves*.

Unfortunately, in Middle Dutch, *quacken* described a vigorous salesman likely to brag or boast. He "hawked" his wares, and a hawker of medicinal salves was a *kwaksalver*. In 1579, the term changed to *quacksalver* and, in 1638, it referred specifically to a medical charlatan. (There is possibly a connection between this charlatan and the miraculous drug, quicksilver.) A *quack* today practices medicine ignorantly or dishonestly or is a person deemed mentally crazy.

The largest public park in the lower forty-eight states, the Adirondack Park and Forest Preserve has the country's largest hiking trail system—it includes the entire western shore of Lake Champlain, which is the geologic result of the last Ice Age, formed roughly ten thousand years ago. If you are the adventurous type, you may want to visit AuSable Chasm, a scenic gorge and bridge open to the public since 1870. Or the High Falls Gorge and the AuSable River Falls, or the ten-million-year-old Howes Caverns and its underground lake. In 1882, the New York State Legislature protected as "forever wild" the six million acres of the park today, which comprise more land than Yellowstone, Yosemite, the Grand Canyon, Great Smoky Mountains National Park, and the Everglades National Park combined.

Adirondack mothers and housewives from pre–Civil War through the early twentieth century kept vegetable gardens and hens for profit: they sold butter, eggs, maple syrup, and boarded their rooms to travelers for pay. Today the region is celebrated as a beautiful protected area for hiking, swimming, boating, climbing, and outdoor enjoyment.

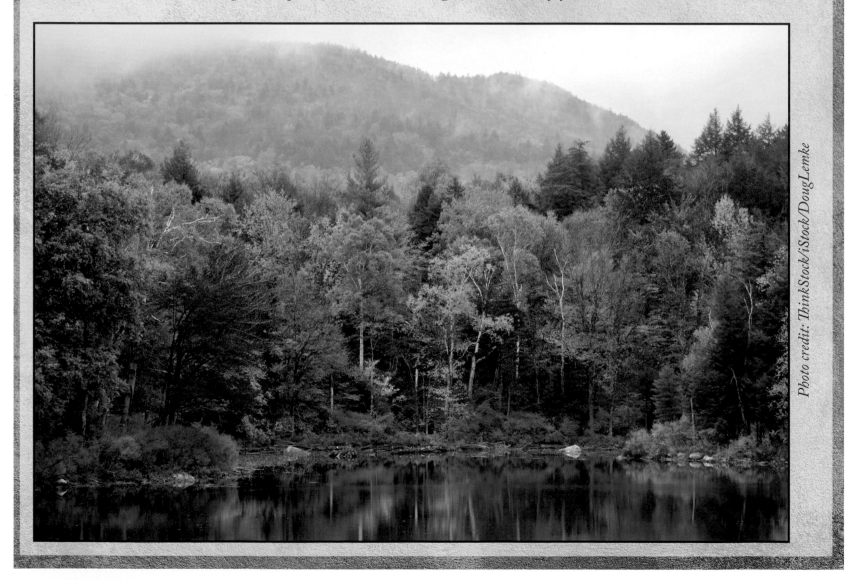

Photo credit: ThinkStock/iStock/DougLemke

HAWTHORN
Crataegus monogyna and other species

Hawthorns, sometimes called red haw or may tree, are trees or shrubs sporting thorns up to five inches in length. Euell Gibbons noted with frustration that the hawthorn is "the most confusing tree in existence" and that there are between two hundred and nine hundred species, "depending on who is doing the counting."

In England, some say Joseph of Arimathea thrust his hawthorn walking stick into the ground where it took root, grew into a massive tree, and thrived for nearly two thousand years. Traditionally associated with the Green Man (as are birch, oak, and holly), hawthorn boughs are traditionally brought indoors and hung above doorways for good luck on Beltane, May 1. Sir James Frazer says in *The Golden Bough* (p.139): "Among ancient customs still retained by the Cornish may be reckoned that of decking their doors and porches on the first of May with green boughs of sycamore and hawthorn."

Prized as a cardiac tonic and for the circulatory system, hawthorn's hypotensive leaves, bark, and tart berries are taken in

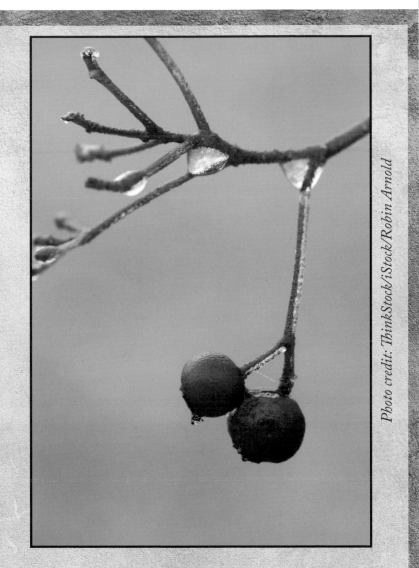

Photo credit: ThinkStock/iStock/Robin Arnold

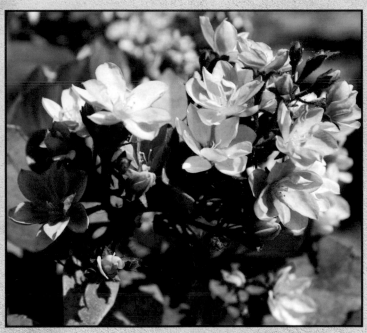

Photo credit: ThinkStock/iStock/Mikhail Ter-avanesov

the form of a tea, tincture, paste, or even jelly to counter high blood pressure and arteriosclerosis. Cherokee herbalist David Winston says hawthorn fruit, leaf, and flower (*Cratagus monogyna*) are useful for weakened heart muscle, venous integrity, and preventing deposits of plaque on arterial walls. Hawthorn is a gentler and more long-term remedy than foxglove and is astringent and useful against diarrhea.

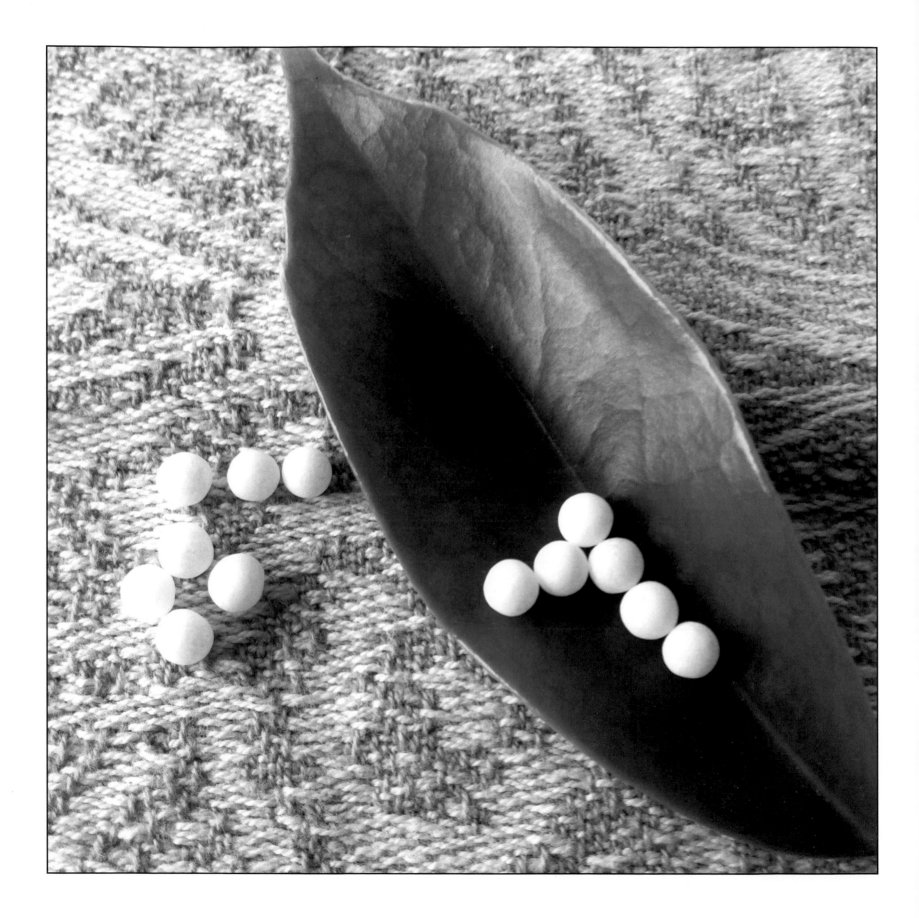

Chapter 12
HOMEOPATHY

Homeopathy is a widely accepted form of treatment that was invented at the turn of the nineteenth century by rebellious German physician Samuel Hahnemann (1755–1843). Beloved in his time and considered "experimental," he dabbled in chemistry and loved linguistics, studying and speaking eight languages by the time he reached age forty-five. Hahnemann loved being a physician but was disgusted by what he observed in his colleagues' daily practice: purgative drugs, bleeding, and blistering techniques that left patients exhausted and frightened. He believed these invasive and counter-intuitive treatments actually made patients much worse than they were before.

While translating the materia medica of Scottish physician Cullen, Hahnemann read of the doctor's praise of *cinchona* (Peruvian bark) in treating malaria. Curious, Hahnemann decided to try the treatment himself, so he experimented with *cinchona* even though he was healthy. He developed fever, a consequence that reminded him of the common Greek and German folk theory "like cures like" and he assumed he had found justification for the theory. Excited, he published the idea that *cinchona* produces an artificial illness in the body that spurs the body's defenses against malaria. His coworkers emulated his experiments but became very sick, so, in his laboratory, Hahnemann reduced the dose to a tiny dilution until the side-effects disappeared. The result was a new method of medicine that he named *homeopathy*.

The "Like Cures Like" Method

Hahnemann applied his research in dilution of substances not only to plants, but also to minerals (such as arsenic and sulphur) and animals (*Apis* is diluted, crushed bees). Many of the plants he used in his ninety-nine remedies were considered toxic in full doses, such as belladonna and poison ivy, but they were healing in diluted doses.

Homeopathy, or *Similus similibus curentur*, meant "let like be cured by like." For example, naturopathic doctors today may prescribe homeopathic *coffea* for a hyperactive child, though in normal doses coffee stimulates hyperactivity. Hahnemann and his fellow researchers at Leipzig University discovered the threshold at which the minute doses caused the action to become the opposite of what was expected; the sedative tincture of opium, for instance, could be used homeopathically to treat lethargy or to reverse near-comas.

Hahnemann's philosophy proved successful; his methods cured Napoleon's army of typhoid fever and his ideas quickly spread across Europe and to North America. The US Food and Drug Administration accepted homeopathic remedies into public health policy in 1938, and today most homeopathic remedies are over-the-counter medicines not requiring a prescription. Because of this, many homeopathic remedies are sold not as health supplements or dietary supplements, but as drugs, and they can claim on the label that they "cure" specific ailments (for self-limiting conditions such as colds and headaches). They are sold with the medical dilution being applied to the exterior of a tiny sugar pill, which is taken by mouth, and they are completely symptom-based, with the determination of proper remedy being based on symptoms expressed by the patient. They differ from herbal preparations in that they are strictly dilutions, whereas most herbal remedies are concentrations or extracts.

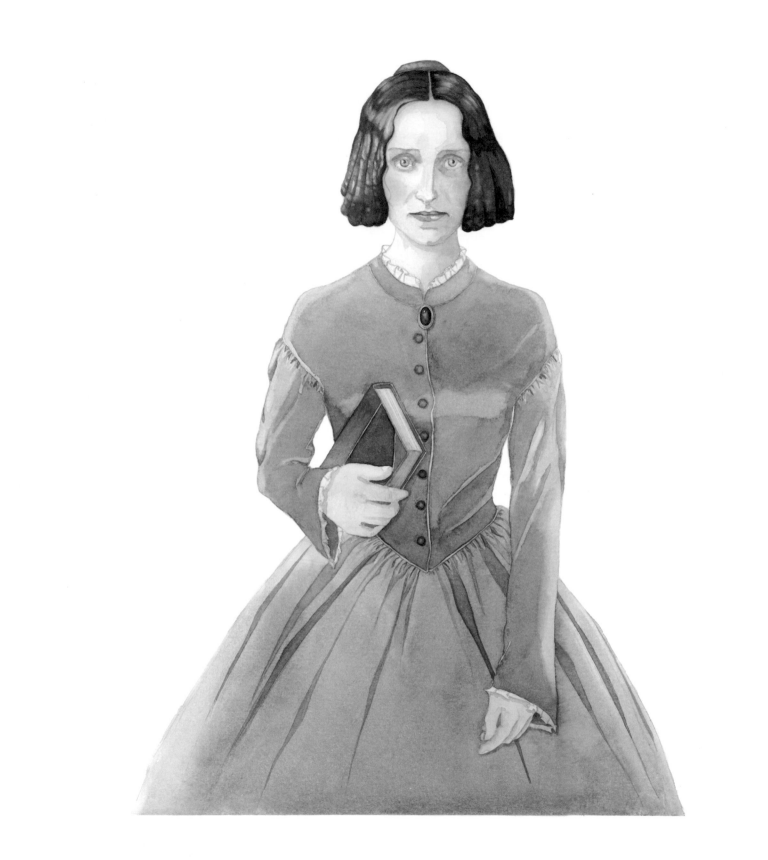

Mary Baker Eddy

(1821–1910)

Born in 1821 in Bow, New Hampshire, Mary Baker Eddy was a formidable and highly controversial woman whose role as a healer won both admirers and enemies, and her controversial life established one of the longest-standing religious groups still practicing today, the Christian Scientists. Mary capitalized on her interest in healing, her strong (almost obsessive) faith in God and Jesus of the Bible, and her determination that neither sickness nor gender would stand in her way of success, and she plowed forward through personal hardship and anguish to establish her own branch of the Christian church—based on healing.

As a child, Mary suffered unexplained illnesses that kept her home from school and awakened her curiosity in the mechanics of the body and mind. As a young girl, she heard voices that she attributed to a divine calling that strengthened her desire to join and participate in the Christian church. But Mary's life was not easy; her illness left her socially lacking and her first husband died before their only son was born. Mary's next suitor died before they could be wed, and she was estranged from her son for years. Still sick in 1853, she married dentist and practicing homeopath Daniel Patterson, who introduced her to the ideas of homeopathic

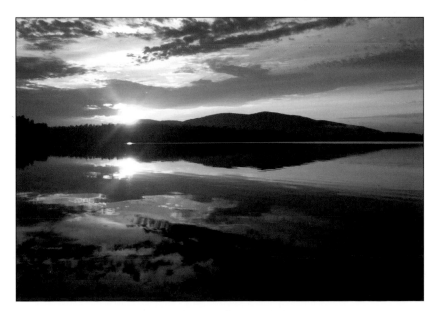

From New England, Mary Baker Eddy's influence stretches worldwide.

healing and the principle that "like cures like." But it wasn't until she consulted homeopathic healer Phineas Quimby that her interest peaked and she turned fully to homeopathic practitioners for her treatments. Always curious, she questioned exactly how homeopathy worked. How was it that an extremely diluted substance can affect the body? How can a near-placebo sugar pill bring about the healing normally achieved with a concentrated medicine? Mary studied with Quimby and, as both patient and student, realized that his ability to heal lay in his training in hypnosis—a concept that stimulated her to ponder the extreme power of thought.

Then, the turning point: Mary slipped on an icy sidewalk in the winter of 1866, and neither physician nor homeopathic practitioner could heal her badly injured back. While bedridden and reading her Bible, Mary repeated a passage of Jesus's healing and miraculously found herself able to walk. Astonished and grateful, she began writing about her experience and, within three years, developed the career and philosophy that would consume the rest of her life. She combined her interest in healing, her semi-clairvoyant ability, her fascination with positive thought, and her devotion to Christianity to produce an entirely new system of medicine: what she termed Christian Science.

To her, this method was completely natural: it showcased the healing of Jesus and trained others to apply this method themselves. Beginning with a handful of devotees (including students as well as patients whom she cured personally), Mary built up her following into the thousands, eventually lecturing at churches across New England and creating the Massachusetts Metaphysical College. She wrote and published dozens of articles, poems, lectures, and books, including *The Journal of Christian Science* (later renamed *The Christian Science Journal*) and *The Christian Science Monitor* (1908), which are still published today.

During a time when medicine was overwhelmingly dominated by male doctors and pharmacists, Mary pioneered the idea that *thoughts* manifested either illness or health in the body, and that simply by thinking, believing, or having faith, one could remove negative manifestations and achieve health. She later abandoned her study of homeopathy and hydrotherapy in favor of powerful positive thinking and Bible study.

It wasn't easy for her. Mary's dominating personality (decades before the liberating years of Women's Suffrage) earned bitter enemies. She didn't see her son for years, her husband Patterson left her, and her third husband, Asa Gilbert Eddy (whom Mary treated for a heart condition) died after only five years of marriage. She was constantly berated by the medical community for her outlandish healing methods and was criticized by the Christian community, who accused her of usurping the established church. Through it all, Mary insisted she was acting on behalf of her beloved church, and she unflinchingly wrote to her parishioners urging them to read her books in their pursuit of Christian healing.

By the time she died in 1910 at age eighty-nine, Mary had seen her opus *Science and Health* translated into German, her curriculum established for colleges and universities, and the edifice of what her followers affectionately called The Mother Church building expanded to hold thousands of people. Near the end of her life, she ventured into new territories in her writing, bravely addressing feminism and politics. Today her book *Science and Health* has sold more than ten million copies and Mary is remembered not only as the founder of the Church of Christian Scientists (Church of Christ, Scientist) with a worldwide membership of approximately 85,000, but more importantly as a faithful advocate for the effects of positive thinking and directed energy toward the illnesses of the body.

GRATEFUL

Already an adjective, *grate* accepted the suffix *ful* to become a double adjective, meaning "agreeable" and "thankful." The word stems from the Latin *gratus*, pleasing, and originally from the Proto-Indo-European *gwere-*, meaning "to favor." Graces, those little prayers said before a meal, appeared in the early thirteenth century. Other meanings for *gwere-* exist, however, including "heavy" and "flood." The connotation *heavy* seems connected since we favor something heavy when we carry it; this meaning also gave Latin *gravis* and lead to *grave*. The connotation *flood* is in the sense of whirlpool or abyss and also carried the meaning "to swallow," hence today's terms *gorge*, *gargoyle*, and *regurgitation*.

ARNICA
Arnica Montana

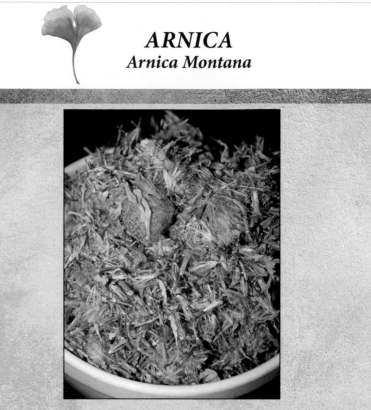

Known as "lamb's skin" for its fluffy aerial parts, especially its dried flowers, arnica is man's best friend for muscle and joint pain, bruising, inflammation, tweaks and twinges, and swelling. It is believed to work by increasing blood flow through affected capillaries, allowing escaped fluids and the blood protein fibrin to be reabsorbed.[1]

Though it appears to have hit the shelves out of nowhere in the last ten years, arnica has been used for centuries—and not only in North America where it grows wild in the Colorado Rockies, the Pacific Northwest, and up through Alaska; worldwide arnica is prized across Europe from the Mediterranean to the Netherlands, in temperate regions with acidic soil or grasslands. Its wide range belies the fact that arnica is overharvested and is losing its habitat to construction and destruction. More abundant anti-inflammatory substitutes can include comfrey, yarrow, mint, and calendula.

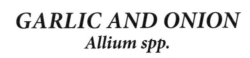

GARLIC AND ONION
Allium spp.

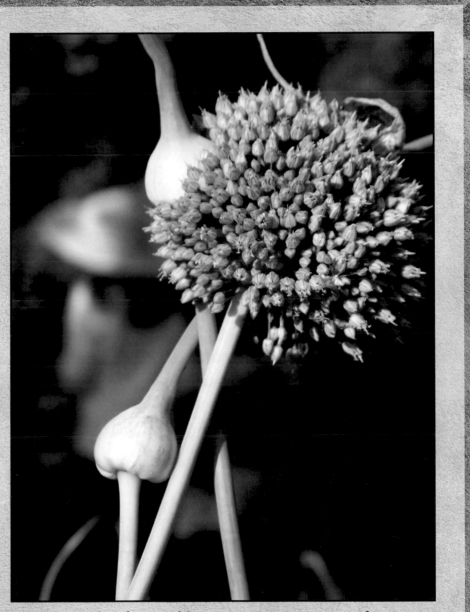

Both our literature and cuisine would be bland without garlic and onion. These two bulbs, in the lily family, have provided taste, healing, and food for thought since the Ancient Egyptian pyramid builders ate quantities of garlic (according to Greek Historian Herodotus) and the Chinese cultivated it for food and medicine since at least 2000 BCE. Ancient Greeks placed cloves of garlic in doorways and crossroads as offerings to their beloved and powerful protector the Goddess Hecate, who was believed to appreciate it. The bulb's role in warding off evil spirits is legendary from the frightened populace of the Middle Ages who hung it outside their doors to ward off the plague to the people of Transylvania who feared vampires.

Though not as mythic, modern scientists have confirmed that eating garlic can significantly reduce blood cholesterol and other fats as well as reduce blood clotting. Western herbalists commonly employ garlic alongside hawthorn to treat hypertension since the bulb has shown a great proclivity for reducing blood pressure in both animals and humans.

Garlic is extremely antiseptic and has been used in military applications for wounds and gangrene throughout America's history. Internally it combats viral and bacterial infections including tuberculosis, dysentery, pertussis, and hepatitis.

Garlic's cousin onion has a folk history of treating upper and lower respiratory infections and has been a staple food in many countries. Because cutting onions causes the nose and eyes to water, it is used homeopathically to treat the same conditions—catarrh, colds, conjunctivitis, hay fever, and laryngitis; its primary use is for upper respiratory congestion (ear, nose, sinus cavity, and throat) in which case it is referred to as homeopathic *Allium cepa*, a major remedy.

Considered a minor remedy in homeopathy, *Allium sativa* or garlic is prepared from fresh minced bulbs and is prescribed for indigestion, dietary changes, pressure in the upper abdomen, colicky pains around the navel, and for "tearing" pains in the hip area and abdomen.

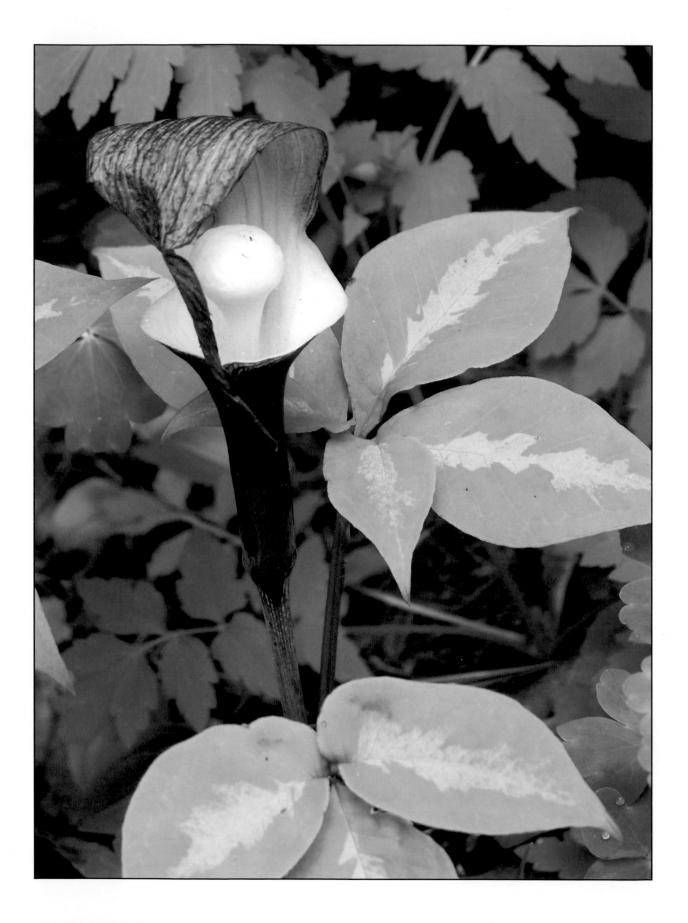

Chapter 13
GAELIC PHARMACY

Of all the world's healing traditions, perhaps none are so charming and rich in nature lore as Gaelic pharmacy, a colorful product of the convergence of Christians and pagans in the windswept, remote regions of Scotland. Gaelic pharmacy closely resembles the Folk Healing of Appalachia and the Bedouin cultures described in Part I: Folk Medicine, Gypsy and Bedouin Traditions (page 52). Yet it is separated here and included in Part IV: Spirit Traditions because of its complete dependence on the strong superstitions of spirits, sprites, elves, and demons. While Appalachian folk healing dealt with Scotch-Irish immigrants using ancient household remedies, objects, and herbs to ward off illness, Gaelic healers of old went further than mere superstition and actually perceived spirits all around them. To a Gaelic practitioner, healing an illness required serious intervention in the spiritual realm to guard against a very real perceived notion of unseen evil spirits snatching babies and causing sickness.

The Ancient Gaelic Culture

The newly converted families of Christian Scots emigrated from Ireland in the late fifth century AD and settled on the western coast of northern Britain in a small kingdom they named Dalriada. These adventurous and hard-working men and women brought with them their Celtic language (called Gaelic) and established communities near the pre-existing pagan Picts (who spoke an early Welsh, later-to-become British, language), the Britons, and the Angles. The arrangement proved destined to bloodshed, however, and the Gaelic Scots, after centuries of war between the four kingdoms, eventually conquered the others and named the newly unified country Scotland.

Over the centuries, the Gaelic culture in the Scottish Highlands flourished into a rich heritage of healing, storytelling, music, legends, and a unique and colorful superstition-laden religious life. The Gaelic Scots were nature lovers who incorporated nature, magic, and myth into their rituals, ballads, and daily life. Healers included white witches who removed evil charms, healed negative magic, and used herbal medicines that were considered valid and efficient treatments for all physical and mental complaints. Other cures involved magic, a sort of supernatural faith (in essence, Folk Healing) involving minerals, metals, animal parts, and other materials in the banishment and deflection of the many evil spirits, fairies, and demons believed to lurk in every meadow, forest, and house. Iron and steel were believed to cast out devilish spirits, so that Celtic smiths who, in addition to being honored for their metal forging skills, were often lauded as important healers. Folklorist Anne Ross describes a sick patient who presented himself at the forge of a metal smithy, asking for treatment. The metal smithy laid the man on his anvil and approached him with his hammer held high, intent to strike him. The patient improved immediately—and, we assume, left.

It was strongly believed that invisible good and evil forces were working for or against people minute by minute, and that every move and word was important in maintaining safety and health. Ghosts and evil forces walked very much alongside the living and were a real menace.

Gaelic Scots practiced the reading of omens and honed their skills to avoid trickery, with the belief that luck, ill-luck, and spiritual pranks by evil forces were constant threats. Times of childbirth, coming-of-age ceremonies, and sabbats of the year were of particular concern, for fairies, witches, and devils were quick to steal children, kill babies, and burn houses. Folk superstitions abounded: one must enter a house from the front door, never the back; iron rods were placed over cradles to protect the baby from thieving

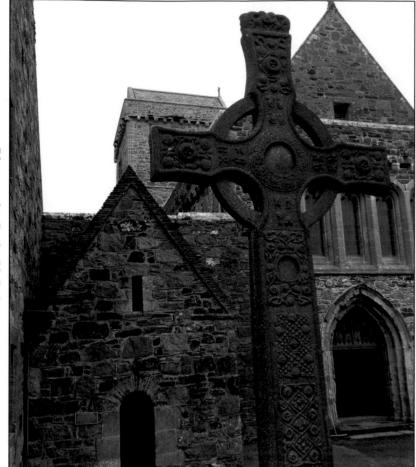

St. Columba's Shrine, Iona Abbey

fairies; warts could be removed with pig's blood; and strangers to a village were never permitted to count one's children, cattle, or sheep lest eavesdropping fairies would overhear the number and decide to steal one of the children. Meddling fairies were particularly despised and could be deterred with iron and holly berries.

Pagan and Christian cures alike were valued by Gaelic Scots until fairly recently. Pagan cures included incantations over knives or burning with fire. Christian cures included fanning a sick person with the pages of a Bible—both methods equally ineffective and superstitious.

Today, Gaelic heritage is experiencing a robust rebirth as people desperately search to rescue their dying and forgotten histories. Considered unworthy and childish during the last few centuries, the Gaelic language is being exhumed from its near-death for study at an academic level, and the entire folk history of Scotland and its early Celtic traditions are being respectfully revisited for understanding and inclusion as important and cherished parts of our world heritage.

Mary Beith

(1938–2012)

At age seventy-three, Scotland's Mary Beith was still a spry and very sharp reporter when I interviewed her via email, learning about her writing that appeared in newspapers across Britain since the late 1950s. It was a complete surprise for Mary to become an esteemed reporter of Gaelic pharmacy, one of the ancient tradition's most renowned chroniclers, and the most sought-after documentarian of Gaelic folk healing. She was born in London and brought up "all over the place," including the West Indies during the late 1940s and early 1950s, and she pursued writing as a career, working in journalism as a staff or freelance writer for national newspapers in Scotland and England until a near-fatal attack of meningitis forced her to quit full-time work. For many years, she contributed a fortnightly column in the *West Highland Free Press* and in 2004 she published *Healing Threads: Traditional Medicines of the Highlands & Islands*.

Her interest in the mysterious subject of Gaelic pharmacy began when a consultant at a Dublin hospital wrote a book on Irish folk medicine that influenced Mary to collect information of traditional Scottish remedies. In 1979, Ronald Black, a lecturer in Celtic Studies at Glasgow University, realized her potential and prompted her to conduct a more thorough investigation, as he was cataloguing the Gaelic manuscripts in the National Library of Scotland in Edinburgh. Black found that the great majority of the pre-eighteenth century manuscripts dealt with medicine, so Mary set to work collecting a hefty supply of traditional remedy information.

It was no easy task: she discovered that the rich tradition of Scottish healing includes a great diversity of plants as well as minerals, insects, animal parts (antlers or goat's blood), and live animals. (It was not uncommon for traditional Gaelic pharmaceutical doctors to prescribe the ingestion of or ritual magic with live mice and spiders.) "I must make clear," she said, "that my researches into the traditional remedies of the Highlands and Islands do not deal only with herbs. The old treatments employed a variety of *materia* and there was a big emphasis on what we may now regard, according to our perspective, as either superstitious, spiritual, or shrewdly psychological approaches involving rituals and incantations." Her collections of traditional remedies swelled with the contributions and recollections of the West Highland Free Press's readers, rural doctors and nurses, historians, archaeologists, sociologists, pharmacists, practicing herbalists, crofters, fishermen, teachers, and poets who sent her their cherished family information or professional folklore. Mary earned a well-deserved reputation as the preeminent chronicler of Gaelic pharmacy and many people traveled to hear her lecture on ancient medicinal history and the magical relationship to the natural world that no longer exists.

I asked her what was difficult about keeping the heritage of Scottish herbal pharmacy alive and she answered emphatically, "It's not really difficult, at all. Highland people are very much aware and proud of so many aspects of their heritage and they have long memories. However, there's always that feeling that the people with firsthand knowledge are forever dying off and if only one had started decades earlier . . . But then, collectors have been making such complaints since at least the seventeenth century. An interesting new development is that the new Centre for Health Science, in the grounds of Raigmore Hospital in Inverness, has a central courtyard where many of the traditional herbs have been planted with brief accompanying notes on how they were once used. Scientists at the Centre have already begun experiments with, and analysis of, some of the old herbal treatments. The Centre, under the leadership of Professor Alasdair Munro, is keen to keep the heritage alive and also hopes to fund the translation into English of some of the medieval Gaelic medical manuscripts held in the National Library of Scotland. In the talks I have given to locals in village halls and schools, and to professionals and students in hospitals and universities, there has been an equal interest from both lay and qualified people. It's *their* heritage!"

Mary kept her collecting of plant information people-based. The late professor Kirsty Larner of Glasgow University's Sociology department stressed to her the importance of combining the social history of the people with their use of remedies—evaluating the medicine and magic of the people only in the context of their social history. The two go hand-in-hand and cannot be separated without losing the importance of one or the value of the other.

The people's remedies naturally reflected their problems at the moment, as well as what was in season and could be gathered, Mary

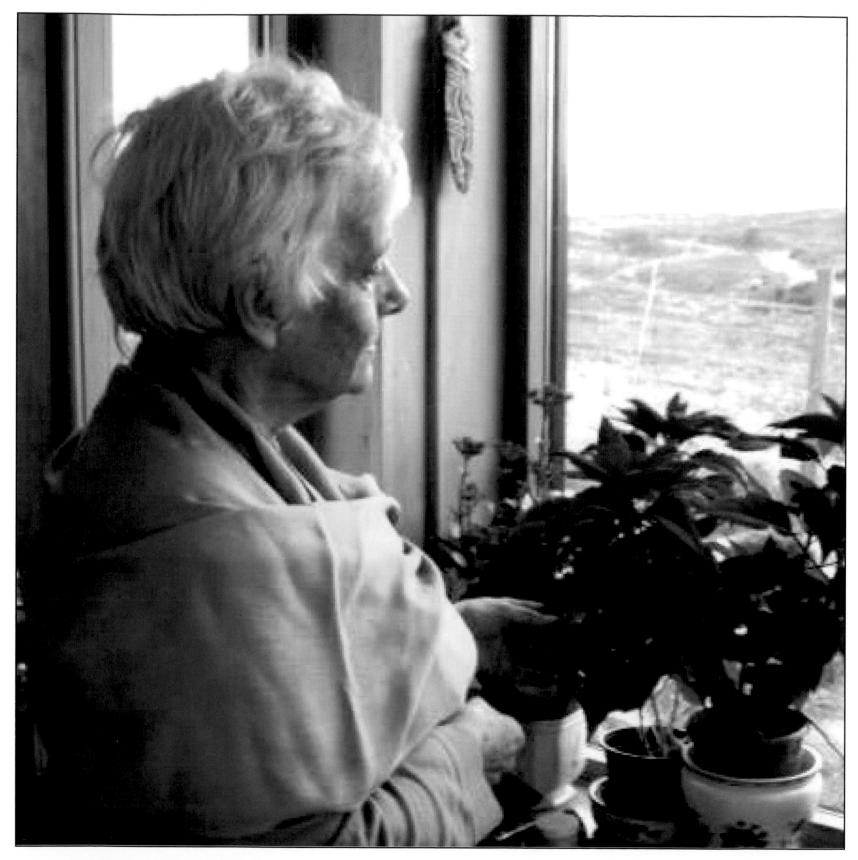

said. "A lot depended on what was available in any particular district. For example, in the Badenoch area of the central Highlands, resin from pine trees was much used, especially in the form of plasters for skin cancers (or what were assumed to be cancerous sores or growths). Wild carrots were similarly used in other areas for such problems. Because of its absorbent and slightly antiseptic qualities, sphagnum moss was extensively used for dressing wounds, for women's periods, and as a forerunner of disposable nappies (diapers) for babies."

Gaelic pharmacy is a rich, vibrant blend of herbal and "other" *materia* that combined to form a cornucopia of healing techniques. The Scots employed a huge range of plants for their traditional remedies: thyme, honeysuckle flowers, St John's wort (external applications only), primrose, eyebright, meadowsweet, betony, dandelion, chickweed, mint, a variety of seaweeds … all these and more were once in constant use, says Mary, so that her only real problem as a chronicler was making sure that people who tell her stories of the old herbal treatments knew exactly which plant they meant. "It's usually best if they can show an example, preferably growing, but a good illustration in a book will do," she said.

"My studies have increasingly deepened my respect for the country people who for centuries and millennia, through trial and error and happy discovery, learned so much about the natural world around them."

Gaelic History

Gaelic pharmacy thrived for centuries, from the center-of-town doctors to the rural country kitchens, and its practices were kept alive through necessity well into the first half of the twentieth century, said Ms. Beith. "Orthodox medicines and treatments were hard to come by in many areas either because of lack of qualified medical people, or poverty, or the difficulties of travel and communication." But the remedies might have endured even if people had greater access to physicians and allopathic medicine, simply because they respected their clan heritage and felt a keen interest in preserving it. "There was a high regard for a number of the old remedies and, perhaps, a lingering memory of the medically trained clan physicians of the middle ages—who combined the official medicine of their day with traditional treatments. It enhanced people's respect for their own ways."

INSPIRE

The breath has had a distinct etymological history in many cultures. Latin gave us *spirare*, meaning "breath," from the PIE (s)peis, "to blow," and it shares this root with *spirit*. Inspire is the combination of *in* + *spirare*, "to breathe" that took on the meaning "to influence or animate with an idea or purpose" by 1390 (Harper, 2008).

An ancient word *wet* meant "to blow, inspire, spiritually arouse," and from this the Proto-Germanic language created *wod-eno* and *wod-ono* to mean "raging mad, inspired." The root *wet* probably led to *Wod-enaz*, later smoothing into Odin or Othin, the Norse God.

From Latin's *aspirare*, "to breathe upon," Old French created *aspirer*, acknowledging when we are breathed upon by the encouraging breath of the spirits to succeed, helping us aspire toward a goal or challenge ourselves.

"I have also learned to respect those plants so often considered as mere 'weeds' that have contributed so much to the practice and knowledge of healing."

Her studies of the Gaelic healing arts combined with her innate passion for writing naturally brought her to study the ancient Gaelic alphabet. To better understand the inherent connection between the spoken (and written) word and the natural world around ancient Gaelic speakers, Mary wrote specifically about the remedies and folklore of trees in *A' Chraobh* (*The Tree*, with Gaelic and English text on alternate pages), a long essay on the old Gaelic Ogham alphabet. Careful to state that she was not a healer, Mary was nevertheless a wealth of information about the vibrant heritage of Gaelic pharmacy, and her lifelong pursuit of the traditional healing methods of Scotland has enriched our study of world heritage.

"I've been interested in plants for as long as I can remember," she said, "but my studies have increasingly deepened my respect for the country people who for centuries and millennia, through trial and error and happy discovery, learned so much about the natural world around them. I have also learned to respect those plants so often considered as mere 'weeds' that have contributed so much to the practice and knowledge of healing."

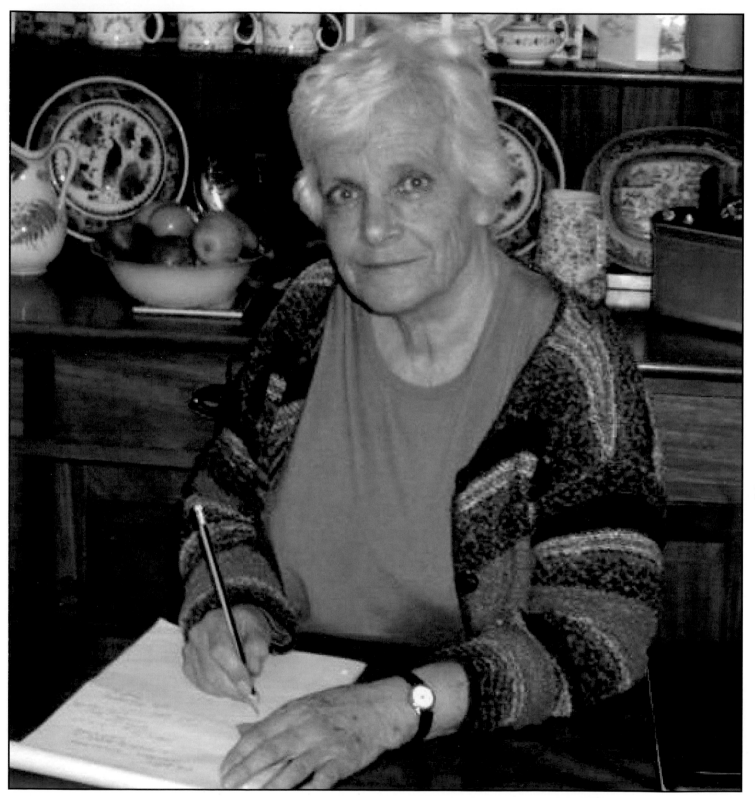

Photo credit: Mary Beith

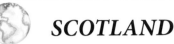

Much of Scotland's forests were cleared by agriculturalists as far back as three thousand years ago, as Bronze Age farm value outweighed forest value. This continued until England's Queen Elizabeth I reserved her country's trees strictly for shipbuilding, forcing England's smelters to harvest Scotland's trees for iron smelting, marking first the decline and then the disappearance of its forest inhabitants: brown bear, lynx, reindeer, elk, boar, beaver, and finally in 1743, the last wolf.[1] The Caledonian Forest once covered more than 1.5 million hectares (almost 3.75 million acres) of the Highlands, but today a mere 1 percent remains.

Naturalist and activist John Muir was born in Dunbar in 1838 and spent his early life in Scotland; he formed the Sierra Club and wrote books about the power of nature's beauty. The Old Physic Garden of Edinburgh was a popular botanist's retreat until it flooded when Nor' Loch was drained in 1689. Today, visitors can visit the Royal Botanic Garden Edinburgh off Princes Street and consume haggis, Angus beef, and farmed venison. Scotland is the proud home of the Highland cattle—long, bushy-haired cows with massive bodies and long, pointed horns, and plenty of sheep whose wool provides for flannels and tartans.

Old herbal recipes call for immersing herbs in whiskey, which began in Scotland as *uisge beatha*, Gaelic for "water of life." Scotland produces two types of whiskey, accounting for 13 percent of its exports: malt (fuller of flavor and more expensive) and grain. Malt is produced by germinating barley seeds in cisterns, then killing the new growth and drying it with peat or oil furnace smoke. Dried sprouts are milled and mashed in hot water to produce a sugary "wort" (see Wort sidebar in chapter 1). Finally, the product is distilled and aged.

Near Inverness lies the Findhorn Foundation, established by Eileen Caddy to connect with "devas" or tree spirits. The community is world renowned for growing extra-large flowers, fruits, and vegetables by speaking and singing to the plants. When I visited in 1996, the majority of community members lived in caravans (trailers) with a few wooden structures, including a beautiful cafeteria and a timber health food store stocked with cheeses, tinctures, and books. Today, the Foundation operates a restaurant, artist studios, and a retreat center.

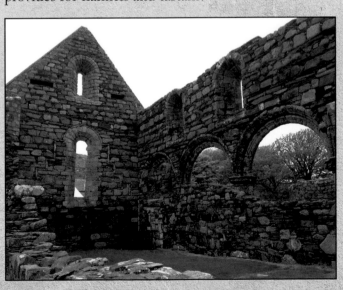

Photo credit: Leslie H. Roberts

Ruins on Iona, Scotland

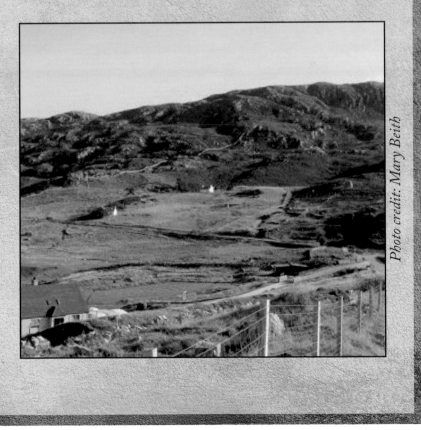

Photo credit: Mary Beith

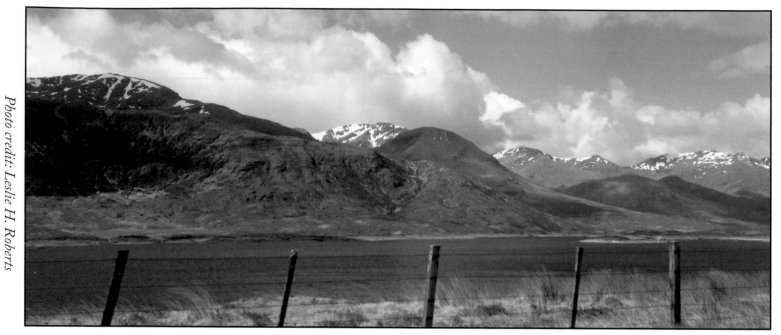

Northern Scotland

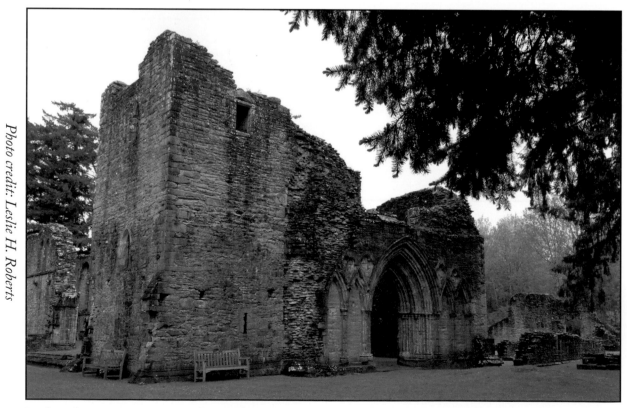

Inchmahome Priory ruins dating from 1238

YARROW
Achillea millefolium

Legend tells us that young Irish girls placed yarrow leaves beneath their pillows to dream of their sweethearts, and brides were given gifts of yarrow to ensure seven years of love. This may stem from a long-recognized ability of yarrow to staunch, or stay, bleeding, and brides wanted their new husbands to stay faithful. Fragrant and bitter yarrow is a magnificent styptic and is frequently used on fresh wounds—just as it has been for centuries by armies across Europe and by native American Indians who both used yarrow to stop nosebleeds, bleeding of wounds and gums, and hemorrhoids.

In southeast Scotland, the Yarrow Water is a river that flows through the Yarrow Valley and passes the settlements of Yarrow Feus, Yarrow, and Yarrowford; William Wordsworth teased his traveling companion by refusing to visit nearby Yarrow, saying, in his poem "Yarrow Unvisited":

"Oh! Green," said I, "are Yarrow's holms / And sweet is Yarrow flowing! / Fair hangs the apple frae the rock, / But we will leave it growing. . . .We will not see them; will not go, / To-day, nor yet to-morrow; / Enough if in our hearts we know / There's such a place as Yarrow."

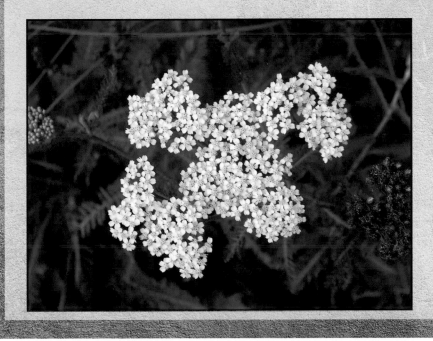

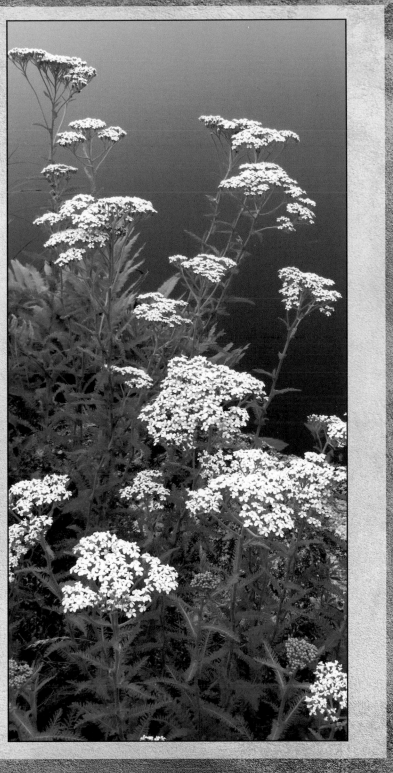

BOGBEAN
Menyanthes trifoliata

Misty Great Britain and Scotland are shrouded with water: bogs, springs, rivulets, and dells, and this abundance of water seeps into healing folklore. People suffering aches and pains often blame their symptoms on rain or simply the thought of a thunderstorm.

Ancient Gaelic pharmacists used the ten-inch-high creeper bogbean to relieve these symptoms. "In very damp and boggy areas—of which there are a lot in the Highlands of Scotland," Mary Beith said, "people used bog bean, or bog trefoil, for a variety of purposes. In the islands, a highly esteemed (but rather nasty-tasting) tonic is still made from the plant." Bitter and diuretic, the leaves and roots of marsh trefoil or water shamrock, as it was fondly called, contain bitter glycosides, alkaloids, flavonoids, and essential oil.

Gaelic healers used the Doctrine of Signatures to identify bogbean as a toxin remover, since its yellow fruit reflected the liver. They used bogbean in cases of jaundice, skin disease, and "gouty rheumatism," as pharmacist Ben Charles Harris describes it. Welsh herbalist David Hoffmann characterizes bogbean tea or tincture as "a most useful herb for the treatment of rheumatism, arthritis, and rheumatoid arthritis," saying it stimulates the digestive tract to produce bile.

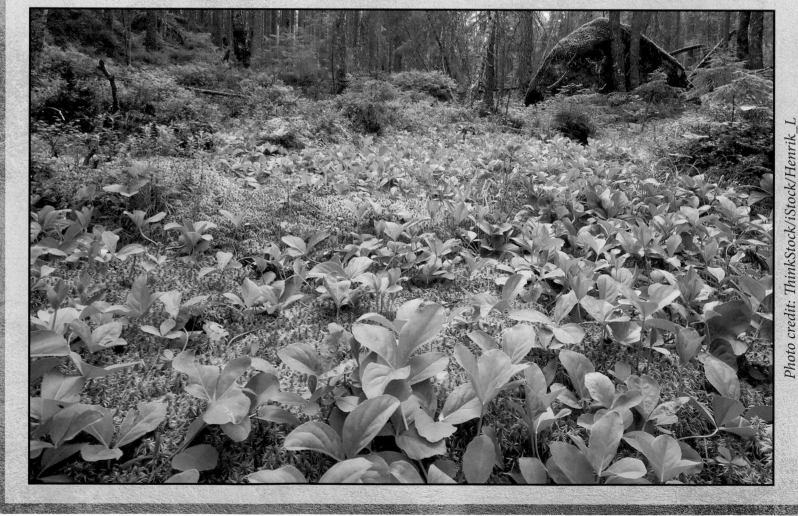

Photo credit: ThinkStock/iStock/Henrik_L

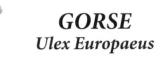

GORSE
Ulex Europaeus

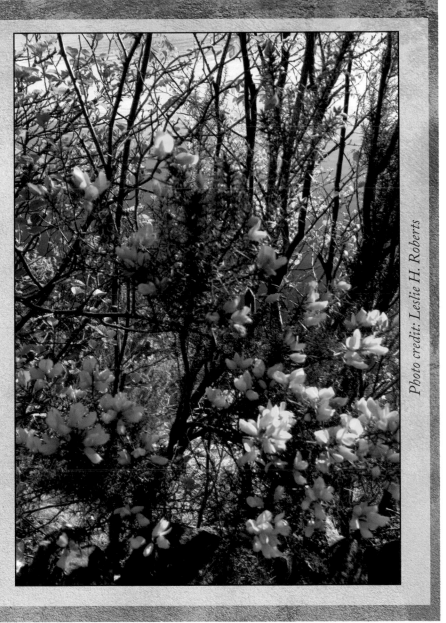

This spiny, dominating shrub is a common sight in heathlands across Great Britain, showing its bright yellow blossoms in dense growths that make perfect small mammal and bird habitat. Gorse, also called broom, whin or furze, this prickly evergreen wild edible produces small buds that make tasty snacks but had few medicinal uses in the Scottish Highlands. Rather, it was important in other pragmatic ways: as a source of fuel, burning hot; as a wine-making ingredient (the perfumy flowers were harvested and fermented into floral wines); in cloth dyeing, gardening, and mite control; and even, according to Pliny, used to collect golddust in the water during gold collection.

Medicinally, the herb seems to have been used as a second-rate plant to resort to when other options are unavailable; *A Modern Herbal* by Mrs. Maude Grieve lists some of the herb's uses as jaundice (likely because of the Doctrine of Signatures); kidney stones; diarrhea; and because of the seeds' alkaloid Ulexine, an obscure use in dropsy.

Photo credit: Leslie H. Roberts

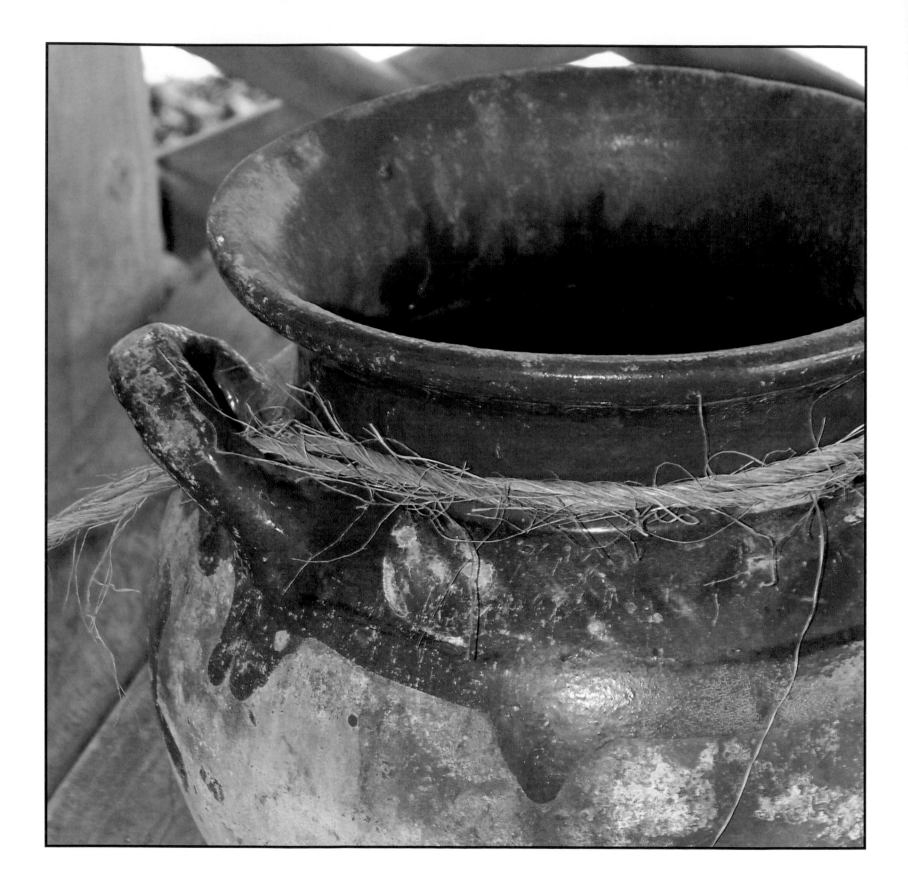

Chapter 14

SHAMANISM AND SPIRIT MEDICINE

To the western medical practitioner, shamanism can seem remote, esoteric, and perhaps even irrelevant. After all, it has nothing to do with pharmaceuticals, surgery, sterilization, or scientific research. Yet shamanism is an ancient and robust form of medical practice very much in use in many parts of the world. Shamans are considered wise intermediaries between the physical and spiritual worlds and, as such, they can access information not available to others. Often considered healers, shamans treat not the physical symptoms of disease but instead focus on the supernatural and spiritual dimensions to address the perceived cause of disease—a source of illness often neglected by allopathic medicine.

Originating in Siberia, the term *shaman* refers to the practitioners of a spiritual experience involving myth, dreamstates, and often the use of mind-altering plants. Ethnobotanists study shamanic medicine because these men and women are the keepers of herbal lore and magical wisdom and, by studying their practice of healing, ethnobotanists can more fully understand ancient cultures.

The difference between shamanic healing and folk healing (*see* Folk Healing, page 52). is that folk healing uses common materials such as foods and household objects to heal the symptoms of a physical ailment. Shamanism, on the other hand, ignores common objects and instead focuses on direct contact and communication with spiritual beings, dead ancestors, or departed shamans to reveal the source of evil that afflicted a person. Then the shaman can banish that evil or can instruct the victim's family in how to proceed with treatment.

Shamans mediate for others, intercepting knowledge sent from spiritual sources and communicating with spirits on behalf of sick individuals or even entire villages. Often considered the Medicine Man or Medicine Woman of the village, the shaman uses supernatural power to access a state of altered consciousness to discover evil influences.

Nearly every culture (European, Australian, Native American, Asian, and African) has some sort of shamanism, faith healing, magical healing, or witchcraft. These ancient, spirit-driven, non-allopathic forms of healing can generally be said to be spirit-based. For this reason, westerners are often uncomfortable with and poorly understand the function of the indigenous shaman, even though this type of healer has existed for millennia. Shamans and spiritual healers, however, serve pivotal roles in their societies, often acting as counsel in government decisions, medic in emergencies, priest in religious ceremonies, wise elder in family discourses, and as doctor.

A shaman is open to what is around her, sees with clarity, speaks with kindness and firm purpose, listens patiently, reveals for others that which they cannot—or do not wish—to see, recognizes and uses the depth of her own power and acts on it fearlessly, and opens others' consciousness to the Eternal. Shamanistic methods are included in a variety of healing traditions, including, as Doña Enriqueta Contreras confirmed, midwifery. "You cannot fend off forces that are invisible to us, that are in other dimensions," she says, without the strength and power of self-confidence—a vital characteristic of the healing shaman.

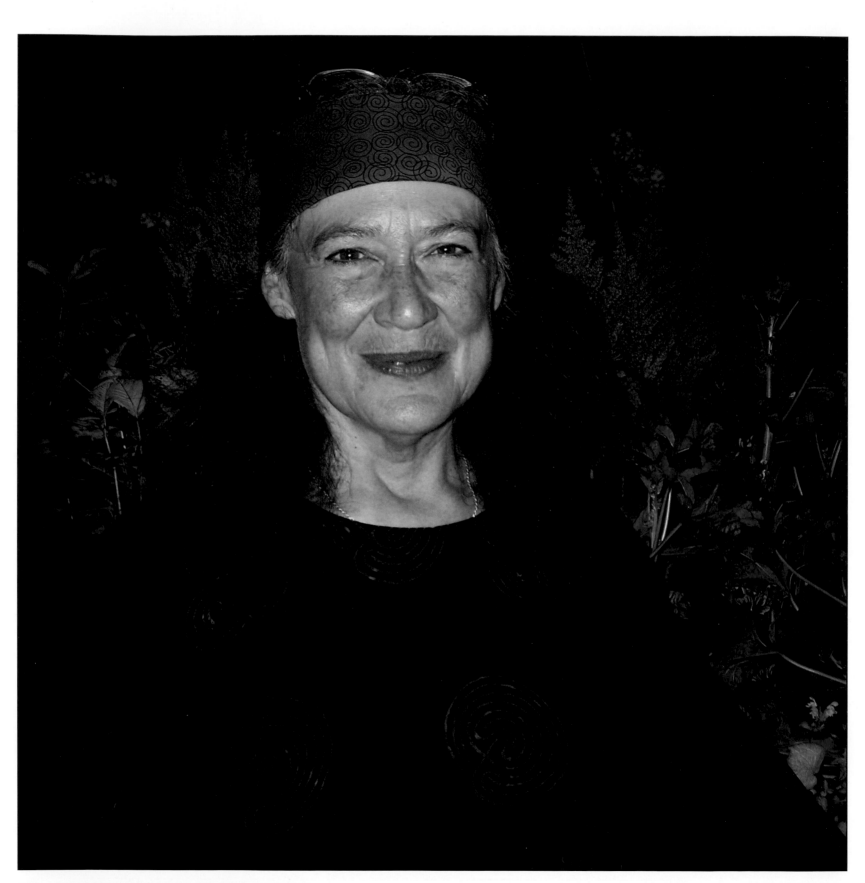

Susun Weed

Susun Weed's enthusiasm makes an impression on you: she's loud, she's smart, and she is spearheading what has become a back-to-the-roots movement in American herbalism. She could be classified as a pastoral herbalist (she raises a herd of goats and produces her own milk, cheese, yogurt, and meat), a chemist (she has painstakingly researched the mineral content of dozens of botanicals to accurately determine the best way to ingest the herbs), an advocate (she teaches at forums and conferences around the world and hosts a live-in apprenticeship program), and possibly a shaman. Susun lists herself as a Priestess of Dianic Wicca and as a Woman of Power she encourages students to find strength both within and outside the natural world of plants.

Appropriately, Susun's first memory was of the scent of lilacs. Born in February on the shores of Lake Erie, her mother took her as a newborn to visit friends and sat her down beside great blooming lilac bushes in April. "I've always connected with plants in a very personal way," Susun told me with a voice that can be breathy and reverent or vehement and forceful. "Plants have been present since the very beginning of my life." Her great-grandmother was her village's herbalist in Switzerland and her family prides itself on a long tradition of nurses and healers.

Her early years would not have suggested her life's passion: she grew up in Dallas, attended UCLA, majored in mathematics and artificial intelligence, was involved in the school newspaper, served as the local news anchor for the national television station at UCLA, and moved to Manhattan. But then—her world changed with the birth of her daughter Justine. She realized she wanted her daughter to spend as much time in nature as she could. "I wanted her to run around naked in the grass," she said, so, in 1968, Susun moved to an area near Woodstock where Justine could fully experience Nature on a broad scale—living, breathing, and harvesting Nature from their own forests and meadows. "How nice to experience our gorgeous planet by foraging from the land!" she recalls.

She coyly describes herself as "an ordinary sixties housewife" (anything but!) and shares that, through her interest in cooking, she learned about culinary herbs, and she planted an herb garden. "A lot of things grew in my herb garden," she says, "some of them might have even been herbs." She had no way of knowing which were her own plantings, however, because she scattered her seeds, and in the spring a whole variety of plants came up that had nothing to do with her. When she read Euell Gibbons's books *Stalking the Wild Asparagus*, *Stalking the Blue-Eyed Scallop*, and *Stalking the Healthful Herbs*, Susun realized the herbs she had planted were "lightweights" compared to the weeds already growing there. "Sure," she says,

"I planted basil and dill, nice and sweet culinary herbs, but right alongside of them grew dandelion and burdock and purslane and lamb's quarter and chickweed! I realized I didn't need to *plant* herbs, that I should have been saying, 'Wow, Nature, you rock!'" Her modest introduction to wild plants germinated into what would one day be a booming international educational venture to teach others the power of wild weeds.

> *"I planted basil and dill, nice and sweet culinary herbs, but right alongside of them grew dandelion and burdock and purslane and lamb's quarter and chickweed! I realized I didn't need to plant herbs, and that I should have been saying, 'Wow, Nature, you rock!'"*

Teaching a cooking class with whole wheat flour at a local community college was what she calls a "fertilizing event." Her course "The Best Bread You Ever Ate: Make It Yourself With Love" was a rebellious subject during the age of white bread and was an instant hit. She taught her students to make wheat flour loaves, rolls, pretzels, crackers, croissants, bagels, English muffins, and chocolate chip cookies, and then she met a woman who taught a course about herbal medicine. "We identified plants, picked plants, made things. We made one soup that turned out to be a great floor cleaner, and people stopped coming around to our houses at dinnertime for fear of what we were brewing." Her friend's fall class was a success, but in the spring she left, saying that Susun needed to teach the class instead. "I can't teach a class on herbal medicine!" Susun protested. "I don't have any degrees or diplomas." Her friend's sage advice: "You know as well as I do that all you need is passion."

She did teach the class, but the community college fired her. "I'd built my own house with hand tools and had no electricity. I heated with a wood stove and cooked with wood, and I had no phone. So they fired me." She rallied her students together and, in an epiphany, asked them to come to her house in the daytime. This novel method of education inspired her: "What a fool I've been! I can teach outside! Of course you have to teach outside."

She began working at a health food store and advised women to take exotic herbs such as dong quai, developing a following of women who relied on her for *Angelica archangelica*. But when the FDA declared Chinese herbs would no longer be available on the US market, her source dried up and her customers were upset, leading her to abandon exotic herbs and return to the roots of herbalism: local wild weeds. "And here I am," Susun laughs, "almost forty years later, still trying to figure out how to teach herbal medicine." Today, Susun is known internationally as the

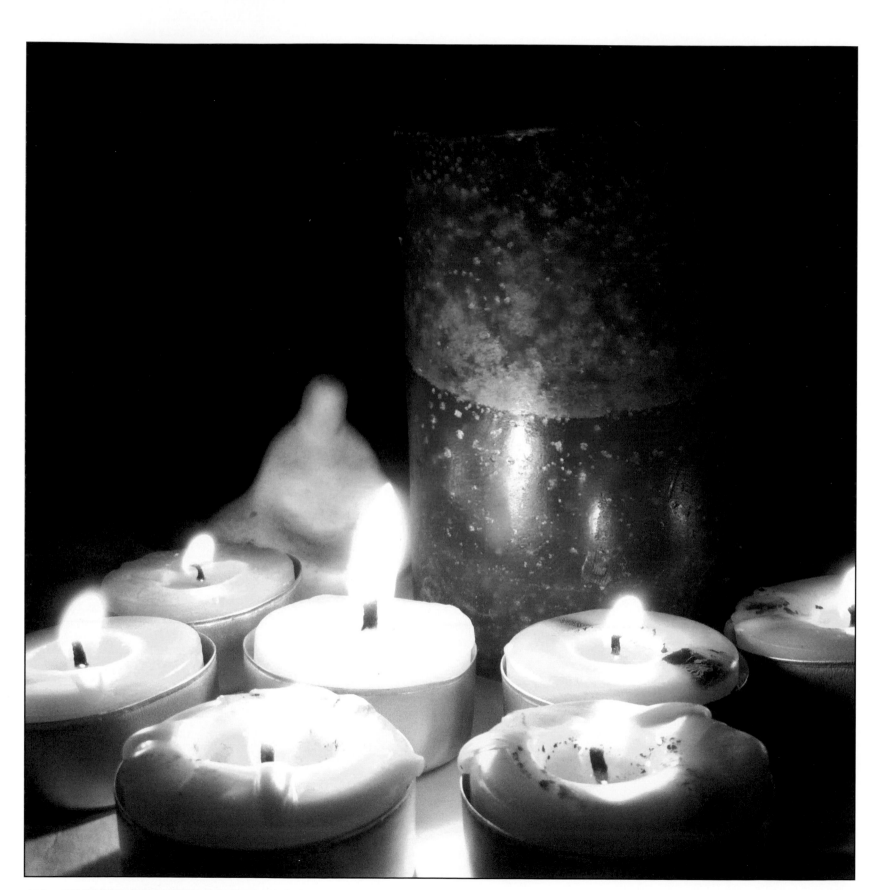

mother of the Wise Woman Tradition and a philosophy that encourages using weeds.

"It was a natural progression," she says, "because I was being mentored by the plants themselves." Hearing laughter outside one day, Susun realized the plants were laughing at her, which was novel enough. But they were laughing at humanity's notion that people learn to use plants through trial and error. In fact, they revealed to her, people learn to use plants by listening to the plants. Susun began to see herself as a simpler. In herbal tradition, a simple is a liquid extract of one individual herb; a compound is an extract of two or more herbs. Susun pledged to use only one herb at a time—a philosophy that honors a reciprocal give-and-take relationship with each plant. "I could learn about their many skills and powers and use them, thereby I could really return to the roots of herbal medicine as people's medicine. It is not a medicine of the elite, but a medicine of the people."

By listening to the plants, Susun drew the uncertainty of other herbalists who claimed it was embarrassing to listen and talk to plants. When she published *Healing Wise* in 1989, fellow herbalists were hesitant to accept her methods. "You'll embarrass yourself and you'll embarrass us," many told her, afraid of the intellectual repercussions from the medical community and elsewhere. But her methodology is now accepted in alternative healing, and she learned firsthand the specific traits of plants that would later become "common" knowledge in herbal medicine.

Take St. John's wort. Since the mid-1990s, *Hypericum perforatum* was used as an antidepressant. Historically, she says, herbals listed it as a vulnerary for treating wounds and even twenty-five years ago, books listed it as *increasing* depression. Susun listened to the plant instead of the books and pioneered the use of *Hypericum* for people who are despondent or affected by Seasonal Affective Disorder. "It's so full of light," she says.

> *"I could learn about their many skills and powers and use them, thereby I could really return to the roots of herbal medicine as people's medicine. It is not a medicine of the elite, but a medicine of the people."*

She calls her tradition the Wise Woman Tradition, and it involves nourishing in an ever-changing spiral. "Many herbalists I know in the United States, Europe, and throughout the world practice the Heroic tradition: poking, puking, purging, and using powerful herbs like cayenne and goldenseal. They use the strongest and most powerful herbs, saying that if it doesn't hurt or taste bad then you aren't doing enough! It's the cleansing crisis, and the Wise

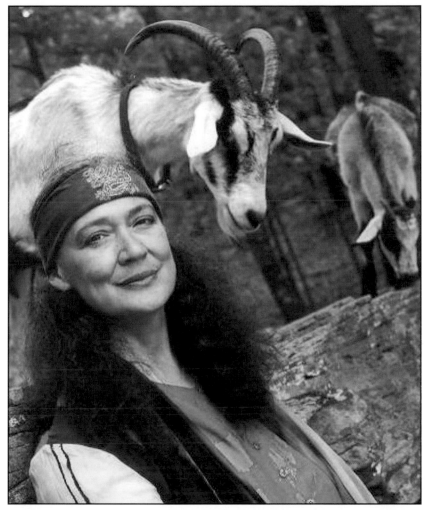

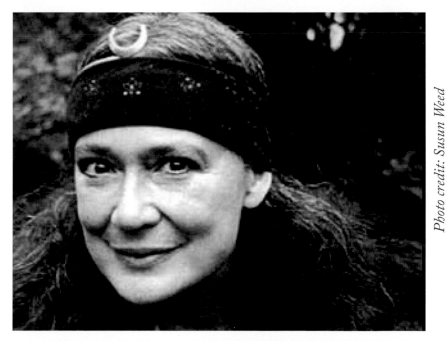

Photo credit: Susun Weed

Photo credit: Susun Weed

Woman Tradition is the direct opposite of that. We are not filled with toxins. Nourishing is what we need and what the planet needs right now. Everything is something else's food. Nothing is waste in nature, nothing is toxic in nature, everything is food. The Wise Woman Tradition is based on nourishment. Nature's way is I eat you and you eat me. I breathe out and the plants breathe in, the plants breathe out and I breathe in. It's a give-away dance. And when I call something dirt and try to throw it away, then I'm taking it out of the dance. In a way I'm stealing it. Be a real citizen of Nature and learn to speak nature's language. I've done my best to live my life by learning from the book of nature, by spending as much time outdoors as I possibly can."

WITCH

The Proto-Indo-European (PIE) word *weg* meant "to be strong or lively," leading to *vegetable* (see Vegetable sidebar) and possibly *wicce*, Old English for "female magician or sorceress." The herbs *Viburnum* and *Verbena* may share etymology with the ancient *witch*.

Gothic *weihs* meant "holy" and German *weihan* "consecrate." The PIE *wid* meant "to see, know, or understand" and lead to our *wisdom* and *vision*. In 1584, Reginald Scot wrote "The Discoverie of Witchcraft" noting with malice, "At this day it is indifferent to say in the English tongue, 'she is a witch,' or 'she is a wise woman.'" This was forty-two years after witchcraft was first criminalized in England; trials lasted almost two centuries and the Witchcraft Act was finally repealed in 1736. It seems *wid* was a predecessor of *wicca* and *witch*. Witch hazel was named in 1541 (the year before official witch persecution commenced), possibly stemming from Old English *wice*, "wych-elm" from *wican*, "to bend."

WITCH HAZEL
Hamamelis virginiana

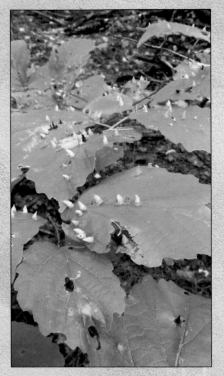

With its curious pointed witch-shaped hats growing on top of its leaves, witch hazel seems to have been named with a straight-forward meaning. But it may not be as simple as that. While the pointed hat-shaped structures atop the leaves, called cone galls, are actually the gall produced by the tiny aphid *Hormaphis hamamelidis*, folklore may have given it the moniker "witch" based on any of a number of stories: the branches have been used for seemingly magical divining; or the slender tree produces flowers only in the winter—distinctly different from any other Eastern United States deciduous tree; or the ear-catching pop as seedpods burst from the branches in the dead of winter sounds ominously like elven-work.

Regardless how it came by the name, witch hazel is a favorite small tree of the woodlands because it is prized for its astringent tannins, gallic acids, and flavonols. Herbalists use the twigs, branches, bark, and leaves of the tree to create rinses and liniments for weepy and oozy sores, both internally and externally. Since Native Americans first used it for swellings and inflammation, it has long been a favorite remedy for hemorrhoids, external infection, poison ivy, acne, and other blisters, and it is even suitable for internal use—but only when it is homemade in the kitchen. The reason? Distilled witch hazel sold at pharmacies always contains 14 percent isopropyl alcohol as a preservative whereas pure water extracts (infusions or decoctions) are safe in small amounts for internal issues such as diarrhea.

MULLEIN
Verbascum thapsus

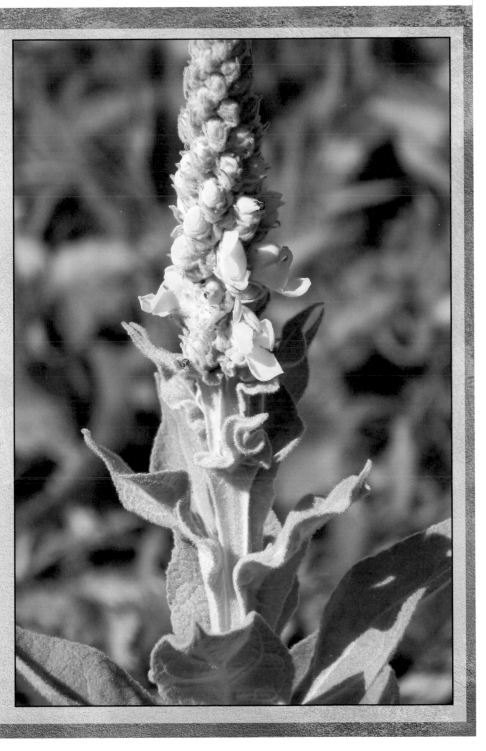

Fuzzy and soft, flannel-leaf or mullein leaves have long delighted children—and they've also delighted their parents who rely on mullein as a gentle and safe remedy for a list of upper and lower respiratory ailments. Coughs, especially, are eased with mullein infusion or tincture, since mullein acts as a gentle antispasmodic and expectorant.

Though native to Europe and Asia, mullein arrived early in North America and native nations began using leaf for cough, lung trouble, and catarrh. The Abnaki made necklaces of the chopped roots that were worn by teething babies, and the Atsugewi pounded the leaves into a poultice for wounds and decocted the leaves for colds.

The polysaccharide-rich flower is commonly used in folk medicine in combination with St. John's wort and garlic for ear infections.

Bernadette Rébiénot

When Bernadette Rébiénot was a child of five years, living on the western coast of Equatorial Gabon, Africa, she was separated from her peers by an occurrence that few children have: she had a vision—what many of us would term an other-worldly experience—that would certainly frighten most five-year-olds. But the vision prepared her in some mystical way for an illness that would strike her later in her youth. For four grueling years, Bernadette suffered a long illness that stole her health (including, temporarily, her eyesight) but which ultimately revealed her life's calling. During her illness, the village doctors were unable to cure her, so young Bernadette's family traveled with her to visit a Pygmy healer near Libreville in the Omyéné linguisitic community of Gabon. The Pygmy master cured Bernadette, but even more importantly he recognized her innate healing abilities and that she would one day be a skilled shaman. He directed her on a lifelong path as a medicine woman.

Bernadette was never officially schooled as a healer. Instead, she possesses that rare innate ability to infer a person's illness and bring relief. When I asked her about this ability, for which she is renowned throughout Gabon, she answered matter-of-factly with great deference to external (often spiritual) forces. In regard to her healing abilities and her use of plants, for example, she said simply that they are a natural gift, adding that "much of my knowledge of traditional medicine was passed on through dreams." Trance states and "alternate" realities, in addition to village teachers, form much of Bernadette's knowledge of shamanic healing, and these are sources of wisdom she taps with great respect.

"At the beginning of my career to heal with plants, my teachers helped me," she says. "But often there were trances that dictated herbal treatment for the healing of sicknesses." After displaying her early talent for spiritual perception, she was formally introduced to Gabonese and African healing traditions at age fourteen, and her grandmother, who became one of her most influential teachers, shared her extensive plant-based knowledge. "In my family," she says, "there is a heredity linked to the plant medicine." In other words, the healing talent is partly genetic and partly cultural, passed down from the women in her family to their daughters and granddaughters.

Bernadette—a tall woman with a round face, a rich, soothing French voice, and brightly colored floor-length traditional African garb—is proud to contribute to the health of her fellow Gabonese through herbal medicine. "Currently," she says, "I work in my country. But I can bring my knowledge to people who ask me everywhere." She is revered in Gabon, where elder men and women are valued for their wisdom and decision-making. In addition to her role as a village elder, Bernadette is a master of the Iboga Bwiti Rites and the Women's Initiations.

The Bwiti religion is a synchretic (blended) religion of African mythology and Christianity, where initiates enter trance states after consuming the powdered root bark of the Iboga tree. Iboga is central to the culture's heritage and is used not only in ritual and ceremony but also, for example, when embarking on a hunting trip or beginning any arduous work, as it is sustaining and energizing (see Iboga sidebar on page 203).

"The most beautiful experience of my life," she says, "the most enriching, is the love that the plants have taught me. To love one's neighbor is to care for them, to attend to their suffering and restore their joy of living. Restoring health is the most essential thing in life."

Formulas for Healing

Bernadette, who has served as the president of the Association of Traditional Medicine Practitioners for Gabonese Health for more than a decade, told me the most difficult thing for her in her work with plants was first recognizing a plant's healing virtues and then retaining them. She was taught that plants are classified into three categories: The first is comprised of healing plants that treat natural diseases such as cough and infertility. The second is made of plants related to spirituality, and the third consists of very sacred plants such as iboga. She notes that the methods of care vary depending on a person's disease.

For instance, Bernadette teaches that there are three forms of illness: "natural illness, supernatural disease, and spiritual disease." In the first case, treatment may be oral (an infusion or a decoction) or through bleeding, inhalation, skin application, washing, or

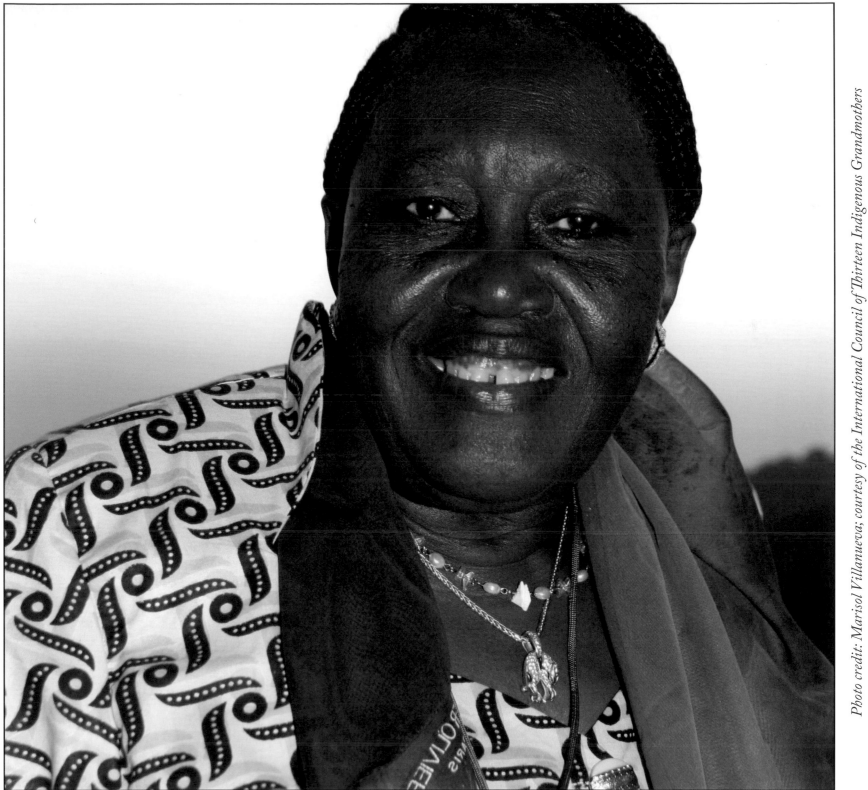

Photo credit: Marisol Villanueva; courtesy of the International Council of Thirteen Indigenous Grandmothers

SPIRIT TRADITIONS   197

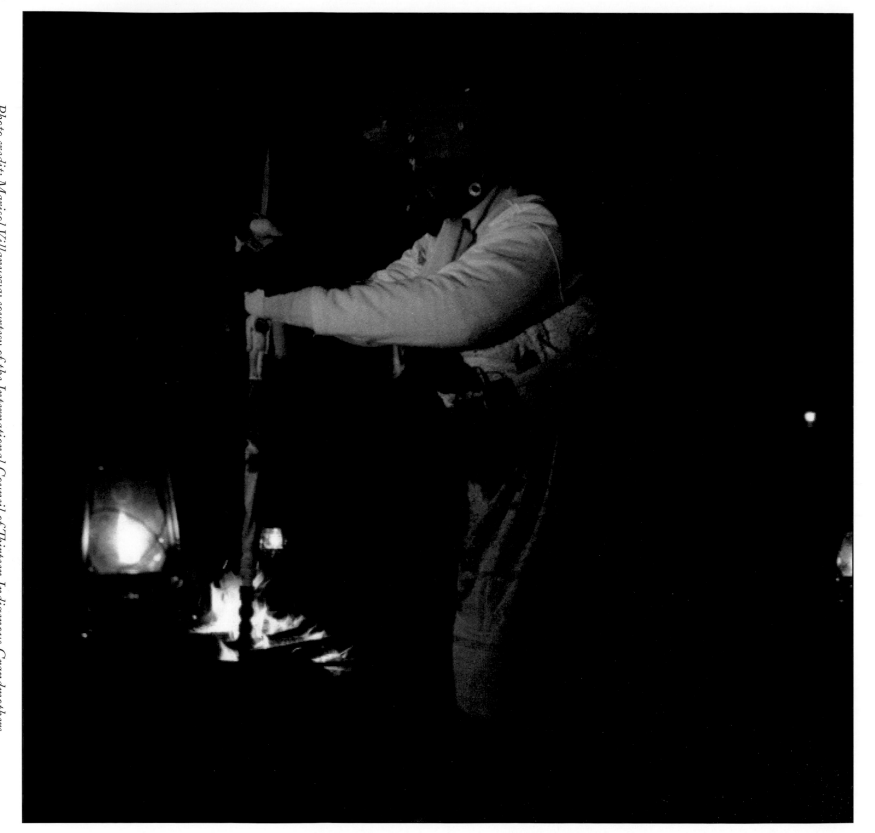

enemas. If these treatments are unsuccessful, Bernadette follows a prescription that takes into account locale, bringing her patient out of the home (or clinic), and placing him or her directly in the forest, under the trees, and in the elements where the person can feel, smell, and hear the forest. She advises "treatment with plants in the forest: steam baths with plants, bathing under a tree, or washing in a river." She'll offer the patient steaming cups of fragrant tea while sheltered beneath the trees, a lovely healing experience that many indigenous cultures remember but "civilized" people have forgotten. In the third case of spiritual disease, treatment (initiation) is offered with the help of sacred plants.

"The most beautiful experience of my life," she says, "the most enriching, is the love that the plants have taught me. To love one's neighbor is to care for them, to attend to their suffering and restore their joy of living. Restoring health is the most essential thing in life."

Bernadette's grandmother reinforced these philosophies of love and service during her youth, teaching Bernadette the special qualities that plants can add to human existence. "My grandmother, in passing to me her ancestral knowledge related to plants, told me it is necessary to respect nature. The stars, like the plants, have life. They talk to us, they can also listen to us, and we can learn many interesting things necessary for humanity. So," Bernadette says, "I'm very in love with nature, especially with forests."

No longer a child of five or fourteen, Bernadette is a wise elder who helped form the International Council of Thirteen Indigenous Grandmothers in 2004, a phenomenal group of women from around the world who convene regularly to offer prayers, wisdom, and direction. The Grandmother's Council members "come together to uphold the practice of our ceremonies and affirm the right to use our plant medicines free of legal restriction. We come together to protect the lands where our peoples live and upon which our cultures depend, to safeguard the collective heritage of traditional medicines, and to defend the earth Herself." Thanks to their efforts and the nonprofit organization Native Village, these remarkable women now travel the world, sharing their experiences and advice with young healers, diplomats, and politicians.

"My grandmother, in passing to me her ancestral knowledge related to plants, told me: it is necessary to respect nature. The stars, like the plants, have life. They talk to us, they can also listen to us and we can learn many interesting things necessary for humanity. So I'm very in love with nature, especially forests."

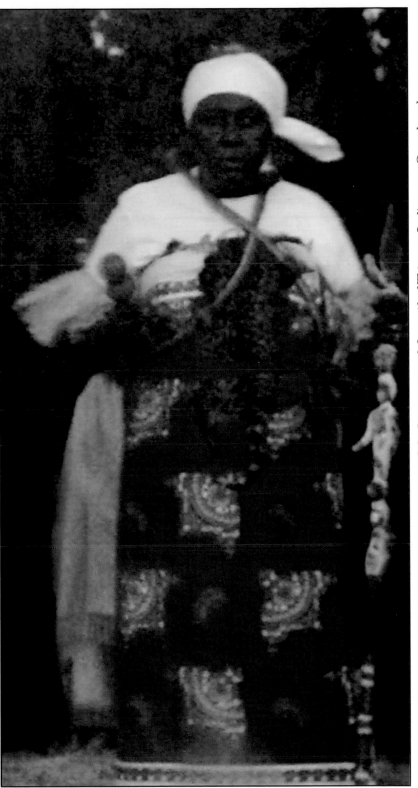

Photo credit: Marisol Villanueva courtesy of the International Council of Thirteen Indigenous Grandmothers

CHICORY AND SUCCOR

In summer, chicory *(Cichorium endiva)* blooms alongside Queen Anne's Lace, dotting roadsides with bright blue blossoms. Except for its roasted root (for a coffee substitute), chicory is generally ignored, but the plant is actually an ancient remedy esteemed as a nutritious edible, a liver tonic, and an emmenagogue.

In biblical times, *chickoryeh* was a salad herb and a cleansing bitter, and according to *A City Herbal* author Maida Silverman, chicory is still included in the traditional Jewish Seder at Passover for its bitterness. The bitter qualities convinced seventeenth-century healers to use it to "cool the heat of the liver."

In the ancient Proto-Indo-European language, *kers* meant "to run" (consider Lithuanian *karsiu* "go quickly"; Old Norse *horskr* "swift"; Middle Welsh *carr* "cart, wagon"). Latin used *kers* to create *currere*, "to run." (Later, this would give way to *current*—of both water and electricity.) *Succurrere* meant "run to help" from *sub* "up to" and *currere* "to run." Anglo French speakers shortened this to *succors*, or succor, the act of healing and giving assistance. The juices of succory would run to the aid of the person who needed them, especially nursing mothers who applied the juice of the crushed herb to their breasts to heal mastitis and sore nipples.

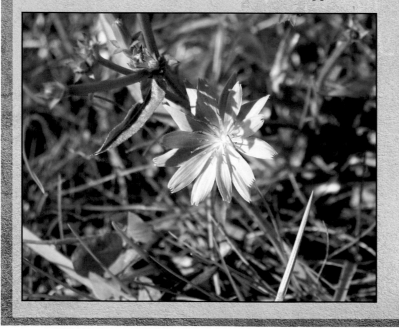

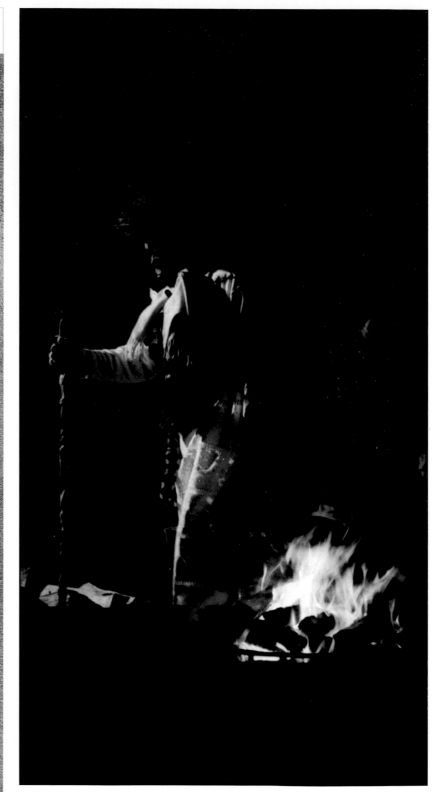

Photo credit: Marisol Villaneuva; courtesy of the International Council of Thirteen Indigenous Grandmothers

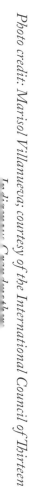

Photo credit: Marisol Villanueva; courtesy of the International Council of Thirteen

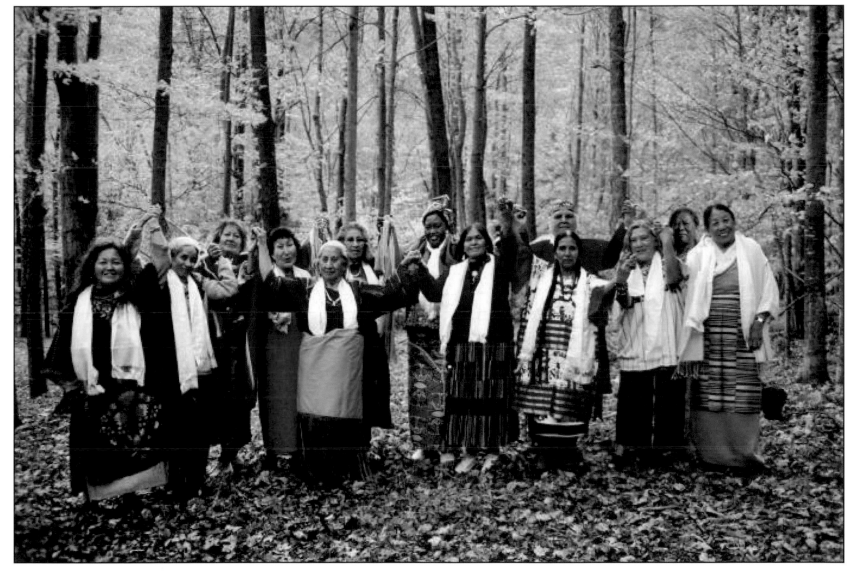

GABON, AFRICA

Nearly bisected by the equator, Gabon is a country of heat and rain, lush green forests, and miles of waterways. The nearly 1.4 million people of Gabon depend on the River Ogooué as transportation to and from the port of Libreville. The wet, hot equatorial jungles provide Gabon exportable resources: sleek mahogany, ebony, and iron. Bordered by Equatorial Guinea, Cameroon, the Congo, and the Atlantic Ocean, Gabon was a French colony before it became an independent republic in 1960, and its official language is French.

Farmers in Gabon harvest many crops, especially the root vegetable cassava, ground nuts and yams, and they export cacao and coffee for the world market.

Grandmother Bernadette Rébiénot's people are the Omyéné, who live along the coast and were the first residents to meet Portuguese sailors, missionaries, and European traders. Other ethnic groups include the Fang, who live in northern and central Gabon, and the Pygmies, who live in the southern forest. Gabonese people are intensely religious, encompassing a variety of beliefs, primarily Christian, animist, and Islamic.

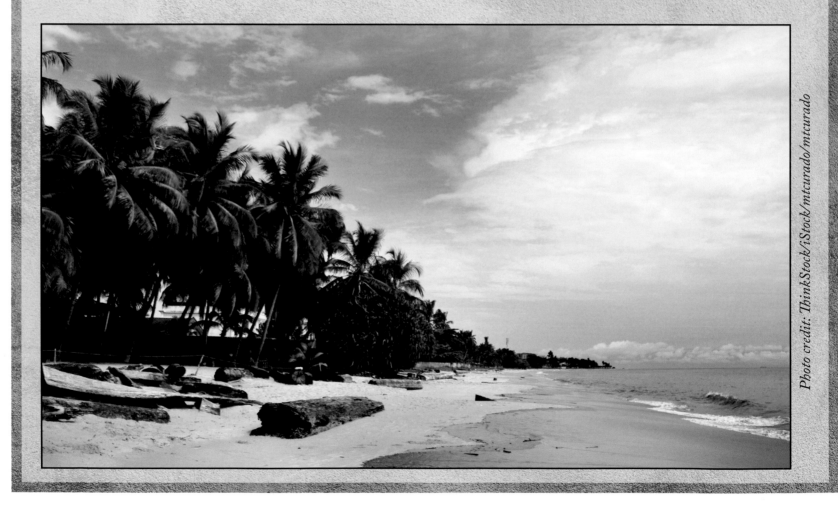

Photo credit: ThinkStock/iStock/mtcurado/mtcurado

IBOGA
Tabernanthe iboga

Iboga is a perennial small tree of the central western African rainforest. Called iboga, eboga, and eboka, its lovely dangling yellow or orange smooth fruits resemble lanterns or long chili peppers. In Gabon, Iboga is used in small doses to resist fatigue and stay alert and is often consumed before hunting trips.

But iboga is also a powerful hallucinogen. Bernadette Rébiénot treasures Iboga for its ritual use in the Equatorial African Bwiti religion, a synchretic religion of Christianity and ancestor worship historically condemned by Catholic missionaries. The root bark is consumed in large doses (as tea or scrapings) by initiates to the religion in Gabon, Cameroon, Zaire, and the Republic of the Congo.

Initiates are given large doses of powdered alkaloid-rich Iboga root bark to stimulate visions. The "father and mother of eboga"—the *essa eboga* and *nyia eboga*—care for each initiate to guard against overdose since more than thirty doses of the powder may be consumed in one night. Though Iboga produces visions, numbs the mouth and skin, and causes vomiting, its spiritual effects are prized: Iboga is believed to loosen the skin so the soul can escape to the spirit world.

Some scholars claim Iboga is the Biblical Tree of Good and Evil as well as the Tree of Life, and indeed, in Bwiti's rituals, the Iboga is respected as if it were the host in a Catholic mass. Renunciation of sins is part of the Bwiti Iboga ritual and many ceremonies take place on Christian holidays.

Under constant scrutiny and the subject of much debate, Iboga was declared a national treasure by the Republic of Gabon in 2000. Clinically, the fragrant alkaloid *ibogaine* in the root bark is under research to combat chemical addictions (particularly to opium, heroine, and alcohol), and the drug is being used in clinical experiments in several countries including Holland.

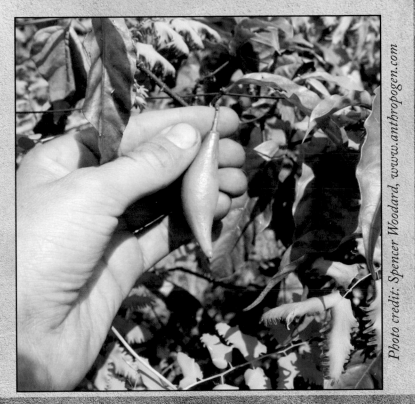

Photo credit: Spencer Woodard, www.anthropogen.com

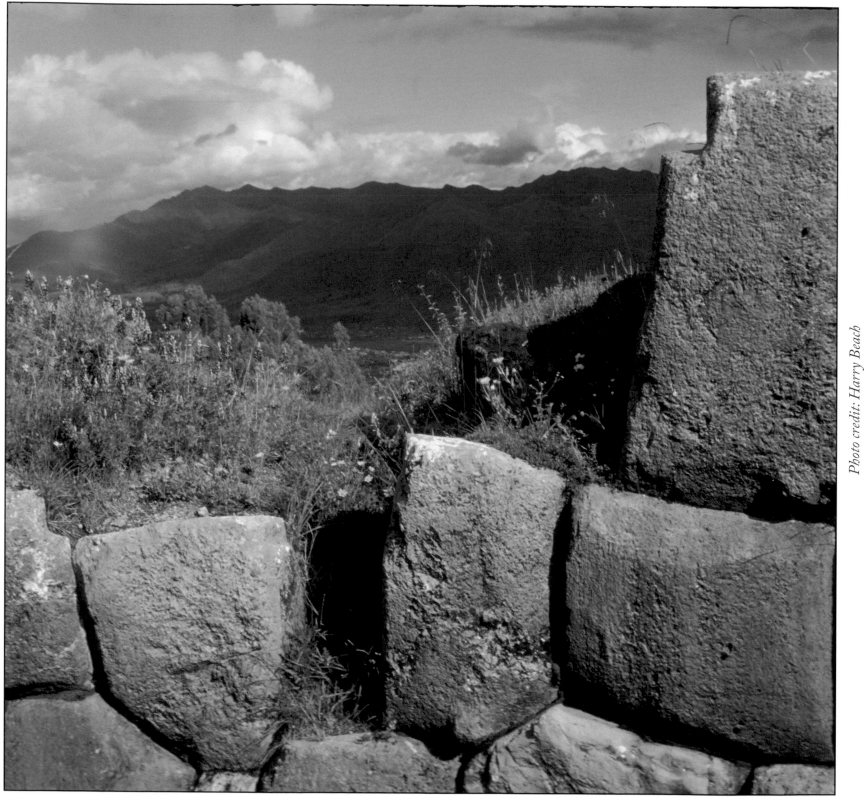

Cusco rock wall

PART IV:
LAND TRADITIONS

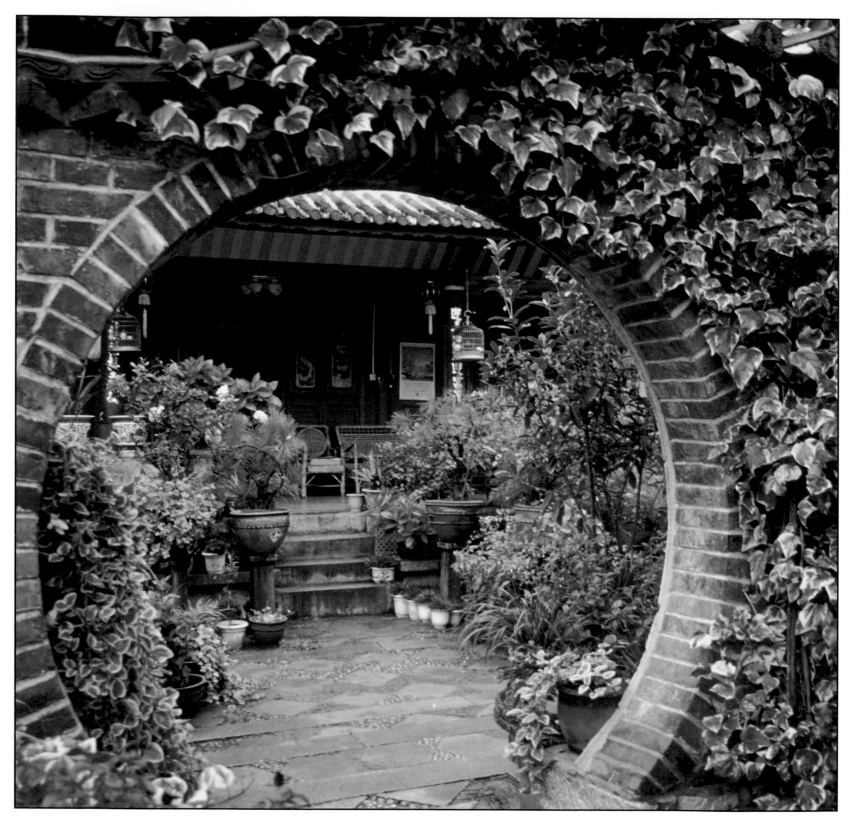

Chapter 15

CONSERVATION AND GARDENING

Our fascination with plants has evolved over the millennia from distant observation and appreciation to a very hands-on practice of manipulation. As a species, we've gone from collective awe and wonder at the marvels of a flower to the commercial exploitation of entire forestlands for individual gain. But it hasn't all been for personal profit; over time, we've gradually grown to understand that our responsibility as a species includes the protection of animals and plants that can't protect themselves.

Conservation in England and Europe was really about replication, with many botanical and research gardens situated in monasteries and in universities by the 1540s. Once new lands were discovered, especially America and Australia, British explorers were quick to identify new plants. In Virginia and the new colonies, for example, botanists and Jesuit priests alike trekked through the forests to gather samples of (or entire crops of) new and interesting plants, including ginseng, bee balm, sassafras, redbud, bloodroot, and tobacco. The most well-known Colonial explorers include John Bartram, whom Linnaeus described as "the greatest natural botanist in the world." Bartram managed to scratch his way into nearly every mountainside and holler from Canada to Florida, in the process collecting plant samples and sending many of them to England. Bartram established what is considered America's first botanical garden near Philadelphia. His son, William Bartram, who had traveled with his father as a child and teenager, struck out on his own, heading south through rugged and isolated lands and recording his journey with more of an artistic perspective, recounting the virtues of plants, vistas and native people through poetry, artwork, and wildly popular and appealing travel books. Other names in the annals of colonial botany include Clayton,

Collinson, Fothergill, Michaux, and even Thomas Jefferson and George Washington.

The people who have gone furthest into the study of plant species tend to be called explorers, botanists, taxonomists, and adventurers of some sort or another. They are sometimes hailed as risk-taking heroes, such as David Burton and Ebenezer Flint, who suffered violent deaths during the course of their explorations in Australia in 1792 and 1874, respectively. Or they are portrayed as stoic or eccentric travelers, such as Asa Gray in the Appalachian Mountains, who traversed insane distances and rugged terrain to explore the deep wilderness and, by collecting samples for herbaria, to provide for those left "back in the city" with a sense of the wonder to be found in the wild.

It's also vital to recognize that all of the names mentioned so far have been men's; women were generally excluded from the annals of history that celebrate human achievement, and usually excluded from lists of botanists or explorers with only a few exceptions primarily for gardeners. For example, Lady Skipwith (d. 1826) is mentioned in Raymond Taylor's *Plants of Colonial Days*, and Philip Short's *In Pursuit of Plants*[1] briefly mentions two women named Marianne North and Ellis Rowan. But Short states that "the fact that only one woman is included in this compilation . . . is primarily due to the fact that the social constraints of the time did not permit women to travel widely, at least not by themselves. Furthermore, married women, often with large families to care for, had limited opportunities even to step out into the local bush and spend time collecting." Women botanists were few and far between; he states that for those born before 1901 in Australia, for every woman there were at least seven men who had collected herbarium specimens.[2]

Conservation or Collection?

Most botanical exploration was for the express purpose of cataloguing species for the new herbaria, the first of which was established in 1570 in Bologna, Italy. And since England's William Withering published the cardiac benefits of foxglove in the late eighteenth century, plant collectors and ethnobotanists have been keenly interested in herbs for medicinal benefit. Later, with the advance of preservation methods of fresh plants, many leaves, flowers, and roots became destined for experimentation in laboratories for the distinct purpose of entering the world medicine supply.

Though their motives may have been noble and their focus on the betterment of their communities, it's key to recognize that the botanists' goals were generally to collect, exploit, and remove plants. Exploration was by and large a commercial endeavor. Nowhere do we find conservation of precious lands and species as a priority until the mid-1800s, when sportsmen advocated for wildlife conservation and advocates such as John Muir worked tirelessly to protect the wilderness of Yosemite and other vast tracts of US lands. Until this time, wilderness held no intrinsic value; rather all plants and animals were deemed "resources" and were available for the taking.

The idea of conservation didn't take hold until US President Ulysses S. Grant and the US Congress created Yellowstone National Park in 1872; the National Park Service would not be created to manage such parks, however, for another forty-four years. These giant land provisions protected large swaths of land, but plants—especially threatened and endangered wild plants—would not find individual protection until 1973 with the establishment of the Convention on International Trade in Endangered Species of Wild Fauna and Flora (CITES).

But even CITES is not the complete answer to plant protection; it governs international trade, largely ignoring domestic use and abuse of plants through cultivation, farming, development, and harvest. United Plant Savers' Richard Liebmann says that in the year 2000, roughly 34,000 plant species (12 percent of plants worldwide and 29 percent of plants in the United States) were "so rare that they could easily disappear."[3] These include edibles, medicinals, wildflowers, and trees, and the United States is not alone—countries from China to India to Europe to Tibet are experiencing firsthand the crushing loss of native edible and medicinal plants.

Conservation at the local levels must be a priority to protect these important plants from extinction. Thousands of garden clubs have sprung up in the past few decades, usually "manned" by women who enjoy their gardens, preserve the food they grow, make medicines from their herbs, and learn and teach on a domestic scale about plants. Hundreds of herbalists have also taken up the call to learn about and protect the green medicines that grow both in our cultivated gardens and also in the wild places typically beyond our reach. Herbalists discuss the benefits and downsides to wildcrafting, with some calling for limits to the numbers of plants collected and others decrying limits but agreeing that wildcrafting needs to be done honorably and ethically. Ginseng growers report their "secret" crop has been discovered and unearthed; herbalists frequently return to their favorite wild herb patches only to find a smaller population than the year before. Local logging and building development plays a huge role in the quick decline of native plants, and thankfully many community planning boards have implemented policies designed to protect sensitive plant systems before building begins, but it is not foolproof.

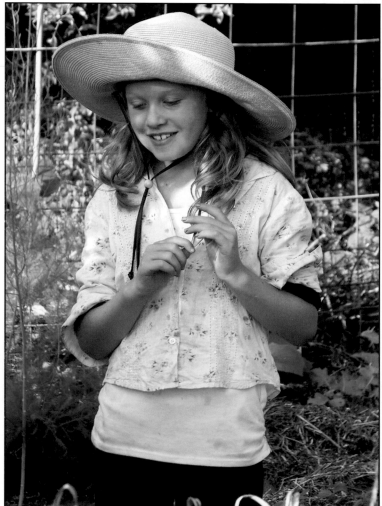

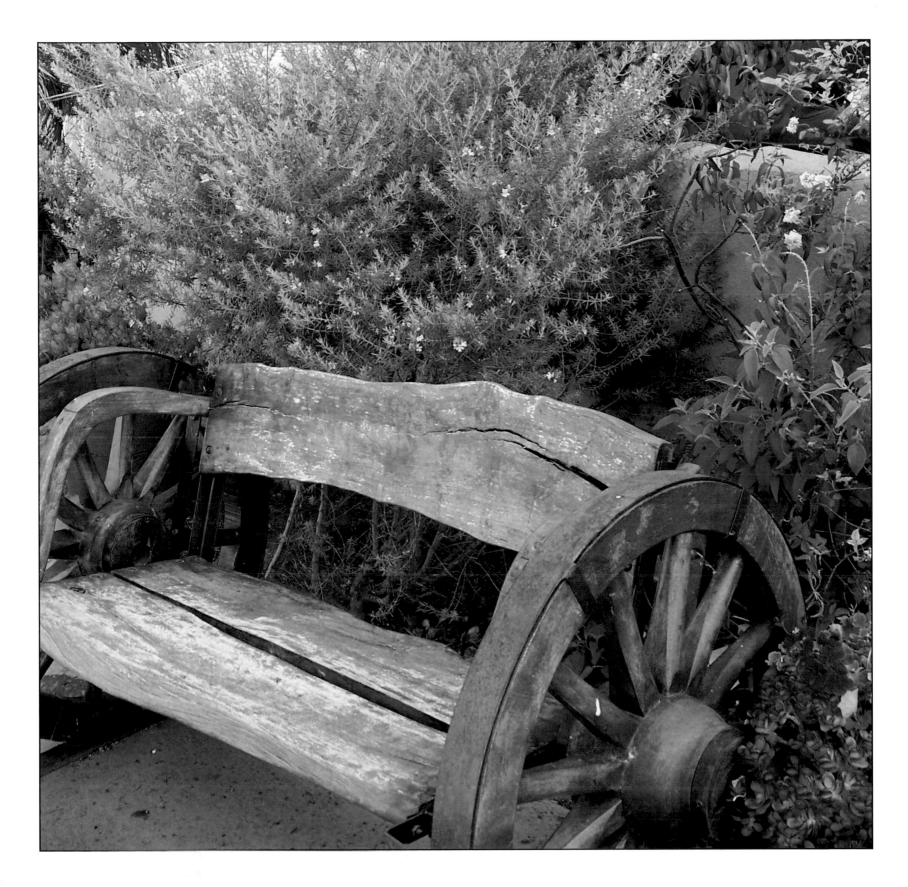

Hatshepsut

(1508 BCE–1458 BCE)

Not content to rule as Queen (and certainly not as regent for her brother or son), Hatshepsut ruled Thebes, Egypt, as a mighty Pharaoh. She was called God's Wife, High Priestess of Amun, and Maat-ka-Ra, names that proclaimed her high status to a country traditionally accustomed to male power-keepers. Gaining authority after the death of her brothers and father, Hatshepsut reigned from 1479 BCE to 1458, presiding more than twenty-one years of peace and prosperity.

Hatshepsut achieved startling results in that time. She is said to have governed her Navy by ordering them to re-open an ancient canal from the Nile River all the way to the Red Sea (near the current Suez Canal), enabling new transportation and exploration. She oversaw the construction of shrines and obelisks, and she ordered the repair of temples. She continued the worship of Hathor and Amun at her temple Djeser-Djeseru (Holiest of the Holy), designing beautiful gardens, fountains, and shrines that flourished in the hot Egyptian desert. Centuries later, her temple was renamed Deir al-Bahari, Monastery of the North, after a Coptic monastery used the site. The original Temple shows evidence of plant worship and plant ritual, with remnants of a grove of trees in the lower court and pools that may have held holy water or sacred milk for Hathor, Cow Goddess of Fertility.

Under Hatshepsut's rule, Egypt exported linen, wheat, and papyrus and imported cedar from Lebanon and ebony from the Sudan. Her most famous act as pharaoh involved international trade and transport: she commanded a three-year expedition to the mysterious land of Punt (possibly Somalia on Africa's eastern coast) to bring back nearly three dozen myrrh trees with roped root balls; the fragrant resin exuded from their trunks would be burned in her temples. She gained fame for sending her naval ships down the Red Sea to Punt in about 1470 BCE to return with spectacular cargoes of elephant ivory, gold ingots, electrum (a naturally occurring alloy of gold and silver), aromatic woods for perfumery, cosmetics, ostrich feathers, leopard skins, baboons, dogs, and even live natives of Punt (their fate remains a mystery). Her scribes recorded the marvelous expedition and all of its bounty in carefully etched bas-reliefs on the temple walls at Thebes.

Hatshepsut is said to have received "daily massages with scented oils," and an inscription on a monument poetically claims "her fragrance was like a divine breath, her scent reached as far as the land of Punt." But she portrayed herself in a masculine way—donning the traditional Pharaoh's beard to convince people of her authority.

Her successor Thutmose III destroyed most of her monuments and images, and though her tomb is the oldest datable tomb in the Valley of the Kings, her sarcophagus turned up empty and archeologists could not locate her mummy. But she was recently "rediscovered" and identified by Egypt's Secretary General of the Supreme Council of Antiquities Zahi Hawass. The clinching identifiable piece proved to be a tooth found in a box engraved with her name. Following X-rays, Hawass determined that the tooth belonged to a mummy that had spent the past century lying unprotected on the floor of a tomb in the Valley of the Kings; he subsequently reunited Hatshepsut with her sarcophagus and accorded her the proper status of Mighty Pharaoh.

VEGETABLE

In the hypothetical Proto-Indo-European language, *weg* meant "to be strong, lively, vigorous, and speedy." Latin coined *vegere*, "to be alive, active; to quicken," and *quick* meant "alive."

Vegere became *vegetus* "vigorous, active" and *vegetare* "to enliven." Middle Latin referred to anything that grew or flourished as *vegetabilis* and Old French coined *vegetable*, "living, or fit to live." Italian and Spanish used *verdura*, "green or growing." By 1400 CE, *vegetable* carried the sense of living and growing specifically as a plant. The celebration that was germination, growth, and reproduction in a plant (eaten for sustenance and life) gave us *vegetable*.

We now see the fruit as separate from the plant itself, as a product. We do not view the full, languid vegetable as having much to do with the strength of the spreading vine. The disappointing phrase "resembling that of a vegetable, dull, uneventful" was first recorded in 1854. Since then, to be likened to a vegetable (i.e., a couch potato) is an insult.

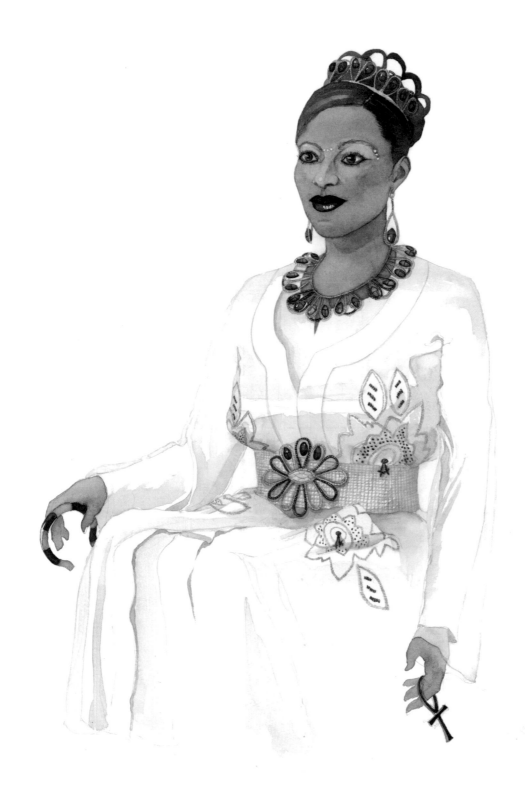

MYRRH
Commiphora myrrha

With an aroma of vanilla, myrrh is one of the most valuable herbs known to history. A shrub native to Yemen, Somalia, and Ethiopia, myrrh's burning resin produces a heavy, sweet-bitter smoke, making it a staple incense ingredient alongside calamus, cinnamon, aloe, cassia, and balm. Unlike other gummy resins, myrrh does not liquefy when burned; rather, it expands into what incense manufacturers term a *bloom*.

Ancient Egyptians employed myrrh as an embalming agent, and both Hatshepsut and (roughly 1,400 years later) Cleopatra imported the resin for perfumery and for ritual burning to honor gods and goddesses. The Magi of the Old Testament bore myrrh, gold, and frankincense for the infant Jesus, and myrrh dissolved in wine was offered to Jesus as he hung on the cross. In the Gospel of John, the women used one hundred pounds of myrrh and aloes to prepare his body for burial.

Myrrh is mentioned four times in the Song of Solomon:

A bundle of myrrh is my well-beloved unto me; he shall lie all night betwixt my breasts.
Song of Solomon 1:13

Who is this that cometh out of the wilderness like pillars of smoke, perfumed with myrrh and frankincense, with all powders of the merchant?
Song of Solomon 3:6

Until the day break, and the shadows flee away, I will get me to the mountain of myrrh, and to the hill of frankincense.
Song of Solomon 4:6

Spikenard and saffron; calamus and cinnamon, with all trees of frankincense; myrrh and aloes, with all the chief spices . . .
Song of Solomon 4:14

Perhaps because of its seductive scent, myrrh became strongly associated with women's sexuality and libido. In Esther's time of the Old Testament, myrrh was a cleansing agent for "unclean" women, and King Ahasuerus, who kept a House of Women from which he would summon concubines, enforced a "cleansing" ritual using burned myrrh.

In Chinese medicine, myrrh is bitter, spicy, and neutral in temperature, and it affects the heart, liver, and spleen meridians. In Ayurveda, a type of myrrh called *guggul* is prized for treating circulatory conditions, nervous system disorders, and rheumatism. Called *Daindhava*, myrrh is used in many Ayurvedic *rasayana* formulas after detoxification or for children, elderly, or pregnant women. *Guggul* is combined with triphala to clear cholesterol and detoxify the body.

Until the fifteenth century in the West, myrrh incense was used at funerals and cremations. Herbal medicine considers myrrh antiseptic, useful in mouthwashes and toothpastes to prevent gum disease. Modern herbalists use myrrh extracted in oil for salves and liniments to kill bacterial infections.

LETTUCE
Lactuca canadensis and L. scariola

With their milky white, latex-like sap, wild lettuces are the ancestors of our culinary lettuces. Ancient Egyptians valued lettuce both as a food and as an aphrodisiac, and they worshipped the fertility god Khem (Min) with bouquets of lettuce leaves since (presumably) the white sap symbolized semen. According to plant archeologists, it appears Pharaoh Hatshepsut grew lettuce in her gardens as a ritual herb, likely because the white sap also represented mother's milk. This imagery led to lettuce being used as a fertility blessing for both men and women and it may have been used in birthing ceremonies, fertility rites, and nursing ceremonies. The milky latex is mildly narcotic and was used in antiquity as a mild substitute for opium.

Wild lettuce is so mild, today it is generally dismissed as a healing herb, and it was dropped from the US Pharmacopoe-

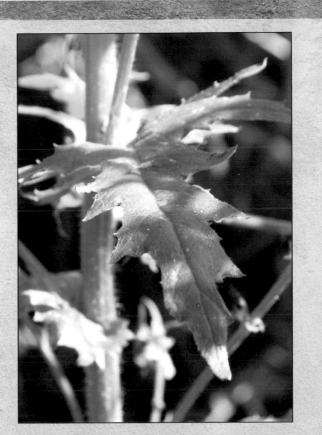

Wild lettuce

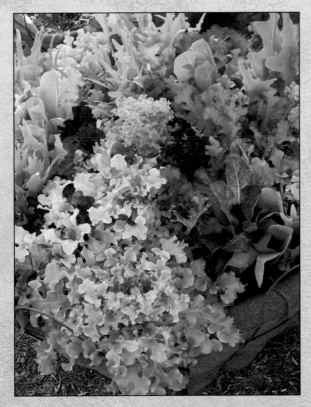

Cultivated lettuce

ia in 1916. It combines well, however, with valerian and other sedative herbs for children as a safe, gentle sleep-inducer.

In the seventeenth century, Nicholas Culpeper declared that lettuce was "owned" by the moon, which explained its cool and moist nature. Lettuce relieved heat diseases, such as headaches, and he advised that "the juice of lettuce mixed or boiled with oil of roses, applied to the forehead and temples procureth sleep …." He noted "the use of lettuce is chiefly forbidden to those that are short-winded, or have any imperfection in the lungs, or spit blood."

When wild foods forager Euell Gibbons ate wild lettuce raw, he found no soporific qualities, but upon eating the greens stewed, "I became aware of a sort of languid drowsiness and feeling of well-being, as though I didn't have a care in the world."

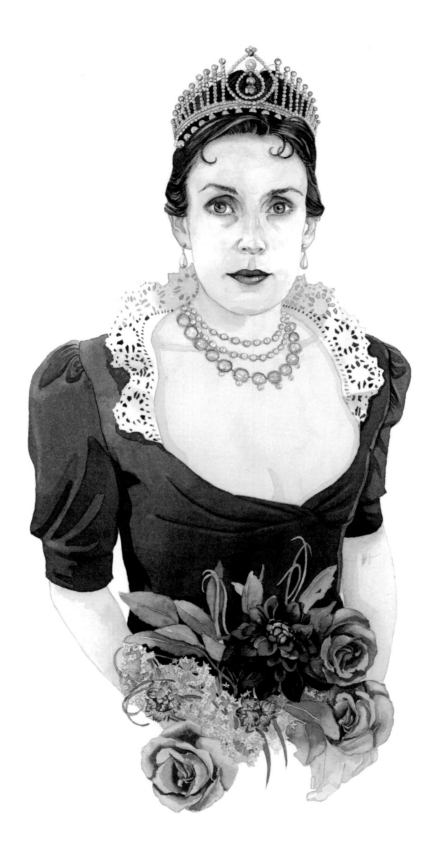

Empress Josephine
(1763–1814)

Though Empress Josephine is often remembered as Napoleon's Queen and jilted lover, she should also be recognized as the foremother of botanical collecting and rose horticulture. Until Josephine's lifetime, upper-class women seldom practiced flower cultivation for enjoyment. Plants and flowers were grown not as ornaments but for their God-given purpose of human service, often only in monasteries. Every flower in a physic garden had been planted by monks for use in their clinics; every flower at a family's cottage for the wife's medicine cabinet. But few were grown simply for their beauty.

Until Josephine. When Napoleon and Josephine de Beauharnais were crowned Emperor and Empress of France in 1804, Josephine discovered the opportunity to garden—and her desire blossomed into one of the most spectacular gardens in Europe and a trove of new plant varieties for gardeners today.

Born Marie Josèphe Rose de Tascher de la Pagerie (affectionately called Rose before her marriage), Josephine delighted in growing scores of exotic species of both plants and animals at her new royal home; she had marvelous coal-heated greenhouses built in which she grew pineapples, tulips, lilies, and peonies, and though she brought in animals from around the world (such as emus, zebras, and ostriches), Josephine became renowned for her cultivation of roses. Until Josephine's time, roses were rather small and unappealing, but under her practiced hand, they grew in stature, color, fragrance, and variety.

But France was at war with every other country in Europe and was isolated by blockades. Any new plant she wished to cultivate required transport from its country of origin. Despite the dangerous state of her country (and her marriage), Josephine networked with travelers, military servicemen, politicians, and even Crusaders from Arabia and Persia to acquire the rootstocks that she planted in astounding numbers at Château Malmaison. During the French Revolution, Josephine's soft influence provided safe passage for her London nurseryman to safely cross battlelines to tend her collection.

Thanks to Josephine, France enjoyed more than two hundred new plants, flowers, and trees, and had she lived longer, she would likely have continued her dream of establishing botanical gardens throughout the country. Several rose varieties have been named for her, including Rosa and Dianthus "Souvenir de la Malmaison," and *Lapageria rosea*.

To satisfy his political ambitions, Napoleon divorced Josephine five years after crowning her empress and wed Archduchess Marie

MUSEUM

The Greek *mouseion* was a shrine to the Muses, the female personifications of dance, music, and literature; its purpose was for study and appreciation of the arts.

The first structure may have been the Museum attached to the Lyceum of Aristotle at Athens, which served as a religious temple to the cult of the Muses as well as a home for teaching and debate. The Museum at Alexandria, constructed for Ptolemy I in about 280 BCE, was linked not with dance or music but strictly to literature.

It may be *amusing* to note that while the Museum was originally built to celebrate the female Muses, it remained in the sole realm of men. In Alexandria, in a large building with a dining hall, men of learning presumably had access to the books and manuscripts kept there, held common property, and utilized a priest appointed by the king. This perhaps advanced the academia of Hellenistic Egypt, but not the creative genius of women.

The nine Muses, daughters of Zeus and Mnemosyne, were:

Calliope	epic poetry
Clio	history
Erato	love poetry, lyric art
Euterpe	music, especially flute
Melpomene	tragedy
Polymnia	hymns
Terpsichore	dance
Thalia	comedy
Urania	astronomy

Louise of Austria; the move was (for Napoleon) politically savvy and (for Josephine) perhaps a relief; it was well-known he had fathered a son with the lovely Polish countess Marie Walewska (whom he also jilted). Josephine remained at Malmaison—and though she was isolated and financially dependent on her former husband, she surprisingly befriended Marie and her son and continued to import, plant, and grow spectacular flowers from around the world. Today, though, they reflect but a fragment of their former grandeur, parts of Josephine's gardens and her former home are a national museum.

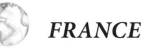

FRANCE

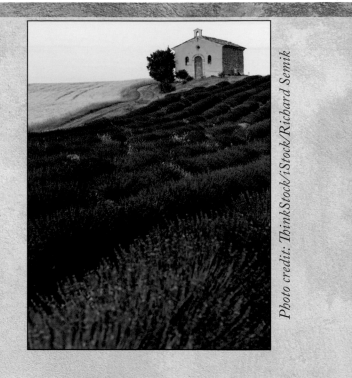

Empress "Rose" Josephine bought Chateau de Malmaison in 1799 during her husband Napoleon's travels to Egypt. The Chateau houses relics of both Josephine and Napoleon, including a glimpse of her once-impressive rose gardens.

In nearby Paris, Josephine and Napoleon were crowned Emperor and Empress of the French in 1804. The grand coronation ceremony was officiated by Pope Pius VII and took place at the Notre Dame de Paris cathedral. Here, French heroine Joan of Arc was captured by the English, tried, and executed at age nineteen in 1431, and it was at the same cathedral in 1455 that Joan's mother, Isabelle Romee, pleaded for the papal delegation to overturn the conviction of heresy. Joan of Arc was beatified in 1909.

Today the French enjoy natural remedies on a great scale—France is second only to Germany in the natural remedies market, although French legislation restricts that the sale of licensed herbal products be sold exclusively in pharmacies. Almost all herbal remedies are classified as medicines and thus are highly governed, instead of being classified as foods or dietary/health food supplements as they are in the United States.

Photo credit: ThinkStock/iStock/Richard Semik

SHAKESPEARE'S ROSE

"What's in a name? That which we call a rose
By any other name would smell as sweet;"

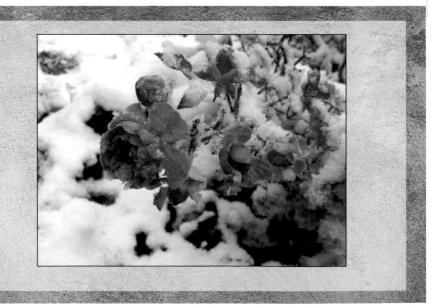

Long revered as one of the most elegant lines in the English language, could this really be a snub at Shakespeare's competition, the Rose Theatre? Shakespeare and Marlowe first performed at the Rose Theatre, but later the Bard formed the Globe. The Rose Theatre suffered the less-than-favorable reputation for its foul, stinking sanitary facilities, and the sardonic Bard may have been joking at the expense of his beloved flower; consider Sonnet #54: "The rose looks fair, but fairer we it deem / For that sweet odour, which doth in it live."

ROSE
Rosa spp.

Roses are called "aphrodisiacs" in reference to the ancient Greek deity Aphrodite, goddess of love, as legend tells us the first rose bloomed when Aphrodite shed tears over the loss of Adonis. Romans conflated Aphrodite with their goddess of sexuality, Venus, whom they symbolized with the red rose, while in Christianity, the Virgin Mary is symbolized by a white rose or a lily.

Hailed by the Greek poet Sappho as the Queen of Flowers, the rose was adored by Shakespeare and Dante Alighieri, who, in his Canto XXX, depicted heaven as a rose, enswarmed by bee-like angels who flew between the rose and the hive, which represented God.

British herbalist Anne McIntyre teaches that rose petals cool the body and clear toxins and heat, just as

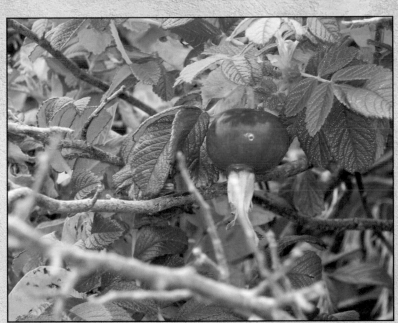

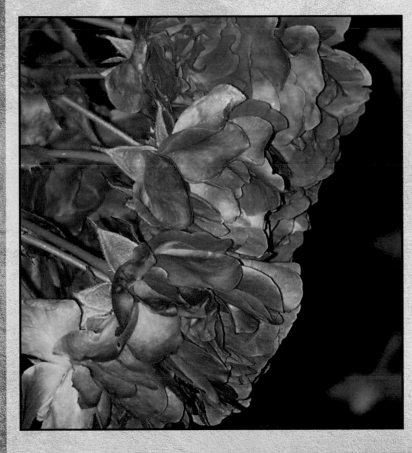

seventeenth-century physician Nicholas Culpeper used the cooling petals of roses with lettuce leaves to ease fevers and headaches—considered "hot" diseases in need of cooling lunar herbs.

Traditional herbalism uses roses as nervine tonics to ease depression, anxiety, premenstrual syndrome, and grief, and the oil counteracts depression, anxiety, cardiac trouble, and lovesickness. Rose tincture or tea is given to ease painful, heavy periods, uterine congestion, infertility, and impotence.

Many herbalists make vitamin C-rich syrups from the rose's fruits, or *hips*, which taste pleasantly tart and are often combined with elderberries and ginger or brewed with cider vinegar and honey.

HRH Princess Basma bint Ali

Picture a doting father leaning over his curious daughter as he shows her how to push a small seed into the dirt: it's an image many of us relate to, as our parents taught us as children to plant seeds. This father, in particular, went further than most: he taught his young daughter not only to cover the seed with dirt and to water it, but also how to collect seeds, cure and germinate them, prune, and even stock and layer plants and trees, as well as to appreciate the different varieties of a single species.

This was no ordinary father and daughter: this was His Royal Highness Ali bin Nayef Sultanzade, son of HRH Prince Nayef bin Abdullah the second son of King Abdullah, the First Founder of Jordan, and Her Imperial Highness Princess Mihrimah Sultana. And the young girl enthralled with the idea that a whole plant sprouts from a single seed was Her Royal Highness Princess Basma bint Ali. Since that fairytale childhood, Princess Basma has figuratively walked in shoes of every stripe and color: those of mother, conservationist, retired military officer, and Princess of Jordan. Her most recent shoes are hiking boots to establish ecological habitats at the new eight-hundred-hectare Royal Botanic Garden of Jordan, which she founded in 2005.

"My father loved geraniums," Princess Basma told me. "He would collect them from all sorts of places, but mostly from Spain. My parents are my mentors, in that they always encouraged and supported me."

Basma also credits her mother with lifelong inspiration for the natural world. Her mother, celebrated artist HRH Princess Wijdan Fawaz Al-Hashimi, PhD, is the president and founder of the Royal Society of Fine Arts (1979) and the National Gallery of Fine Arts (1980) Amman, Jordan, and she is currently the Jordanian Ambassador to Italy. She would insist her children spent the majority of their time outdoors around the capital city of Amman, in the Hashemite Kingdom of Jordan. "She would always have us gather whatever we could find from the garden," Basma says, "and use it for making arts and crafts. In so doing, she made us see the beauty in the simplest things, be it a rock, twig, or an ordinary flower."

Basma's childhood was joyfully filled with the collection of seeds, and her father taught her how to cure and germinate her finds. "He even helped me set up a solarium in the balcony of my bedroom. I remember distinctively when eating fruits I would collect the seeds and then propagate them. The one seed which stood out was the date seed because we had to place it in the freezer for nearly two weeks before seeding it. The very idea of which I found to be quite absurd, since dates came from the date palm which stereotypically meant it came from the desert."

"I was in awe of [my father's] ability to navigate the desert. Trying to emulate him I started to look for the minutest details in the landscape and see beyond the surface. It forced me to feel the soul of the earth."

Growing up in a desert climate seemed particularly harsh for eight-year-old Basma, until her father's keen eye taught her a patient wisdom. "I used to view the desert as a hot and unforgiving climate. But my father made me realize that if we re-create the in-situ conditions we are more likely to succeed in our efforts [of seed germination]. This led me to become more observant and sensitive to the bio-geographic conditions surrounding the plants and species associations as well as the climatic changes during the seasons and how important it is to observe them." On weekend picnics in the desert, her family would glide across the sands in convoys of four or five cars, passing dunes, curves, and topography that appeared nearly featureless. "At first it's a monotone of yellow beige, then suddenly out of nowhere we would arrive at a Bedouin tent where our lunch was waiting for us. To the untrained eye, one would assume we were traveling haphazardly, but my father knew exactly where we were. I was in awe of his ability to navigate the desert. Trying to emulate him, I started to look for the minutest details in the landscape and see beyond the surface. It forced me to feel the soul of the earth."

Pastime to Profession

Princess Basma joined the Jordanian Armed Forces (JAF) after graduating high school and then attended the Royal Military Academy, Sandhurst (RMAS) in the United Kingdom. She later graduated from Boston College in 1993 and, upon returning to Jordan, she resumed her military service.

It was in this unlikely career that her childhood environmental passion was allowed to flourish. While parachute training with the Special Forces in 1993, and serving as a platoon commander to the Royal Military Academy at Zarka, Basma was challenged by a

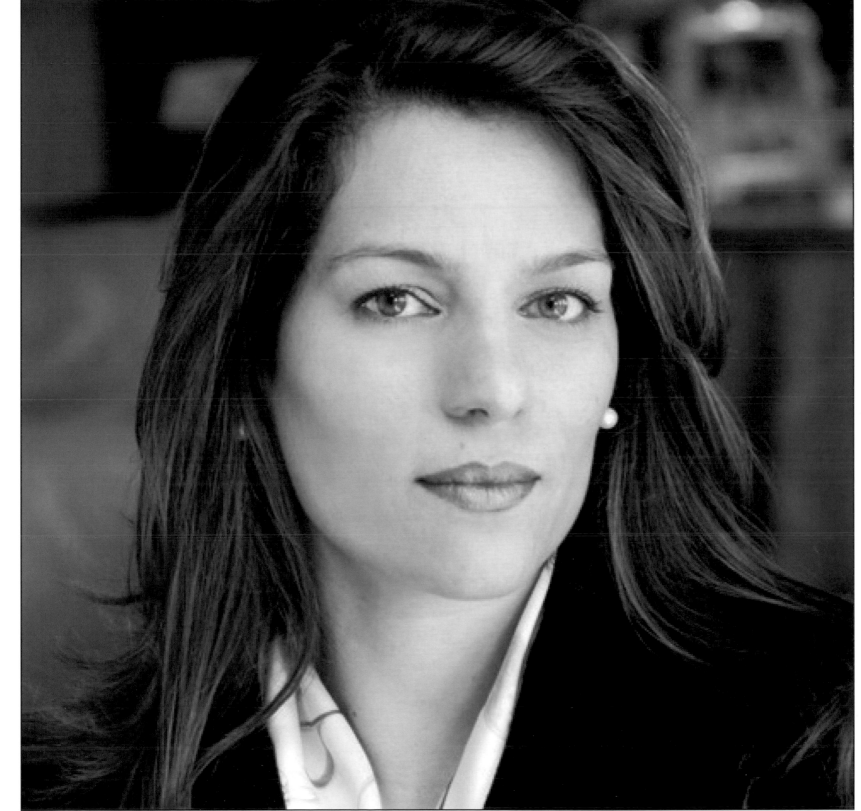

commanding officer to attempt the scuba diving course. But she was petrified of the sea, and the officer knew it. Always one to rise to a challenge, she decided to prove him wrong. To this end, she and her cousin completed the course, becoming in the process the first two female officers in JAF to achieve it. "That is when I completely fell in love with the sea," Basma says, "which lead me to join Sea Education Association in Woods Hole [Massachusetts] and do a semester at sea in 1994." Incorporated in 1930, the Woods Hole Oceanographic Institute is the world's largest nonprofit oceanographic institution.

The sea dives opened up an alarming world for her. "I could see the destruction and neglect that our coral reef was under. I knew I had to take action or it would be too late. So I started to mobilize anyone who would listen by conducting clean-up dives; of course, that would be the military. At one point, I even had over two hundred US marines conduct a clean-up dive since they were on exercise in Jordan. But I felt my efforts were only scratching at the surface." In 1995, she was instrumental in the creation of the Royal Marine Conservation Society of Jordan (JREDS).

"Plants still had a special place in my heart, and whenever I traveled I made sure I visited gardens. For me, that was my indulgence, and I must admit Kew stood out of them all. I always longed to have such a garden in Jordan not only to just visit but to teach me about our native plants, of which I knew very little. It frustrated me that I had no references or places to tell me about my plants. So I decided if no one has done it yet, I may as well do it myself." And she did. In 2000, Basma retired from the military to create the Royal Botanic Garden at Tel Al Rumman.

The Royal Botanic Garden

In association with England's Botanic Gardens Conservation International, Basma established the eight-hundred-hectare Royal Botanic Garden (RBG) above the King Talal Dam, a scenic yet remote area of Jordan. The preserve includes natural habitats, an herbarium, themed gardens including a medicinal herb garden, and an Islamic garden with an Andalusian irrigation system independent of electricity. The Royal Botanic Garden offers public access, education, scientific research, conservation for Jordan's endangered plants, as well as a visitor's center, an exhibition hall, conference facilities, and even eco-lodges and hiking and horseback-riding trails.

Sprouted from Princess Basma's idea in the 1990s, the Royal Botanic Garden of Jordan first saw progress in 2004 and already

nearly five hundred species have been catalogued. Once this area flourished with oaks and understory plants, but the region was denuded by centuries of intensive grazing and agriculture, as well as invasive species such as eucalyptus and even catfish in the waterways. Princess Basma aims to educate local shepherds in sustainable grazing management to regenerate the cypresses, oaks, olives, pistachios, and native almond trees. And the Botanic Garden is participating in the Medicinal and Aromatic Plant Research Study. "It has been identified that Jordan holds 1 percent of the world's total population of some 310,000 vascular plant species," she says.

Conservation

Educating people about the importance of environmental preservation has been a constant challenge. "The most difficult thing about our work in marine conservation is peoples' attitude toward environmental issues," Basma says. "This applies to all levels of the socio-economic strata. When I first started in the very early nineties, people would humor me because I was a Princess, but not because they believed in the cause. I took advantage of that and kept going. But it was always an uphill struggle and at times very discouraging. For example, I was still working in the military when I got a call from a botanist telling me that one of the last two remaining clumps of *Hyphaene thebaica*, gingerbread tree or *thebaica*, Doum Palm Trees, in Aqaba were in danger of being uprooted due to the development that was taking place. He was fraught with anxiety and fear for those poor trees. So, immediately, I jumped into my car and headed off on the three-hour drive south to see for myself. To save time, and ensure the safety of these trees, I called up the Commander of the Southern Forces. On the phone, I was talking in a very serious manner, telling him we had an emergency on our hands and he had to take immediate action to ensure the safety of the Doum. And how important this was and that I am on my way to ensure everything would be taken care of properly. Now all along he was serious and hanging on to every word I was saying. He kept reassuring me that things will be handled appropriately and how he will not let anyone harm 'the Doums.' Then he asked a very simple question, 'Who are these Doums? Where did they originally come from?'

"The minute I mentioned that they were not people but trees, I heard him muffle the phone and burst into laughter. He kept saying

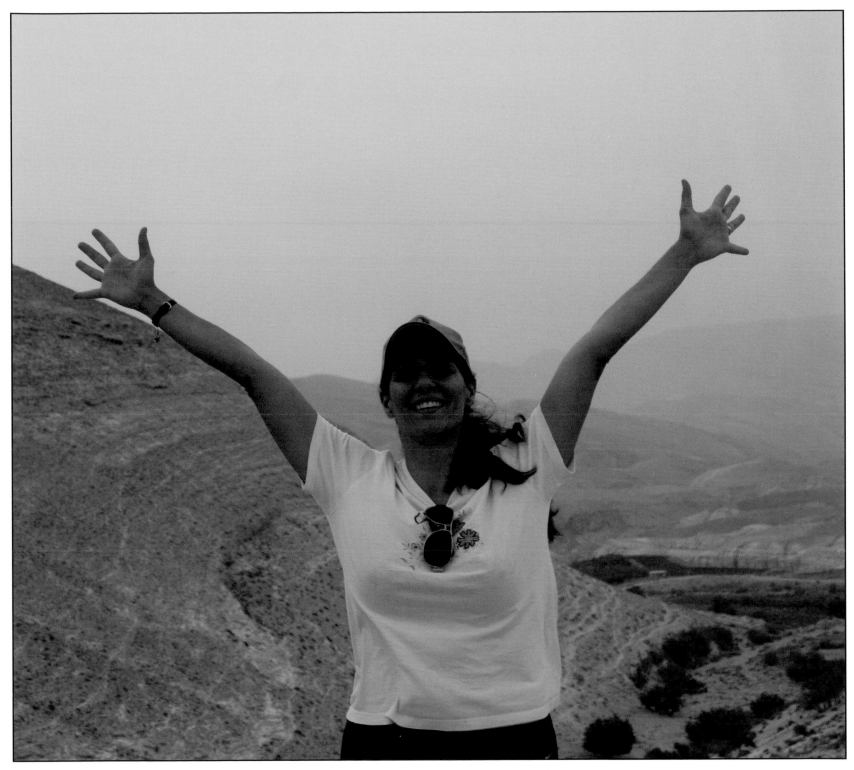

Princess Basma at Tel Al Rumman, Jordan

yes, of course, we will do our utmost to protect them, but finally he blurted out how he thought we had an International Security issue at hand, and how amusing it was for him that 'it's just a bunch of palms.' I took it with a pinch of salt, and explained to him the significance of his actions, after which he started to come around. They are still there, being the northernmost-found Doum trees.

"I have faced many such situations where people I am dealing with have absolutely no idea of the ramifications of our failure to protect our ecological resources. However, over the years, this attitude has begun to change with the guidance of His Majesty King Hussein bin Talal and HRH Prince El Hassan bin Tallal. They brought attention and importance of environmental protection to the forefront of public policy."

"I have faced many such situations where people I am dealing with have absolutely no idea of the ramifications of our failure to protect our ecological resources and services."

Herbs for Food and Medicine

The majority of Jordanian cuisine has long been based on whole grains, cereals, dry legumes, dark greens, low-fat dairy foods, "lots of herbs," and heart-healthy fats. "Now doctors around the world are recommending the very same principles," she says.

Princess Basma routinely uses herbs in her kitchen as well as for medicinal purposes. One plant in particular, *Paronychia argentea Lam.*, commonly known as Silvery Whitlow-wort or "foot of the pigeon" in Arabic, is commonly used for painful kidney stones. "I use this plant very often, when I am out in the country and far from an herbalist or in desperate condition due to my kidney stones and need it immediately. I gather it myself from wherever I may be in Jordan. All you have to do is gather a handful, rinse the dust and dirt with cold water, then add boiling water and steep for a few minutes, then drink it. No matter how agonizing your pain is from the kidney stones or uric crystals, within ten to fifteen minutes, it's all gone. Whenever my daughter is out and about, she spots it immediately and always picks some up for me, which I find quite endearing.

"I try to use plant-based remedies for my children. Especially in winter, Chamomile essential oil plays a vital role in our flu/cold/sore throat therapy. I dab a tiny drop on their collar, by the time evening comes the infection is almost all gone."

CONSERVATION

Today *conservation* implies keeping lands or species safe, through the original Proto-Indo-European (PIE) *solwos* is from *sol*, "whole." Latin formed *solidus*, "solid," Sanskrit formed *sarvah*, "uninjured, whole"; and Greek used *holos* for "whole." Old French took *solwos* to form a number of words, including *salus*, "good health," and *salvus*, "healthy, safe." Latin used *servare*, "to keep safe," which gave rise to *preservare* and Old French's *preserver*. The word *safe* appeared in English in 1280 CE, and a hundred years later, *preserve* appeared. About the same time, *conserve* was formed from Latin's *conservare* and meant "to keep, preserve" or to "keep watch, maintain." Old French used *salve* and *garde*, "a keeping," to produce *sauvegarde*, which entered English in 1421 as *safeguard*. The idea of a *conservationist* protecting the environment entered English in 1922 and a *preservationist* to protect historic property became vogue in 1927. Today, we eat preservatives in our food and spread conserves on our toast.

She also brews mint for her children's tummy upsets (as an herbal infusion or with regular black tea), as well as thyme, wild or cultivated. "Thyme is used as a remedy for upset stomach and is drunk as an infusion. But those with low blood pressure must take care since it brings it down. However, we also use it as a dry spice mix that is served most usually as a breakfast or dinner in a small plate. Then one puts a small amount, approximately a teaspoon or two in their own plate, then drizzles olive oil just next to it on the plate. Tear a piece of local bread and dip it first in the oil, then in the dry mix. The other way is we make a sort of pizza of it called manageesh (plural). Basically, it is a bread-like dough that has been rolled open just as a pizza, but not too thin, then heavily sprinkled with the Za'tar mix that's basted in olive oil. It is then baked and eaten fresh out of the oven. It is a very popular weekend brunch dish and children love it as a snack food. It is hot and fresh from the local bakery, its sweet yet spicy and warm aroma is absolutely impossible to resist. An utter comfort food."

Basma inspires others in the same spirit in which her father introduced her to the world of Islam as a source of scientific knowledge. "Islam is more than just a religion that details how people should conduct themselves," she says. "It holds the sacred knowledge, the Truth. I have since learned to observe how this truth is evident in God's creation. Such examples are as simple as looking into the geometric design of a seedpod, flower dimensions, even the spiraling growth of a plant or even snail. I am in total awe of the Majesty, Totality, and Unity of Creation of God and it only re-enforces the notion that man has just begun to scratch at the surface of this knowledge. The only way I can describe my amazement is in three words: the Unity of Diversity. I really feel both blessed and humbled at what is around me."

"If you are true to yourself, the potential is limitless."

These lessons have guided Princess Basma in her pursuit of environmental conservation and fulfilling her dreams. "Always believe in your potential no matter how small or insignificant others may perceive you to be," she says. "It only takes one person to make change, and if you are true to yourself, the potential is limitless. But you have to do it with true conviction, no matter how overwhelming the matter may be, no matter how long it may take. If you are true and honest, then you will be successful."

JORDAN

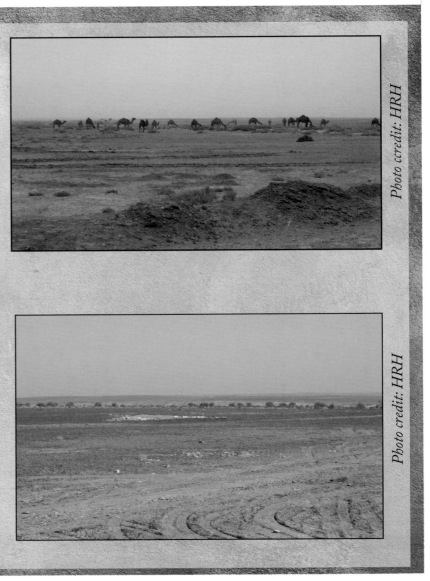

Photo credit: HRH

Photo credit: HRH

Vivid with colors of ochre, sand, and butter—occasionally punctuated by a burst of red Oleander blossom—the landscape of Jordan is a living reflection of its ancient desert history. Its population of 5.3 million mostly Arabic-speaking Sunni Muslims shares its borders with Saudi Arabia, Iraq, Syria, and Israel's West Bank (Palestinian National Authority), as well as the vast Dead Sea, into which the Jordan River empties itself. The lowest body of water in the world, the Dead Sea is landlocked and is seven times saltier than an ocean.

Jordan is ruled by King Abdullah II Ibn-al Hussein, who governs in the parliamentary monarchy and is known as a reformer and advocate for Middle East peace. Among the Arab, Circassian, Armenian, Kurdish, and Bedouin residents, there are many well-versed in the plantlife that flourishes in Jordan's arid deserts. Along rock walls, ancient stone towers, snow-covered roads, high-elevation dry grasslands, and rugged canyons, drought-tolerant plants live in colorful bounty beckoning travelers.

The native wildflowers of Jordan include eleven species of iris, as well as the common giant fennel (*Ferula*), spurge (*Euphorbia*), wild thyme (*Coridothymus*), Palestine Pheasant's Eye (*Adonis palaestina*), hollyhock (*Alcea setosa*), and squill (*Urginea maritima*). There are also the coveted caper bushes from which chefs pluck edible buds—careful to avoid the backward facing spines—as well as the poisonous Oleander (*Nerium oleander*). Jordan's great biodiversity thrives despite—or perhaps because of—its arid temperatures, and many of its flora are brightly colored. Many boast sharp thorns and spines, as well, to protect them from goats and other desert herbivores.

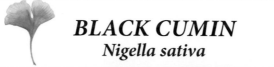

BLACK CUMIN
Nigella sativa

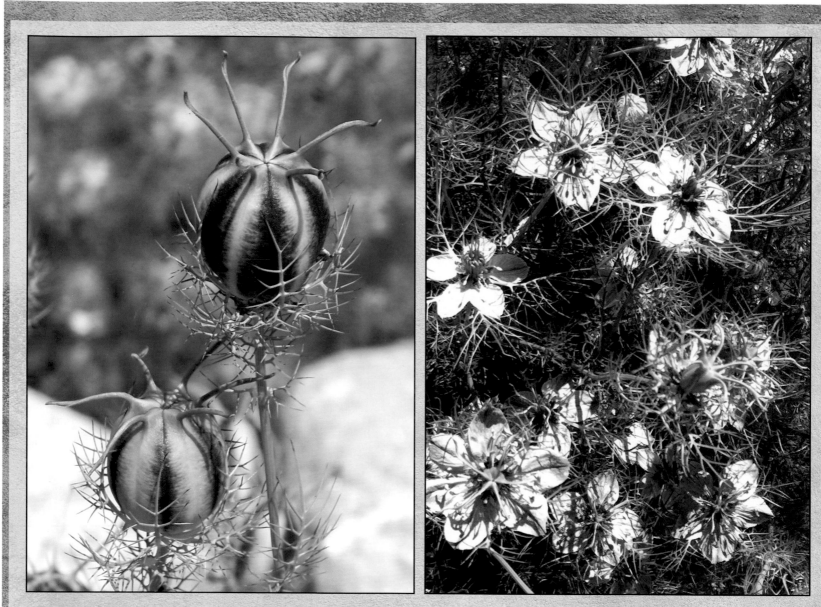

lso called black caraway and black coriander for its tiny black seeds, *Nigella* seeds have been discovered in archeological digs in Egypt, indicating it was used in antiquity as medicine and/or food. Folklore holds that black cumin can treat a variety of diseases from eczema to indigestion to food allergies, and modern medicine credits the steam-distilled essential oil with a potentially powerful analgesic action based on tests in animals. Tests have also shown that extracts of *Nigella* seeds reduce or eliminate bacterial outbreaks of *Staphylococcus aureus*, reflecting its popular antibacterial folk use and a treatment for yeast infections.

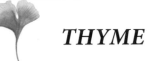

THYME

Throughout India, thyme is a trusted culinary herb to flavor and preserve meat, fish, and poultry. High in volatile oils and bitters, thyme is a common remedy for asthma, whooping cough, spasm, and irritable bowel symptoms. It combines with elecampane, peppermint, and wild cherry to ease spasmodic coughing and promote ease of respiration. It's easy to prepare a quick antiseptic oil from the leaves to treat external wounds, and for this purpose it pairs nicely with St. John's wort and yarrow.

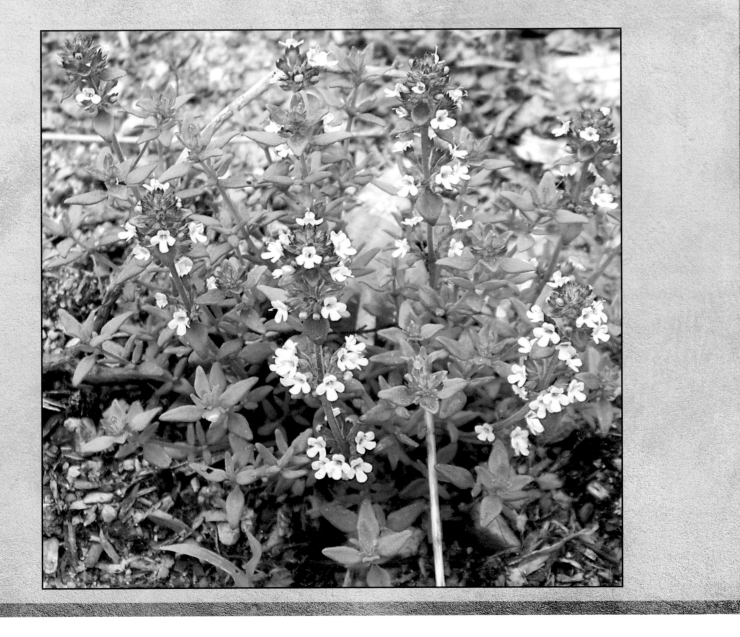

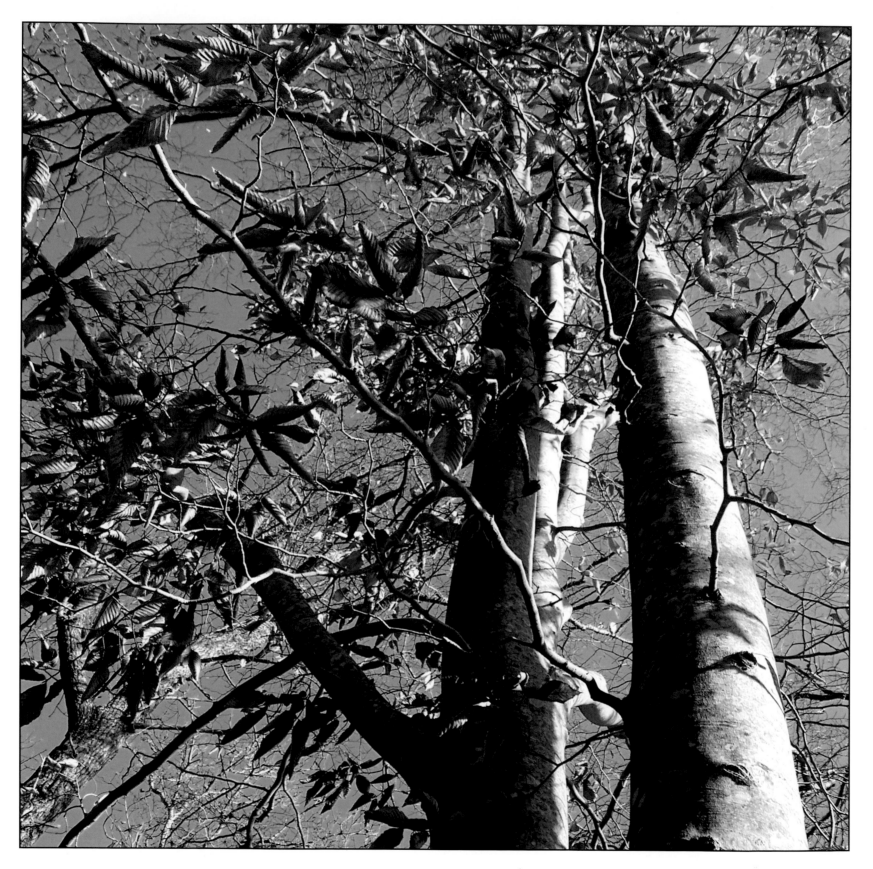

Chapter 16

ETHNOBOTANY

Put simply, ethnobotany is the study of the relationship between people and plants. Scientists want to learn how people (usually native tribes, aboriginal peoples, and indigenous cultures) interact, relate with, and use their native plant species. How do we use them? How do we honor and celebrate them? While it is a science as much as any other, ethnobotany is much more people-centered than, say, chemistry.

The term *ethnobotany* was first coined in 1895, though the study of people's relationship with plants goes back millennia. At the dawn of humanity, our interaction with plants was strictly for a handful of purposes: food, shelter, hunting, protection, and, perhaps most importantly, art and magic. The use of plants for healing apparently did not surface until much later, when humankind began noticing how plants affected the body, rather than the spirit (Naranjo, 362). The celebrated "herbals" of ancient cultures (notably Greece) were compendiums of knowledge about specific plants and how they healed illnesses; these early herbals from authors such as Dioscorides (and later from Gerard) included much of the information ethnobotanists collect today: particulars of biology, agricultural and growing requirements, folklore from within the culture, and—especially—economic opportunities available for pharmacology and science.

Within ethnobotany, it is impossible to separate the person (or the tribe or community) from the plant, which is central to indigenous existence. Consider the remarkable variety of uses of plants for which humankind should be very grateful: preservative, drug/medicine, food and food thickener, fiber, veterinary medicine, dyes, cleaners, containers, ceremonial uses, tools, weapons, lighting, paint, musical instruments, lubricants, magic, insecticide, paper, smoking tools, snuff, soap, stable gear, toys and games, water indicator, water-proofing agent, clothing, furniture, fuel, incense, jewelry, fragrance and perfume, cosmetics, and building materials. These ideas stem from ethnobotanist Daniel Moerman, but a high school class I taught quickly created a similar list with only a little brainstorming. Ethnobotanist G. T. Prance divided tree use by Amazonian tribes into the following basic categories: food, construction material, technology, remedy, commerce, and other.

People are beginning, in the last century, to construct a more two-sided relationship with plants—whereby we acknowledge plant resources and give back in addition to taking. We've constructed national and state parks to conserve land and international governments are working to stop the extinction of endangered plants. In third-world countries, people rely almost solely on plant medicines, while people in developed nations often use herbal medicines to supplement conventional health care and (increasingly) to enhance their relationship to the natural world.

Much of university-level ethnobotany involves folk classification of plants, researching how various segments of a community's population gather and use plants, and how communities and tribes plan to survive famine or disease, etc. The science also promotes biodiversity, domestication, and the discovery of new fuels, foods, and medicines from cultures long accustomed to the use of what we consider "new" and "exotic" plants.

The most rewarding aspect of this changing science will likely be greater appreciation for the earth's bewildering diversity of plants and humanity's comfort level in connecting with those plants, both physically and spiritually. With the growing Slow Food Movement and school garden initiatives, the study of ethnobotany will surely expand to include a greater esteem for the cultures whose heritage has protected these plants and their uses for us to study and (respectfully) use today.

Rocío Alarcón

etite and slender, Ecuadorian native Rocío Alarcón is a fierce proponent of protecting and promoting the age-old relationship between people and plants. She is one of those mystic revolutionaries who encompass two different realms within the world of plants: in one, she is the knowledgeable ethnobotanist who has pushed her way into the typically male-centered academic arena with persistence and true ability. In the other, she is the quintessential feminine teacher who guides her class in learning a distinct, hands-on approach to herbal healing, primarily with what she terms "spiritual massage" or "spiritual bathing."

Born in Quito, Ecuador, Rocío first learned about plants from her grandmother, whom she considers her mentor. "Her knowledge and her relationship with the plants were the inspiration for my future," Rocío says. "My grandmother was a healer and during her life she depended on the plants for the maintenance and survival of her seven children. All my life, I saw my relatives and people in different regions of my country using plants for different situations and conditions. My great-grandmother, grandmother, and mother were my first instructors since I was a baby. Later, healers of the tropical forest taught me the different ways to love, respect, and use the plants from those regions." Sharing daily activities with her grandmother and the locals in the Andes, *cordillera* gave Rocío the opportunity to learn and practice many uses for the astonishing abundance of plants that grew near her.

Rocío has since collaborated with a number of international organizations to research economic opportunities for locals using products of the rainforest, working with the Wildlife Conservation Society, Care, The Nature Conservancy, Sage Mountain, and the Eden Project. She has worked with many Amazonian indigenous communities, including the Huaorane, Quichua, Cofan, Shuar, and in the Chocó region with the Chachi and with the Afro-Esmeraldeños (the black community). In the Andes, Rocío's focus is with the Quichuas and Mestizos. She is renowned for her good word among the Quichua peoples, and ethnobotanist Christopher Joyce writes in *Earthly Goods: Medicine-Hunting in the Rainforest* that it was Rocío's strong reputation among the locals that allowed ethnobotanist Brad Bennett to conduct his studies there. Joyce describes Rocío as possessing a "rugged constitution and determination that has earned her the respect of the Quichua," and he praises her for knowing "more about the indigenous population of the country than most anyone in Ecuador." At the Jatun Sacha biological station in the Ecuadorian Amazon, Rocío helped Bennett catalog five hundred tree species.

As a teacher, Rocío has captured the hearts of thousands of women with her guidance in spiritual bathing, a technique new to western herbalists but familiar to Rocío from her childhood. "I received my first bathing when I was born and later many times, so my first memory about my bathing was in the middle of aromatic waters covered with white petals and my body was massaged with a handful of soft plants. Later when I had fever, I remembered to bathe with fresh aromatic water from wild plants and I felt in my body the process of healing, energy coming into my body, serenity, and my muscles feeling a big relief and no more pain."

Spiritual bathing, she says, is a normal daily practice in the Andes Mountains. "We prepare different kinds of bathing depending on the situation and the condition of each individual. People with experience in this ritual are in charge of advising and offering this knowledge to the population."

"The most rewarding experience was living in the middle of the forest and seeing people using plants for each activity in their lives: health, food, shelter, healing ceremonies, etc."

The process involves determining which plants should be used for a certain condition, gathering the plants, and brushing the plants across the skin in quick successive motions across certain "energy fields" of the body. During an intensive workshop with Rocío in 2007, I learned the differences between sweet and bitter plants, partly in taste but especially in their energy. Bitter plants were to be used to clear away negative energy, and sweet plants were to sustain good energy; she demonstrated her method of using the plant as a broom across the skin. I had half expected her to gently sweep the plant bundles across the skin in a manner similar to pulling a sweater off—nothing too gentle, but a simple, rote exercise. Instead, Rocío invigorated the class by demonstrating firm, quick brush strokes that whisked across her arms and down her legs—broad energizing strokes accompanied by her emphatic chants and loud prayers for the energies to be swept along their paths. She was pushing the energy out with the bundle of herbs—taking charge of her body's energy with a positive force and character. The class sat spellbound, watching and listening to this petite woman as she thundered with power before us. Rocío demonstrated when to use gentler methods for healing for children, when to collect bitter or pungent herbs, and when to collect sweet and fragrant herbs.

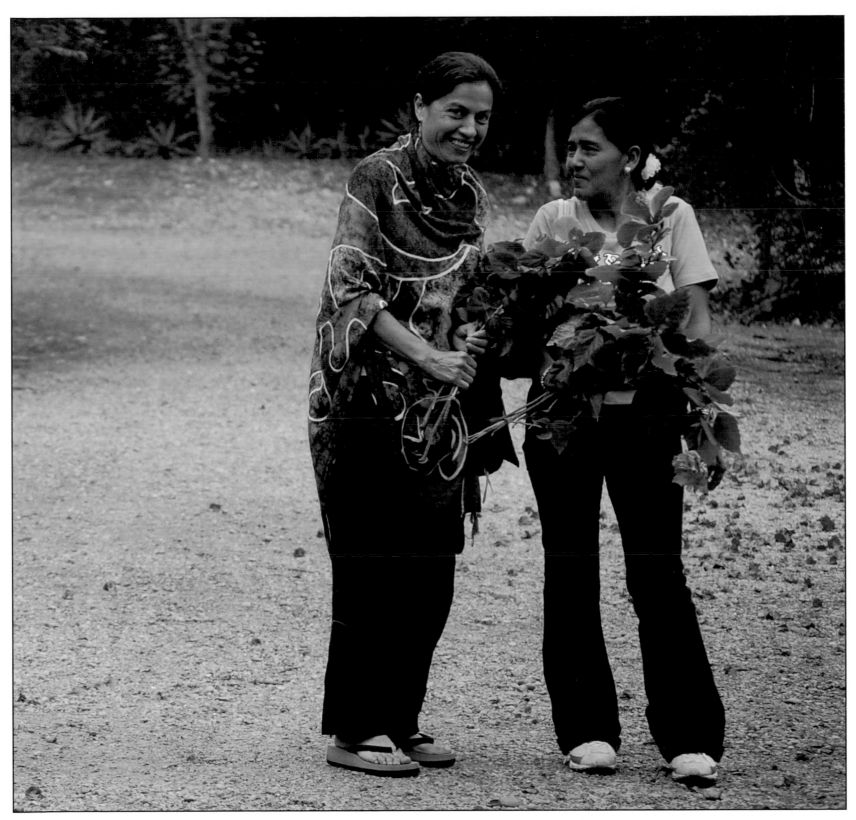

"All these types of experiences are kept in my memory and I wanted to share them with other people. People in stress and anxiety can find a better quality of life using simple resources easy to find in the garden or in a pot or forest."

For her *la limpia* ceremony, which means *clean*, Rocío uses aromatic plants such as eucalyptus, chamomile, sweet thyme, calendula, laurel and nogal (see Walnut sidebar). "These plants are very simple to find and use for this ceremony that makes people feel less stress," she says. But in her travels to more temperate climates, it has been difficult for her to find her beloved plants—in countries with four seasons, the winter plants are "dry." She also laments that not all people have a special relationship with plants and many think "all problems in their health can find solutions in the western medicine."

The healing traditions of Ecuador are ancient and remarkable, as each ethnic group performs its own ceremonies. "They are unique to each individual, and the person treated is not just treated physically," says Rocío. "The body is split into spiritual and emotional, those bodies are the ones the ceremony focuses on. Behind each healing, there is a 'healing celebration,' which is always linked to specific plants, for a specific individual and their ailments."

EARTH

Our planet has had many names. The ancient Proto-Indo-European language (PIE) used *er* to refer to land. Proto-Germanic people used *ertho*, Old Norse *jörd*, Middle Dutch *eerde*, and Old High German *erda*. Old English *eorde* meant "ground, soil, or dry land."

To the Greeks, *ge* or *ga* referred to land, *genomos* "earth dweller," *Gaia* "earth," and *Pangaea*, the name given in 1924 to the late Paleozoic era supercontinent. Geomancy and geometry mean "earth-measure."

Finns called the earth *maa*, which lead to the Russian *mammot* and, in 1706, *mammoth*, "the animal of the earth." Another PIE word *ters* meant "dry," similar to Sanskrit *tarsayati*, "dries up," Avestan *tarshu*, "dry, solid," Greek *tereses-thai*, "to become dry or thirsty." Latin derived *terra*, "earth," giving us *terrain* and *terrestrial*.

Even the herb turmeric has earth roots: in Middle Latin *terra merita* literally meant "worthy earth."

DESIRE

To desire something is to await the fortune of the stars, from the phrase *de sidere* "from the stars," as *sidus* means "star or heavenly body." The word entered English about 1230 AD and, 150 years later, *consider* was first written in English, literally "with the stars," especially as pertained to decision-making. Nearly all decisions of ancient cultures were made under the perceived direction of the stars and especially with the goddess Venus. The ancient Proto-Indo-European *wen* meant "to strive after, wish, desire." Sanskrit used *vanas* and Old English used *wyscan* to express the idea of wishing or desiring. The Egyptian goddess Hathor and the Greek Aphrodite were both renamed Venus by the Romans, and astronomers named that famous bright wishing planet Venus in about 1290 AD.

Rocío has enjoyed living among these native peoples. "The most rewarding experience was living in the middle of the forest and seeing people use plants for each activity in their lives: health, food, shelter, healing ceremonies, etc." She rejoices that "where there are not doctors, there are plants to save the lives of people."

The most basic precept of ethnobotany—the relationship between people and plants—is central to Rocío's work. She obtained a diploma as a practitioner of Holistic Therapies and a PhD at the University of London's School of Pharmacy Centre for Pharmacognosy and Phytotherapy, then she researched plants as medicine and food in the Basque Country of Spain, a topic close to her heart. "The history of human health is linked to plants," she says, "so today it is more important [than ever] to protect nature. Humans need to find new elements in the plants to improve their quality of life, such as better quality food and medicine. Food is medicine, and probably many plants around the planet have many substances to offer humans. We are all connected in the world, today more than before, so we can share the experiences with plants because they are guiding us to find a healing path.

"The young generation, especially women," Rocío says, "need to find inspiration in plants for a better future for humanity."

WALNUT
Juglans spp.

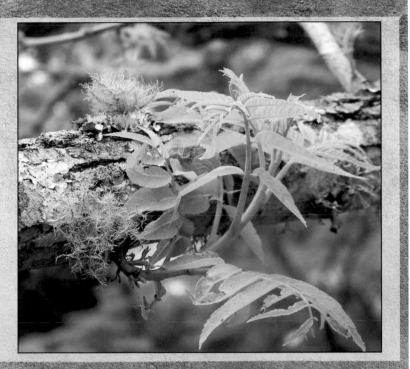

The black walnut can grow one hundred feet high, with scanty leaves and sturdy timber. Woodsmen consider the pest-resistant wood stronger than white oak and use it for furniture and cabinetry. The walnut earned its genus name from the god Jupiter (*jovis*) and *glans*, referring to the acorn or nut, so named in Greece when men ate acorns but gods dined on walnuts.

Its close relative the South American Nogal is commonly called Peruvian or tropical walnut. Nogal nuts are used in candies, confections, and baking; many South American stews are thickened with sautéed nogal nuts and mushrooms.

Versatile walnut trees can be used for timber, dye, medicine, and food, though black walnuts frustrate gardeners because their roots produce juglone, a toxin that thwarts the growth of herbs and vegetables growing nearby.

Medicinally, nogal and all walnuts are prized for their outer hulls, which are green, bitter, antiparasitic, and used to treat amoebic dysentery. The bitter hulls kill pinworms, tapeworm, and other intestinal parasites and are valued as a dye.

ECUADOR

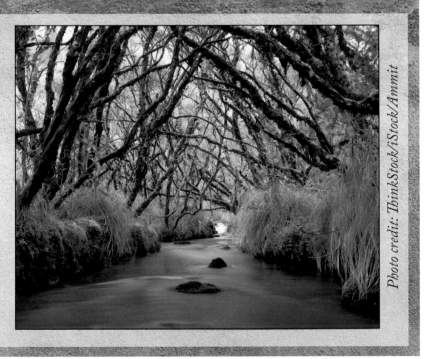

Imagine traveling approximately four hundred miles—roughly the length of Kansas—and discovering mangrove forests, rainforests, high-altitude grasslands, semi-desert scrublands, and miles of sandy Pacific beaches. This is Ecuador: the smallest country in South America and botanically the richest. Ecuador, home to nearly fourteen million people, is a world-center for biodiversity, boasting more than twenty-five thousand plant species, or 10 percent of the world's total. All of North America, by comparison, holds only seventeen thousand plant species (Ades, 2003). The Galapagos Islands are part of Ecuador, contributing to the country's vast biological wealth.

The people of Roman Catholic Ecuador, who are mostly *mestizos*, speak either Spanish or Quechua, the language of the ancient Incas. They export petroleum, but they also send to the world their natural jewels in the form of cut flowers, coffee beans, bananas, shrimp, cocoa beans, and Pacific Ocean fish.

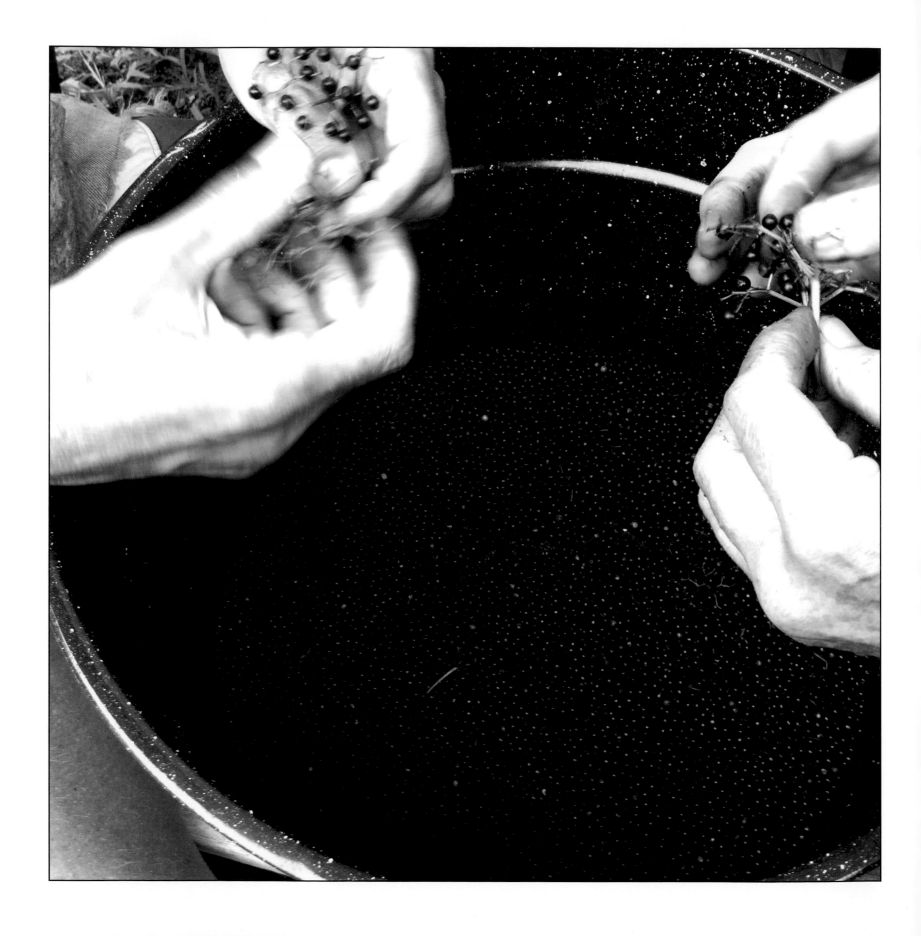

Part V:
HANDCRAFTING TRADITIONS

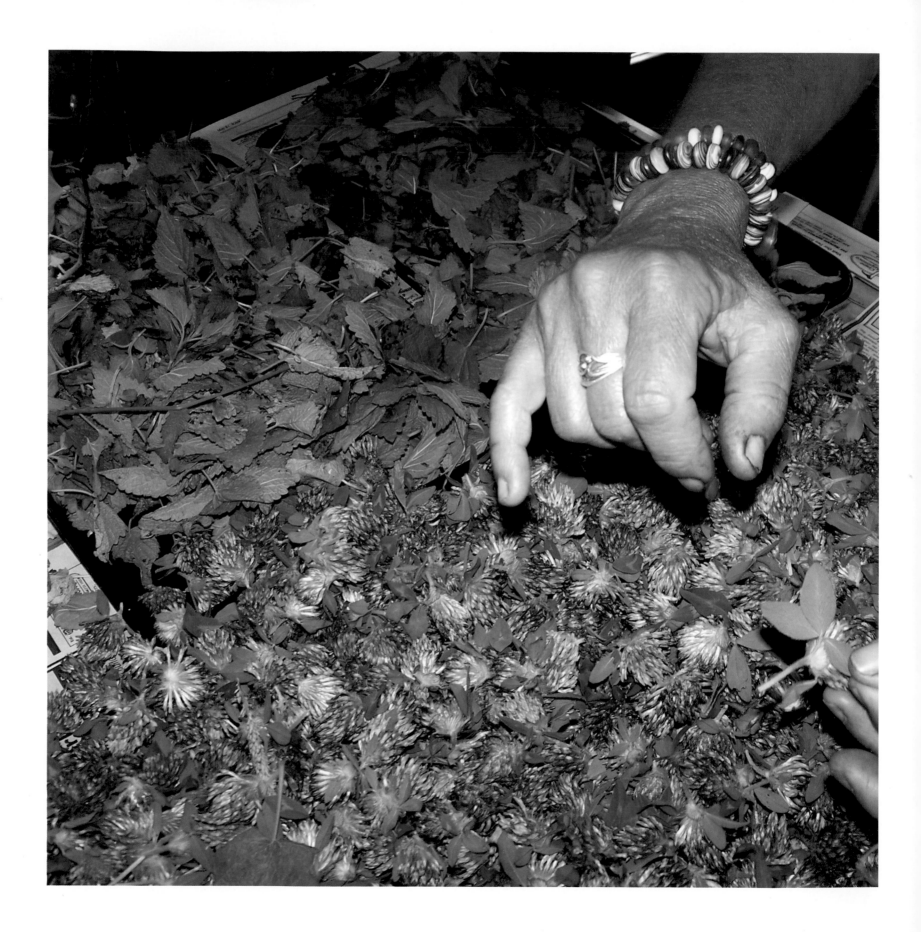

Chapter 17

How to Make Herbal Remedies in Your Kitchen Inspired by World Traditions

Original recipes by the author inspired by the women in this book

IN THIS CHAPTER, YOU'LL FIND:

Introduction

Just like every country and culture has its own distinguishable cuisine, its own heritage about marriage, and its own myths and religions, so does each culture create its own traditional remedies. The world's healing traditions vary in taste, texture, intent, ritual, scale, and time-to-heal, but—interestingly—they almost always involve the use of plants. How fascinating that people throughout the world have placed green plants at the center of their quest for health! It speaks to people's experience with not only the chemistry of plants, but also to the spiritual nature of relating to a great life force.

Every world tradition handcrafts remedies with the plants—some on a grander scale than others. Oriental medicine, for example, may incorporate multiple plants and ingredients in very complex formulae, while flower essences and homeopathy are simple and singular. Most remedies are part chemistry and part intuition, made with a consciousness and respect that "infuses" a certain energy into the final product.

From the wide range of remedies found in the world's traditions, I've selected a representative sample that are safe, fun to make, and effective to use. The following oils, pastes, salves, tinctures, bitters, tisanes, steams, soaks, sprays, baths, face lotion, smoke blend, spice blend, and even fertilizer are all easy to make at home and will instill a creative sense of connection with the healers profiled here, since each remedy is inspired by a woman in this book.

While the methods are derived from my nearly twenty years' experience crafting traditional plant remedies, each recipe reflects the work of the women here and the experience of their cultures and heritage. Feel free to substitute herbs that you can grow or harvest yourself—adapting and sharing these handcrafting arts are the best ways to further our incredible heritage of plants and healing.

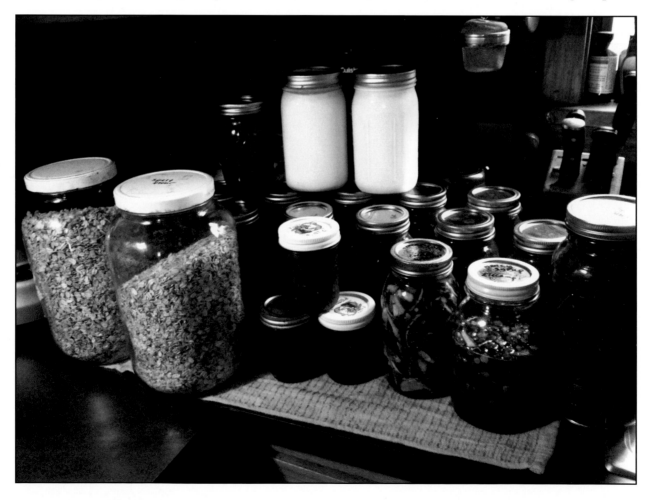

Oil Recipes

O ils have been pressed from the fruits, nuts, and seeds of various plants for millennia, yielding thick and aromatic juices that make their way onto our tables and our skin. Many oils such as flaxseed and hemp contain omega-3 fatty acids that may reduce the risk of coronary heart disease, while olive, sweet almond, apricot kernel, grapeseed, pumpkin seed, pomegranate seed, and borage seed oils (known as carrier oils) are renowned for their skin-softening properties and their ability to "carry" plant ingredients through the dermal layers to nourish deeply beneath the skin.

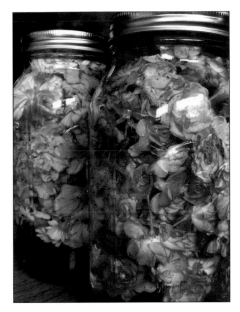

Using oils as carriers is one way to apply them; another effective way is to use oils as a menstruum, or medium, in which you extract an herb's vital healing qualities. An herb is macerated and steeped in a jar of oil, then strained; the resulting nutrient-rich oil is used topically to treat skin, muscle and joint issues, and it can be added to beeswax to create yet another remedy: the salve, or ointment. The following recipes all combine oils that can be applied topically to enhance the skin or penetrate below the surface for deeper action.

Topical Oil

Warming Arthritis Oil

T he Ayurvedic tradition (see chapter 6, "Ayurveda") reveres the use of sesame seed oil, a high-fat oil that is excellent for the skin and very nutritious in Indian cuisine. This recipe is inspired by the rejuvenating Ayurvedic herbs cinnamon and ashwagandha, as well as bitter fennel that has traditionally been used to stimulate digestion. Arnica is a renowned anti-inflammatory herb, though it is at-risk in the wild. Use it respectfully; to learn more about arnica, see chapter 12, "Homeopathy." Topically these herbs combine to provide relief for inflammation and stimulate blood flow to sore joints and muscles.

Ingredients

¼ cup dried ashwagandha root, chopped
¼ cup dried arnica flowers
½ teaspoon cinnamon powder

1 cup sesame seed oil
½ pint glass jar

To Make

In a small saucepan, combine the herbs with the oil. Heat very gently for 20 minutes, stirring frequently and being careful not to let the mixture simmer. Strain, pressing out as much oil from the plants as possible, and reserve the liquid in a glass jar leaving a half inch of headspace at the top of the jar. Use immediately if you wish while it is still warm, then cap, label, and store the jar in a dry place on a dish or plate as oils have a tendency to ooze out of their containers.

To Use

With clean fingers, rub the warm or room temperature oil into the skin, directing it over sore muscles and joints. Avoid cut or broken skin.

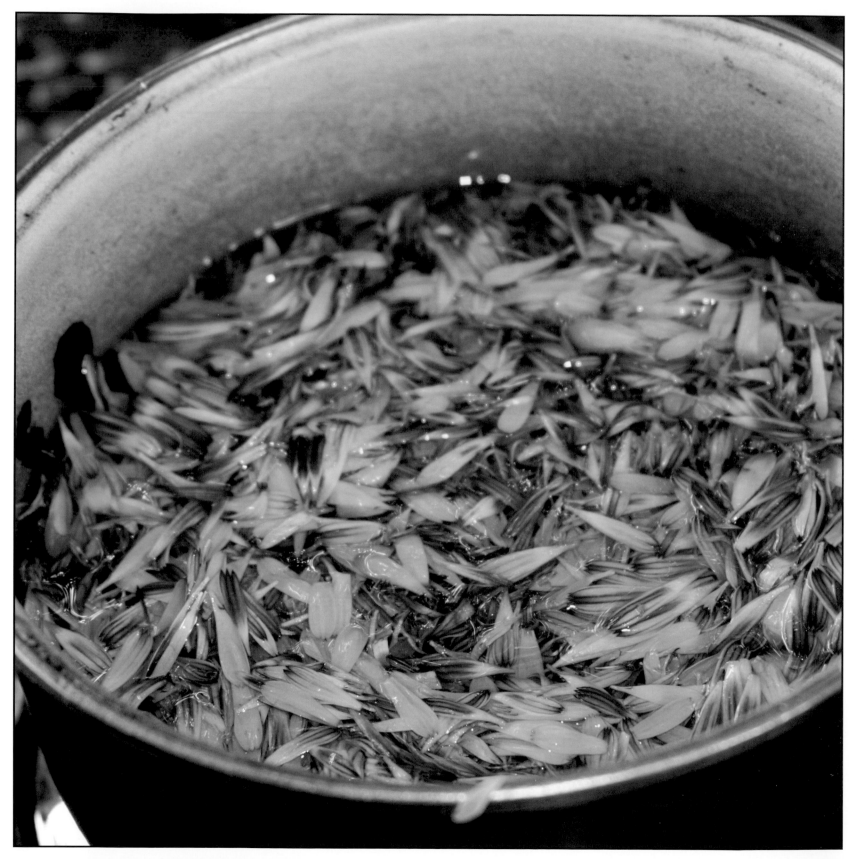

Pastes

A paste is simply a liquid and a solid mixed together to form a thick mass that can be applied to the skin. Pastes have a long history because they are easy to make, require little preparation, and can be made effectively with either fresh or dried plants. Most people are familiar with pesto, a culinary delight made from basil leaves and oil. But did you know a paste is an ancient remedy suitable for the first aid cabinet?

Here we feature two types of paste—the first is a beauty mask for the face made with argan oil, inspired by the work of Moroccan chemist Dr. Zoubida Charrouf and her work to protect the argan trees and create women's cooperatives (see her profile in chapter 10, "Pharmacology"). This is a lovely mask applied wet onto the face, allowed to dry, and rinsed off. The second paste is a first aid remedy for bee stings, which is quick to use in emergency situations.

Face Mask with Argan Oil

Ingredients

¼ cup oats
¼ cup seeds (sunflower, sesame, poppy, cranberry, etc.)
1 tablespoon argan oil (or olive, sweet almond, apricot, etc.)
1 teaspoon plain yogurt (optional)
½ teaspoon aloe vera gel (optional)

To Make

Grind oats and seeds in a food processor or blender until a fine powder is achieved; you'll have some coarse bits as well, and these make a good exfoliant for the skin.

To Use

In the palm of the hand, blend 1–2 teaspoons of this oat-seed powder with the oil, yogurt, and aloe vera, if using, until you have a smooth paste. Add more oat/seed powder if needed. Pull back the hair and apply to the face in smooth, circular motions. Allow to lightly dry, then rinse. Follow with a clay mask or a moisturizing cream.

Wound Paste

Ingredients

1 cup plantain leaves (you can find plantain in your yard; see chapter 4, "Folk Medicine," for a detailed profile of plantain)
2–4 teaspoons olive oil

To Make

Coarsely chop the fresh plantain leaves and place in a mortar and pestle. Grind, drizzling in oil, until you form a thick paste. Alternatively, spin leaves and oil in a food processor until you form a paste. Store in a tiny jar in the refrigerator; use within a couple of days.

To Use

Apply directly to bug bites, bee stings, and splinters.

Salves and Ointments

A salve, also called an ointment or a balm, has historically been a blend of oil and fat, such as lard. Today, many salves are made with beeswax (which is clean-smelling and easy to work with), but people around the world still use rendered lard to great effect and even hydrogenated oils such as Crisco will work. The oil (or lard) is infused with fresh plant material so that the chemicals of the plant are extracted into the oil, which is then heated and mixed with chips of wax to create the ointment. The recipes here honor the Western herbal medicine tradition (see chapter 1, "Western Herbal Medicine") and can be made with a wide variety of plants.

St. John's Lip Balm

Though St. John's wort is often used as an antidepressant, it is also a wonderful skin healing herb and folklore suggests it might be helpful for sunburn and even as a skin-protectant from sun exposure. See chapter 1, "Western Herbal Medicine," for more details about St. John's wort.

Ingredients

1 cup olive or canola oil
1 cup fresh St. John's wort flowers and/or leaves
¼ cup beeswax, grated or shaved
15–20 drops mint essential oil (optional)
7 or 8 2-ounce glass jars

To Make

Pour the oil into a saucepan. Add the chopped flowers or leaves, making sure they are not wet—excess water will spoil a salve! On a very low heat, gently warm the leaves with the oil for 20 minutes, being careful not to simmer. Strain lightly and pour the oil back into the pot. Add the beeswax. As soon as the wax melts, add the essential oil, if using, and pour into the glass jars. Cap immediately and allow to cool.

Yield: about seven 2-ounce jars.

To Use

Apply to the lips (or any dry skin) as needed.

Sage Wound Ointment

There are dozens of wildflowers, weeds, herbs and trees that are valued as "vulneraries," or plants that heal wounds. Instead of or in addition to sage, you could also use red clover blossoms, violet flowers and leaves, comfrey leaves, yarrow leaves, St. John's wort flowers, pine needles, hemlock tips, witch hazel bark and twigs, plantain leaves, oregano/thyme/marjoram leaves, and many more. These plants are detailed throughout the book; for more information about sage, see chapter 2, "Native Nations Medicine."

Ingredients

1 cup olive or canola oil
1 cup fresh sage leaves, chopped
¼ cup beeswax, grated or shaved
15–20 drops lemon, sage or thyme essential oil (optional)
7 or 8 2-ounce glass jars

To Make

Pour the oil into a saucepan. Add the chopped leaves, making sure they are not wet—excess water will spoil a salve! On a very low heat, gently warm the leaves with the oil for 20 minutes, being careful not to simmer. Strain and pour the oil back into the pan. Add the shaved beeswax. As soon as the wax melts, add the essential oil, if using, and pour into the glass jars. Cap immediately and allow to cool.

Yield: about seven 2-ounce jars.

To Use

With clean fingers, smear the ointment onto fresh wounds, cuts, scrapes, infections, rashes, etc., avoiding deep punctures. Use as needed.

Extracts and Concentrate Recipes

An extract or concentration is a remedy in which the plant has been steeped in a liquid such as wine, port, or witch hazel for a period of time and then the remaining fibrous matter (marc) is strained off. This results in a very strong extract that contains most of the alkaloids, essential oils, resins, glycosides, flavonoids, sugars, tannins, and other plant chemicals. One of the few things not extracted into the liquid is the fiber, which makes these remedies highly digestible and easy to consume. Extracts can be added to massage oils or pastes for external treatment, or they can be diluted in water or juice for taking internally. Extracts can also be made with apple cider vinegar and vegetable glycerin. Extracts made with commercial witch hazel can only be used externally, as liniments.

Bitters

Inspired by folk healers and the knowledgeable gypsy and bedouin healers (see Juliette de Bairacli Levy's profile in chapter 4, "Folk Medicine, Gypsy, and Bedouin Traditions") of Europe, these bitters

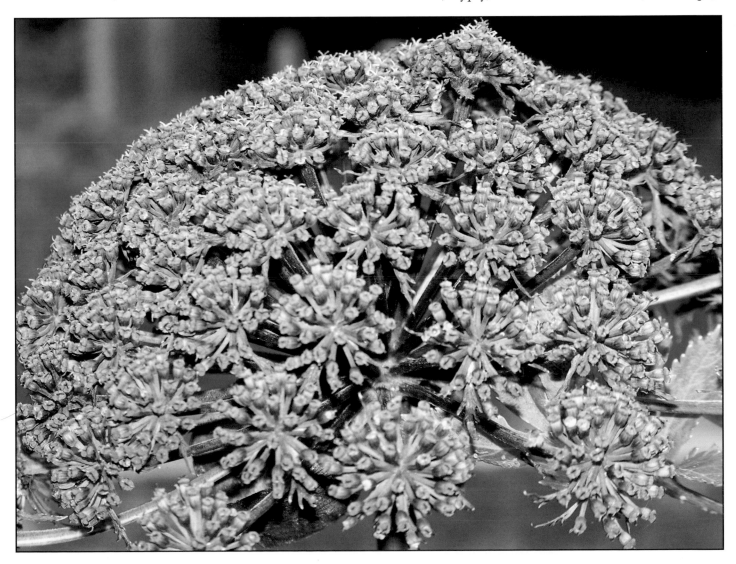

are fantastic digestive aids. We are blessed with many herbs that ease digestive upset—they are called carminative herbs that work by stimulating gastric juice and bile production to relieve a variety of gastric conditions such as peptic ulcer, bloating, gas, diarrhea, and heartburn. The aromatic oils present in many herbs are pleasant to consume and many "old-fashioned" candies and syrups have been made with them. Bitters can be taken before or after a meal, in water or tea, or they can be "dressed up" and drizzled on fruit or ice cream for a memorable dessert.

Angelica-Orange Bitters

Ingredients

1 cup dried orange peel, chopped
¼ cup gentian root
¼ cup angelica seeds
1 teaspoon fennel seed
½ teaspoon coriander seed
½ teaspoon gingerroot, chopped
1 pint red or white wine

To Make

Heat Method: In a large saucepan, combine all ingredients and pour over them the wine. Very gently simmer 20 to 30 minutes, stirring occasionally. Remove from the heat and strain, collecting the water in a jar or bottle. Cap, label, and store in a cool, dry place.

No-Heat Method: In a glass pint jar with a tight fitting lid, place all the fresh and/or dried ingredients. Cover with the grain alcohol,

cap, and shake. Steep for 2 weeks. Strain, reserving the liquid and storing in an attractive bottle.

To Use

Take by the drop or the quarter-teaspoon to aid digestion, or warm slightly and sip from a tiny glass as an aperatif; alternatively, add to syrup, ice cream toppings, or confections.

Witch Hazel Liniment for Rashes

Ingredients

1 handful chopped plantain, red clover, sage, ladies mantle, pau d'arco, rosemary or other healing herb
1 cup commercial witch hazel extract

To Make

In a glass pint jar with a tight fitting lid, place all the fresh and/ or dried ingredients. Cover with the witch hazel, cap, and shake. Steep for 1 to 2 weeks. Strain, reserving the liquid, and store in an attractive bottle.

To Use

Use this liniment externally only. With clean fingers and a clean cotton ball, apply gently over rashes such as eczema, psoriasis, and poison ivy and oak.

Tinctures

Tinctures differ from the extracts described previously because they are extracted into hard alcohol such as vodka. The handcrafting of tinctures may be the closest herbalism comes to pharmacology and the laboratory production of isolates. By tincturing an herb, we get the most concentrated form of it without distilling it. There is quite a debate now regarding "whole plant" medicines versus isolated "active" compounds, since scientists now have the ability to extract single chemicals from a plant believed responsible for healing. Whole-plant advocates, however, maintain that we truly don't know which chemicals do what, and also that this type of behavior is foreign to the spiritual nature of working with plants for health. For more details, see chapter 10, "Pharmacology."

To tincture a plant, harvest it fresh and process it immediately; have a glass pint jar ready along with grain alcohol—Everclear, vodka, or brandy (listed here in order from strongest to weakest). Generally we tincture hard plant matter such as roots and seeds in Everclear or vodka, saving brandy for soft matter such as flowers, but there is no hard-and-fast rule. Feel free to experiment with different liquids and plants to determine the intensity of extract you desire. Tinctures are designed to be used for acute health situations (short term of, say, 2 to 3 weeks or fewer). Chronic illnesses respond better to using water-based remedies such as teas and tisanes.

Menorrhagia Tincture

Astringent herbs are useful for drying things up; topically astringents are applied to wounds to act as a styptic to stop the bleeding. Internally, tinctures of astringent herbs can be helpful for acute conditions of excess flow, particularly heavy menstrual flow. Herbs such as ladies mantle, shepherd's purse, raspberry, yarrow, and wild cranesbill are useful for women with excessively heavy periods. See chapter 5, "Alchemy and Aromatherapy," for more details about ladies mantle, and chapter 13, "Gaelic Pharmacy," for details about yarrow.

Ingredients

1 cup fresh yarrow leaf
1 cup fresh ladies mantle leaf
1 pint vodka

To Make

In a pint jar with a tight-fitting lid, combine the plant ingredients and pour over them the vodka, filling to within ¼ inch of the top. Cap, shake, and steep for 2 weeks to 4 months. Strain, reserving the liquid. Cap, label, and store in a cool, dry place.

To Use

A typical dose is ¼ to ½ teaspoon every 3 to 4 hours for heavy bleeding. Use for a maximum of 5 days, then discontinue until the next menstrual cycle.

Pain-Relieving Tincture

Herbs such as meadowsweet, willow, and wintergreen contain pain-relieving salycilates. Because there is a risk that these phytochemicals can act like aspirin and cause Reye's Syndrome, do not give this tincture to children or teens who develop fevers with colds or flu.

Ingredients

3 tablespoons dried meadowsweet
3 tablespoons dried willow bark
8 ounces vodka

To Make

In a pint jar with a tight-fitting lid, combine the herbs and pour over them the vodka, filling to within ¼ inch of the top. Cap, shake, and steep a minimum of one month. Strain, reserving the liquid. Cap, label, and store in a cool, dry place.

To Use

Take ¼ teaspoon every 3 to 4 hours for pain such as headache or muscle and joint pain.

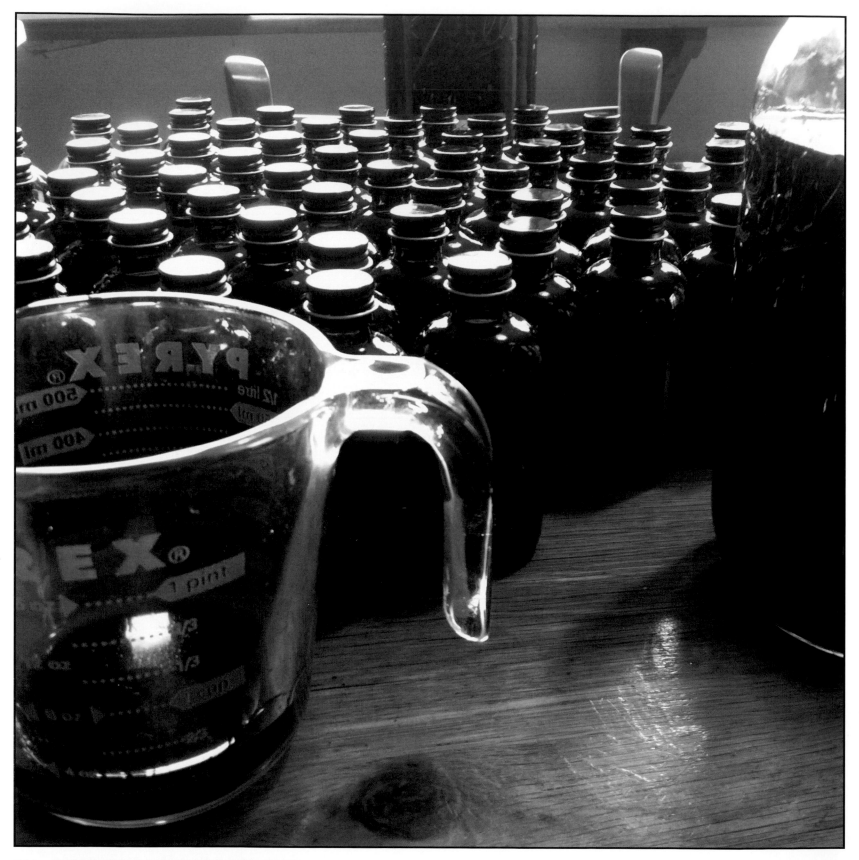

Water Remedies: Of and For the Water

Infusion

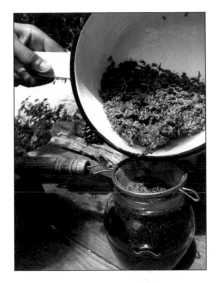

An infusion is one of the simplest remedies to make with plants, often with beautiful results. Probably every culture in the world makes infusions, which is the steeping of plant matter in water. Different cultures use hot or cold water, they steep for minutes or days, they use one herb or dozens, and they drink the infusion plain or they add all sorts of ritualized ornaments, including milk, cream, honey, sugar, vanilla, bitters, lemon, spices, and more.

Water is the key element, which must be clean and fresh. It does not matter if the water is distilled, spring, or from a faucet, though you do not want to use carbonated or chlorinated water. Choose an enamel, crockery, or stainless steel pot, but avoid aluminum. Experiment with steeping times with the various herbs you choose.

An infusion of herbal matter is properly called a tisane or an herbal tea; an infusion made with the tea plant *Camellia sinensis* is properly called tea (see chapter 7, "Eastern Oriental Medicine"). The following infusions (tisanes) honor the Western Herbal Tradition (chapter 1) and Oriental traditions since infusions are an important method of delivery of botanical medicine in both cultures. Hibiscus tea is also popular throughout South America and Jamaica, where it is served as a chilled beverage with meals. See chapter 7, "Eastern Oriental Medicine" for more information about hibiscus.

Hibiscus Tisane

Ingredients

1 teaspoon dried hibiscus flowers
1 teaspoon lemon peel (optional)
1 cup boiling water

To Make

Place flowers and citrus in a teapot and pour boiling water over them; steep for 6 to 8 minutes. Strain and sweeten if desired.

To Use

Serve iced with lemon slices or hot with small stevia leaves.

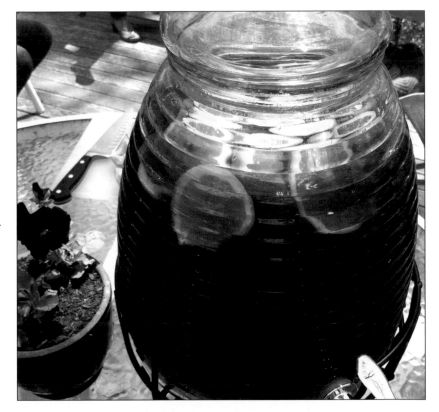

Steam-Inhalation

Take advantage of the volatile, strong-smelling essential oils present in many plants. These fragrant oils can be used in a variety of ways; by mixing with hot water, an effective steam can be obtained that is useful in cases of bronchial congestion, asthma, sinusitis, and sore throat. Fresh plants can be left in the bowl for beauty and to infuse further, or they can be strained. This easy home remedy is inspired by Middle Eastern remedies with Polynesian plants and is often used in Western herbal traditions. See chapter 3, "Polynesian Medicine," for more details about eucalyptus.

Eucalyptus Respiratory Steam

Ingredients

1 cup dried eucalyptus leaves
3–4 cups boiling water

To Make

Prepare a large, shallow pan or salad bowl and a thick bath towel. Place the leaves in the bowl and heat a pot of water to boiling.

To Use

Sitting by the bowl, pour the water into the bowl. Lean your head over the bowl, pulling the towel over your head to capture the steam. Be sure to close your eyes! Breathe through the nose and/or mouth. Have a tissue nearby so you can blow your nose as the steam helps clear mucous and nasal passages.

Body Soak

Make a tea and, instead of drinking it, soak the body in it; that's the basic premise behind a soak. It's a nutrient-rich, healing infusion of herbs in water that heals from the outside in. Soaks can be useful for the whole body in a tub of water, or for areas of the body that need a little extra attention, such as the feet, the hands, or in the case of the following recipe: the postpartum perineum.

Midwives' Perineum Sage Soak

A popular remedy used by midwives around the world, a sitz bath or perineum soak can easily be made at home to speed the healing of perineal tissues and to counter infection. Inspired by renowned herbalist Doña Enriqueta Contreras and the world's midwifery traditions (see chapter 8, "Midwifery"), this astringent soak can contain herbs that are naturally antiseptic, such as sage, oregano, calendula, yarrow, red clover, and comfrey. They fight bacteria at the same time they astringe—or tone—stretched or torn tissues. Red clover and calendula are also emollient—soothing and moisturizing to aid in skin regeneration.

Ingredients

1 cup dried sage or rosemary leaves, chopped
1 cup dried yarrow leaves, chopped

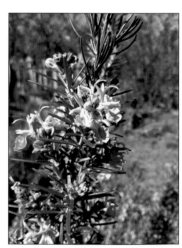

To Make

In a saucepan, steep the herbs with 2 cups just-boiled water for 20 to 30 minutes. Strain and reserve the tea in a jar.

To Use

Pour the hot tea into a bath and immerse the body; alternatively, pour the warm tea into a sitz-bath tray fitted onto the toilet to immerse the perineum, sitting and relaxing 5 to 10 minutes. Gently pat dry. Repeat several times daily.

Sprays

A spray or mist is made of water and essential oils for quick use as a light fragrance. This is a fun and easy project for children as several spritzers can be put together quickly, they smell great, and they can be confidently sprayed almost anywhere (avoiding the eyes). These make a lovely party project and take-home-gift for a girl's birthday party. Using essential oils honors alchemy and aromatherapy (see the profiles of Mary Prophetissa and Cleopatra in chapter 5, "Alchemy and Aromatherapy"), two world traditions that are credited with scientifically discovering essential or volatile oils and promoting their use in health and body care. Most essential oils are clear, but to experiment with color, choose blue-hued chamomile and yarrow (they get their color from the presence of azulene). For simple fragrances in body and bath products, use lavender, mint, lemon balm, sweet orange, or sage; for more exotic fragrances, select cardamom, ginger, ylang ylang, lemon verbena, balsam fir, or vetiver.

Soothing Balsam Spray

Ingredients

1 cup water
20–30 drops Balsam Fir essential oil

To Make

Simply pour the water into the spray bottles you wish to use and divide the drops of essential oil between them. Cap.

To Use

Spray on the skin, the hair, linens and pillows, and in the air.

Seaweed Bath

An authentic bathing technique that is beneficial for the skin and is a strong connection to plants is to bathe directly with seaweed fronds. This is inspired by chapter 3, "Polynesian Medicine," and also chapter 14, "Shamanism and Spirit Medicine," and is adapted from the author's article "Taking the Sacred Waters" in *Taproot Magazine*, Issue 6.

Kelp Spirit Bath

Ingredients

Several fresh kelp or dulse fronds, or 2–4 tablespoons dried flakes

To Make

Using fresh fronds: Place the fronds in the tub while the water is running as hot as possible. Enjoy, then remove fronds before draining water.

Using dried seaweed: Fill a large pot of water on the stovetop and bring it to a boil. Add the seaweed strips or flakes (using a large infuser makes this easy to clean up) and simmer for 15 minutes.

To Use

Pour the hot seaweed tea into the bathtub, straining if necessary. Enjoy.

Milk Recipes

Just as we can infuse herbs into water to make tisanes and washes, so can we use milk, which in many parts of the world is more accessible than fresh water. Farming and nomadic cultures throughout history have steeped their herbs in milk for both internal and external remedies. Feel free to use cow, goat, soy, rice, almond, or buttermilk.

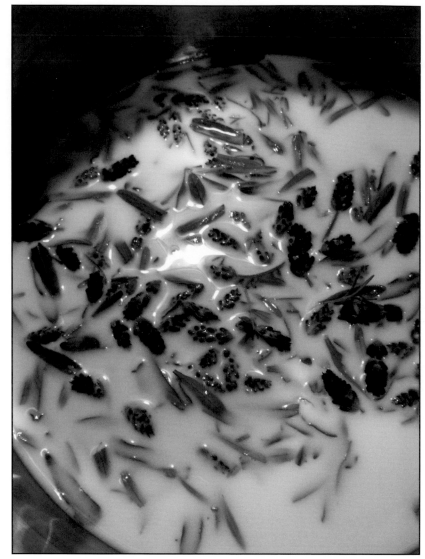

Creamy Face Smoother

Tansy, though not an herb you want to take internally because of its potency and its potential for being too intense (especially during pregnancy), is an herb widely used topically to clear the skin. Many old herbals extol the virtues of buttermilk infused with tansy as a beauty aid; it is soothing in cool, creamy milk lightly rubbed onto the face. See chapter 10, "Pharmacology," for more details about tansy.

Ingredients

1 cup fresh tansy flowers
1 cup fresh milk

To Make

In a saucepan, gently combine the flowers and milk and stir over very low heat. Allow to barely simmer, stirring constantly, for 15–20 minutes. Strain, reserving the liquid in a shallow bowl.

To Use

When cool, dip a small cloth into the milk and apply lightly to the face, or simply splash on using both hands. Rinse with cool water.

Spiritual Bathing

Inspired by ethnobotanist and healer Rocio Alarcon's teachings (see chapter 16, "Ethnobotany") and also by intense shamanic ceremonies (see chapter 14, "Shamanism and Spirit Medicine"), this method actually involves no water and is not a bath at all, but is part of a powerful engagement of the mind and the plant world. Alarcon recommends using sweet or bitter plants in quick sweeping motions across the body in an energetic cleansing of the aura. Tall wildflowers with stalks work best for this ritual.

Shamanic Herbal Energy Ceremony

Ingredients

Collect sweet herbs: sacred basil (Tulsi), lemon balm, red clover, goldenrod, Sweet Annie, hyssop, etc.

Collect bitter herbs: mugwort, yarrow, St. John's wort, pine branches, etc.

To Make

As part of your cleansing ritual, carefully select the herbs that you intuitively feel drawn to. Collect several branches or stalks, enough that you can hold in one hand comfortably.

To Use

Take a deep breath and, with full intention, quickly brush the branches over your body starting at the head and working your way down the neck, shoulders, arms, torso, and legs. Repeat on the other side. Visualize the aura releasing negative energies and shedding "hooks"; use this opportunity to be vocal, inviting the plant spirits to participate and remove negative energies. In her practice, Rocio is very loud with grunts, shouts, and prayers. This is an intense shamanic cleansing ceremony and is best performed on sacred days and full moons.

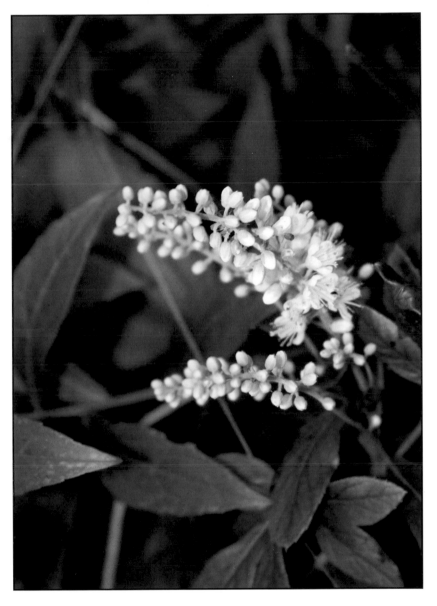

Smoke

Cultures throughout history have indulged in smoking herbs, often in a ritual or community setting. America's native nations crafted intricate rituals with carefully made pipes from sacred woods and harvested special herbs for use in their ceremonies. Kinnikinnick means "mixture" in Unami and Ojibwe; rarely is one single plant, such as tobacco, used in the smoke. Tobacco has many cousins that are considered sacred smoking herbs; in fact, as Michigan herbalist Jim McDonald warns, people today are paying tobacco a disrespect with our flagrant disregard of this sacred herb. "Smoking tobacco as an act of prayer," he says, "has been practiced as long as tobacco has been available to our kindred, and throughout all the lands where tobacco has since traveled. It is an entirely different practice than habitual smoking, which is properly characterized as the abuse of tobacco: we are abusing it. And if we abuse it, the way it tells us that this is wrong is by making us sick. It will do this until we learn to listen."

There are scores of recipes for a delicious and sacred smoking mixture that can be made from a variety of herbs, most notably mullein, sage, bearberry (*Arctostaphylos uva ursi*), Indian tobacco (*Lobelia*), black birch (*Betula nigra*), cherry bark (*Prunus* spp.), red sumac, red willow (Red Osier Dogwood), and many more. Smoking mullein has been used to ease respiratory congestion and soothe spastic coughs. This recipe is inspired by chapter 2, "Native Nations Medicine."

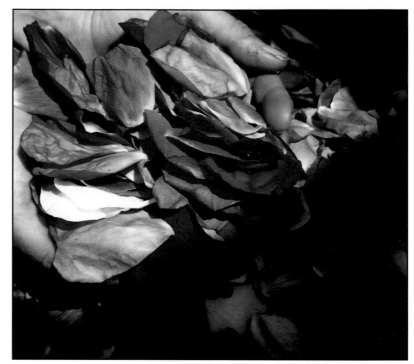

¼ cup dried black birch leaves, shredded
¼ cup dried rose petals, crumbled

To Make

Combine the herbs and store loosely in a leather pouch in a dry space.

To Use

When ready to smoke, pack a wooden pipe with ¼–½ teaspoon herbs; light and inhale gently.

Mullein Smoking Blend

Ingredients

½ cup dried mullein leaves, shredded
½ cup dried sage leaves, shredded

Za'Atar

Sumac yields clusters of very tart berries that can be roughly stripped from the stem and easily dried. Your fingers will taste incredibly tart after handling the berries; be careful and don't get the mix in the eyes. For this recipe, the sumac should be lightly or completely dried, which can easily be done on a screen, on a sheet of newsprint, or in an oven.

HRH Princess Basma bint Ali (see chapter 15, "Conservation and Gardening") shared her family's Za'atar traditions with me, adapted here, noting that they eat Za'atar most often as a breakfast or dinner in a small plate, and that she and her daughter prefer wild thyme because it is spicier. They love to tear pieces of their local bread and dip it in a bit of oil and then the Za'atar mix.

Za'atar Mix

Ingredients

2 teaspoons dried wild thyme, chopped
2 teaspoons dried marjoram
2 teaspoons ground sumac berries
2 teaspoons dried oregano
2 teaspoons sesame seeds
1 teaspoon cumin
½ teaspoon cinnamon (optional)
1 teaspoon coarse salt (not fine)

To Make

In a cast-iron skillet, gently roast the sesame seeds until warm and fragrant, just a few minutes. Quickly remove seeds to a bowl, cool, and add all other ingredients, stirring well. Store tightly lidded.

To Use

Sprinkle the mixture on a shallow dish and drizzle olive oil into it. Pull pieces from a freshly baked baguette and dip into the mix.

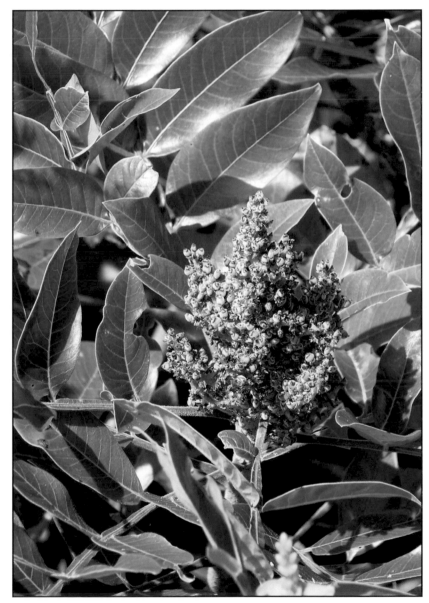

Fertilizer

As a gardening aid, nothing beats nettle "tea." It is popular for feeding both garden and house plants because a water extract of nettle plants is incredibly mineral-rich, which is also why it's a time-tested medicine and food for people, as well. Part of the tenets of feeding the land and conserving natural resources is to use what is available, and if there is nettle growing nearby, you can easily maintain the health of a garden with a minimum of labor. Another favorite fertilizer herb is comfrey; both comfrey and nettles are high in nitrogen, chlorophyll, magnesium, iron, and sulfur.

Garden Feeding Fertilizer

Ingredients

1 bucketful fresh nettle plants (leaves, stems, flowers, seeds), preferably in the later part of the season after they're no longer ideal for eating, or

1 bucketful fresh comfrey leaves
1 bucketful fresh water

To Make

Place the nettles or comfrey leaves whole into the bucket, keeping it loose and not compacted. Pour in the water, add a wide thin rock or iron grate to keep the plant matter submerged, cover with a lid or a sheet of wood, and place in the sun. Allow the "tea" to steep 1 to 2 weeks. The water will begin to ferment, froth, and sour; this builds beneficial bacteria and extracts nutrients and minerals from the nettle.

To Use

Strain off into another bucket or wheelbarrow and dilute with water, generally 10 parts water for every 1 part tea. Gently pour onto the ground around the base of tomatoes and fruit trees. Compost the leftover plant matter or bury where you will plant tomatoes next season.

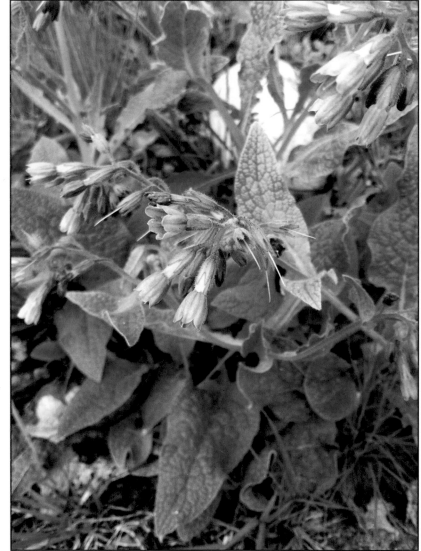

ORGANIZATIONS & RESOURCES

Please support the following nonprofits, organizations, and businesses with which the women herein are associated:

Kia Ingenlath: Casa de Milagros and The Chandler Sky Foundation, http://www.ninosdelsol.org

Isla Burgess: Viriditas, Centre for Plant Directed Learning and Participatory Science, www.viriditas.co.nz

Bernadette Rebionot: Center for Sacred Studies, http://centerforsacredstudies.org

Rosemary Gladstar: United Plant Savers, https://www.unitedplantsavers.org

Dr. Chang Yi Hsiang, The World Medicine Institute, Honolulu, www.wmi.edu

Bernadette Rebionot: Native Village, http://www.nativevillage.org

Dr. Phuntsog Wangmo, The Shang Shung Institute of America, http://www.shangshung.org/home/

Dr. Tieraona Low Dog, Arizona Center for Integrative Medicine, http://integrativemedicine.arizona.edu/index.html

Dr. Zoubida Charrouf, Targanine Cooperative, http://www.targanine.com/

Inez White, Australian Bush Flower Essences, http://ausflowers.com.au

Kate Gilday, Woodland Essence, http://www.woodlandessence.com

Mary Baker Eddy, The Mary Baker Eddy Library, http://www.marybakereddylibrary.org

Mary Beith, The West Highland Free Press, http://www.whfp.com

Susun Weed, http://www.susunweed.com

HRH Princess Basma bint Ali, The Royal Botanic Garden of Jordan, http://royalbotanicgarden.org

Holly Bellebuono, The Bellebuono School of Herbal Medicine, http://www.vineyardherbs.com

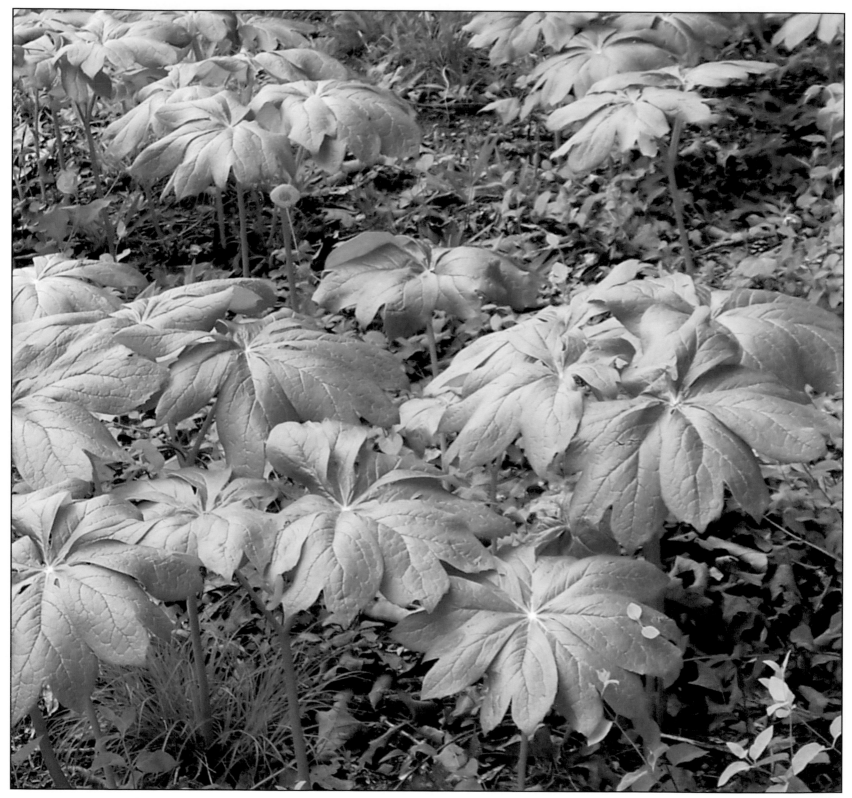

Mayapples

BIBLIOGRAPHY BY CHAPTER AND SIDEBAR

Part I: Plant Traditions

Chapter 1: Western Herbal Medicine

"Nurse" sidebar:
"Online Etymology Dictionary." *Online Etymology Dictionary.* Douglas Harper, 2001-2013. Web. <http://www.etymonline.com/>.
Stearn, William T. *Stearn's Dictionary of Plant Names for Gardeners: A Handbook on the Origin and Meaning of the Botanical Names of Some Cultivated Plants.* Portland, Or.: Timber, 2002. Print.

"Frome, England" sidebar:
Guralnik, David B. *Webster's New World Dictionary.* Cleveland: World Pub, 1959. Print.
Tourtellot, Jonathan B. *Discovering Britain & Ireland.* Washington D.C.: National Geographic Society, 1985. Print.
Snelling, Rebecca. *The Second Touring Guide to Britain.* Basingstoke, Hampshire: Publications Division of the Automobile Association, 1981. Print.

"St. John's wort" sidebar:
Grieve, Mrs. Maude. *A Modern Herbal: The Medicinal, Culinary, Cosmetic and Economic Properties, Cultivation and Folk-Lore of Herbs, Grasses, Fungi, Shrubs & Trees with Their Modern Scientific Uses.* Dover, New York: 1971; pg. 707.
Wheatley, David. "Safety of St. John's Wort (Hypericum Perforatum)." *The Lancet* 355.9203 (2000): 576. Print.

"Demeter" sidebar:
Frazer, James George. *The Golden Bough; a Study in Magic and Religion.* New York: Macmillan, 1951. Print.

Guthrie, W. K. C. *The Greeks and Their Gods.* Boston: Beacon, 1962. Print.
"Online Etymology Dictionary." *Online Etymology Dictionary.* Douglas Harper, 2001-2013. Web. <http://www.etymonline.com/>.

"Cusco Province, Sacred Valley, Peru" sidebar:
Hubbard, Ethan. *Journey to Ollantaytambo: In the Sacred Valley of the Incas.* Vermont: Chelsea Green Publishing, 1990.

"Calendula" sidebar:
Hoffmann, David, and David Hoffmann. *The Herbal Handbook: A User's Guide to Medical Herbalism.* Rochester, VT: Healing Arts, 1988. Print.
Sanders, Jack. *The Secrets of Wildflowers: A Delightful Feast of Little-known Facts, Folklore, and History.* Guilford, CT: Lyons, 2003. Print.
Rickett, Harold William. *WildFlowers of the United States.* New York: McGraw-Hill, 1966. Print.

"Vermont" sidebar:
Farewell, Susan. *Hidden New England.* Berkeley, CA: Ulysses, 2007. Print.

"Rebel" sidebar:
"Online Etymology Dictionary." *Online Etymology Dictionary.* Douglas Harper, 2001-2013. Web. <http://www.etymonline.com/>.

"Oregon and the Pacific Northwest" sidebar:
http://www.oregon.com/history/oregon_trail/timeline_1792_to_1815

"Bearberry" sidebar:
Foster, Steven and James A. Duke. *A Field Guide to Medicinal Plants and Herbs of Eastern and Central North America.* Boston: Houghton Mifflin, 2000. Print.

Kloss, Jethro. *Back to Eden: A Human Interest Story of Health and Restoration to Be Found in Herb, Root, and Bark.* Loma Linda, CA: Back to Eden, 1982. Print.

Meyer, Joseph Ernest. *The Herbalist and Herb Doctor.* Hammond, IN: Indiana Herb Gardens, 1918. Print.

"Innovate" sidebar:

"Online Etymology Dictionary." *Online Etymology Dictionary.* Douglas Harper, 2001-2013. Web. <http://www.etymonline.com/>.

Chapter 2: Native Nations Medicine

1 *Minority Health.* Centers for Disease Control and Prevention, n.d. Web. Dec. 2013.

Moerman, Daniel. *Native American Ethnobotany Database.* University of Michigan–Dearborn, n.d. Web. Dec. 2013.

U.S. Department of the Interior, Bureau of Indian Affairs

"Cherokee" sidebar:

1 Mooney, James. King, Duane (ed.). *Myths of the Cherokee.* Barnes & Noble. New York. 1888 (2007).

2 Davis, John B. "The Life and Work of Sequoyah." *Oklahoma Historical Society's Chronicles of Oklahoma*, Volume 8, No. 2. June 1930. Accessed online November 9, 2013.

"Georgia and South Carolina" sidebar:

Personal interview with Jody Noe, October 2013.

"Welcome to the Website of the Cherokees of South Carolina!" *The Eastern Cherokee, Southern Iroquois and United Tribes of South Carolina, Inc.* Cherokees of South Carolina, n.d. Web. 01 Dec. 2013. <http://www.cherokeesofsouthcarolina.com/>.

"Cedar" sidebar

The University of Michigan Native American Ethnobotany Database of Daniel Moerman provided the following ethnobotanical studies:

Rousseau, Jacques. 1945 *Le Folklore Botanique De Caughnawaga.* Contributions de l'Institut botanique l'Universite de Montreal 55:7-72 (p. 35).

Herrick, James William. *Iroquois Medical Botany.* State University of New York, Albany, PhD Thesis, 1977; (p. 270).

Mechling, W.H. "The Malecite Indians With Notes on the Micmacs." *Anthropologica*, 1959; 8:239-263 (p. 247).

Smith, Huron H. "Ethnobotany of the Ojibwe Indians." *Bulletin of the Public Museum of Milwaukee*, 1932; 4:327-525 (p. 380).

Fernald, Merritt Lyndon, and Alfred Charles Kinsey. *Edible Wild Plants of Eastern North America.* Harper and Row Publishers, New York: 1958.

Claus, Edward P., and Varro E. Tyler. *Pharmacognosy.* Philadelphia: Lea & Febiger, 1965. Print.

"Prayer" sidebar:

"Online Etymology Dictionary." *Online Etymology Dictionary.* Douglas Harper, 2001-2013. Web. <http://www.etymonline.com/>.

"Milkweed" sidebar:

Gladstar, Rosemary, and Pamela Hirsch. *Planting the Future: Saving Our Medicinal Herbs.* Rochester, VT: Healing Arts, 2000. Print.

Foster, Steven, James A. Duke, and Steven Foster. *A Field Guide to Medicinal Plants and Herbs of Eastern and Central North America.* Boston: Houghton Mifflin, 2000. Print.

Chapter 3: Polynesian Medicine

Gutmanis, June, and Susan G. Monden. *Kahuna La'au Lapa'au: The Practice of Hawaiian Herbal Medicine.* Norfolk Island, Australia: Island Heritage, 1976. Print. Mala Laau: *A Garden of Hawaiian*

Personal interview, Waianae Coast Comprehensive Health Center, 2009

Personal interview with Rosanne Harrigan, University of Hawaii at Manoa, 2009

"Question" sidebar:

"Online Etymology Dictionary." *Online Etymology Dictionary.* Douglas Harper, 2001-2013. Web. <http://www.etymonline.com/>.

"Olena/Turmeric" sidebar:

Castleman, Michael, and Michael Castleman. *The New Healing Herbs: The Classic Guide to Nature's Best Medicines Featuring the Top 100 Time-tested Herbs.* Emmaus, PA: Rodale, 2001. Print.

Loewenfeld, Claire, and Philippa Back. *The Complete Book of Herbs and Spices.* New York: Putnam, 1974. Print.

Teiten, Marie-Hélène, Simone Reuter, Stéphane Schmucker, Mario Dicato, and Marc Diederich. "Induction of Heat Shock Response by Curcumin in Human Leukemia Cells." *Cancer Letters* 279.2 (2009): 145-54. Print.

Whistler, W. Arthur. *Polynesian Herbal Medicine*. Lawai, Kauai, Hawaii: National Tropical Botanical Garden, 1992. Print.

Personal interview with Auntie Velma DelaPena, February 2009.

"Eucalyptus" sidebar:

Harris, Ben Charles. *The Compleat Herbal: Being a Description of the Origins, the Lore, the Characteristics, the Types, and the Prescribed Uses of Medicinal Herbs, including an Alphabetical Guide to All Common Medicinal Plants*. Barre, MA: Barre, 1972. Print.

Pratt, H. Douglas. *A Pocket Guide to Hawai'i's Trees and Shrubs*. Honolulu, HI: Mutual Pub., 1998. Print.

Pukui, Mary Kawena, Samuel H. Elbert, and Esther T. Mookini. *New Pocket Hawaiian Dictionary: With a Concise Grammar and Given Names in Hawaiian*. Honolulu: University of Hawaii, 1992. Print.

Tierra, Michael. *The Way of Herbs: Fully Updated–with the Latest Developments in Herbal Science*. New York: Pocket, 1990. Print.

Whistler, W. Arthur. *Polynesian Herbal Medicine*. Lawai, Kauai, Hawaii: National Tropical Botanical Garden, 1992. Print.

Chapter 4: Folk Medicine, Gypsy, and Bedouin Traditions

Simpson, Bernadette. *Wandering Through Wadis: A Nature-Lover's Guide to the Flora of South Sinai*. Dahab, Egypt: NimNam, 2013. Print.

Elliman, Wendy. "Israeli Researchers Explore Secrets of Natural Remedies." *JWeekly* 22 June 2001: n. pag. Web.

Hildegard von Bingen

1 Hildegard, and Priscilla Throop. *Hildegard Von Bingen's Physica: The Complete English Translation of Her Classic Work on Health and Healing*. Rochester, VT: Healing Arts, 1998. Print.

2 Flanagan, Sabina. *Hildegard of Bingen, 1098-1179: A Visionary Life*. London: Routledge, 1998. Print. p. 97.

3 Throop, 1998.

4 Hozeski, Bruce W. *Hildegard's Healing Plants: From Her Medieval Classic Physical*. Boston: Beacon, 2001. Print.

5 Ibid

6 Review of Higley, Sarah, Hildegard of Bingen's Unknown Language: An Edition, Translation and Discussion. (The New Middle Ages series.) Palgrave Macmillan, 2007 (reviewed by S.B. Straubhaar, UIOWA, 2008)

"Germany" sidebar

A Guide to the European Market for Medicinal Plants and Extracts. London: Commonwealth Secretariat, 2001. Print.

"Lavender" sidebar:

A Guide to the European Market for Medicinal Plants and Extracts. London: Commonwealth Secretariat, 2001. Print.

Claus, Edward P., and Varro E. Tyler. *Pharmacognosy*. Philadelphia: Lea & Febiger, 1965. Print.

McVicar, Jekka, and Jekka McVicar. *The Complete Herb Book*. Richmond Hill, Ont.: Firefly, 2008. Print.

Juliette de Bairacli Levy

1 Puotinen, C.J. "A History of Holistic Dog Care: A Profile of Juliette De Bairacli Levi, Pioneer of Natural Rearing Methods." *The Whole Dog Journal*, July (2006): n. pag. Print.

2 Ibid

3 *Juliette of the Herbs*. Dir. Tish Streeten. N.d. DVD.

4 Puotinen, C.J. "A History of Holistic Dog Care: A Profile of Juliette De Bairacli Levi, Pioneer of Natural Rearing Methods." *The Whole Dog Journal*, July (2006): n. pag. Print.

5 *Juliette of the Herbs*. Dir. Tish Streeten. N.d. DVD.

6 Bairacli-Levy, Juliette. *Herbal Handbook for Everyone*. London: Faber and Faber Limited, 1966. Print.

7 *Juliette of the Herbs*. Dir. Tish Streeten. N.d. DVD.

8 Bairacli-Levy, Juliette. *Herbal Handbook for Everyone*. London: Faber and Faber Limited, 1966. Print.

"Heal" sidebar:

"Online Etymology Dictionary." *Online Etymology Dictionary*. Douglas Harper, 2001-2013. Web. <http://www.etymonline.com/>.

"Greece" sidebar

1 "The History of Western Herbalism." *Christopher Hobbs – The Virtual Herbal*. Christopher Hobbs, n.d. Web. 01 Jan. 2013. <http://www.christopherhobbs.com/>.

Chapter 5: Alchemy & Aromatherapy

1 Ebbell, B., and Leon Banov. *The Papyrus Ebers: The Greatest Egyptian Medical Document*. Copenhagen: Levin & Munksgaard, 1937. Print.

León, Vicki. *Outrageous Women of Ancient Times*. New York: Wiley, 1998. Print.

Skipper, Cathy, and Patrice DeBonneval. "Making and Using Hydrosols—Home Distilling." *The International Herb Symposium Proceedings: Celebrating the Healing Power of Plants* (2013): n. pag. Print.

Queen Cleopatra

1 Anderson, Jaynie, and Giovanni Battista Tiepolo. *Tiepolo's Cleopatra*. Melbourne: Macmillan, 2003. Print. p. 81.

2 Davis, William Stearns, and Willis M. West. *Readings in Ancient History: Illustrative Extracts from the Sources*. Boston: Allyn and Bacon, 1912. Print.

3 Ibid, pg. 162

4 Ibid, pg. 163

5 Schaalje, Jacqueline. "Ein Gedi." *The Jewish Magazine* April (2002): n. pag. Web. <http://www.jewishmag.com/54mag/ein-gedi/ein-gedi.htm>.

6 Hasson, Nir. "After Repeated Failures, New Effort to Revive the Legendary Balsam Plant Shows Promise." *Haaretz* Sept. 2 (2010): n. pag. Web. <http://www.haaretz.com/print-edition/news/after-repeated-failures-new-effort-to-revive-the-legendary-balsam-plant-shows-promise-1.311617>.

7 Jones, Prudence J. *Cleopatra: The Last Pharaoh*. London: Haus, 2006. Print.

"Kore" sidebar:

"Online Etymology Dictionary." *Online Etymology Dictionary*. Douglas Harper, 2001-2013. Web. <http://www.etymonline.com/>.

Starhawk, Diane Baker, and Anne Hill. *Circle Round: Raising Children in Goddess Traditions*. New York: Bantam, 2000. Print.

"Alexandria, Egypt" sidebar:

"History of Egypt." *HistoryWorld.net* (2002): n. pag. Web. Jan.-Feb. 2009. <http://www.historyworld.net/index/sitesearch.asp?cx=partner-pub-6806100451075168%3Ap3uag0k4vwf&cof=FORID%3A10&ie=ISO-8859-1&q=egypt&x=-948&y=-81>.

"Cinnamon" sidebar:

Stearn, William T. *Stearn's Dictionary of Plant Names for Gardeners: A Handbook on the Origin and Meaning of the Botanical Names of Some Cultivated Plants*. Portland, Or.: Timber, 2002. Print.

Loewenfeld, Claire, and Philippa Back. *The Complete Book of Herbs and Spices*. New York: Putnam, 1974. Print.

Claus, Edward P., and Varro E. Tyler. *Pharmacognosy*. Philadelphia: Lea & Febiger, 1965. Print.

Tierra, Michael. *The Way of Herbs: Fully Updated—with the Latest Developments in Herbal Science*. New York: Pocket, 1990. Print.

Maria Prophetissa
"Mer, Mary" sidebar:

Raver, Miki. *Listen to Her Voice: Women of the Hebrew Bible*. San Francisco, CA: Chronicle, 1998. Print.

Stone, Merlin. *Ancient Mirrors of Womanhood: A Treasury of Goddess and Heroine Lore from around the World*. Boston: Beacon, 1984. Print.

"Tansy" sidebar

Krochmal, Arnold, and Connie Krochmal. *A Field Guide to Medicinal Plants*. New York, NY: Times, 1984. Print.

Kennett, Frances. *Folk Medicine: Fact and Fiction*. New York: Crescent, 1976. Print.

Claus, Edward P., and Varro E. Tyler. *Pharmacognosy*. Philadelphia: Lea & Febiger, 1965. Print.

Macinnis, Peter. *Poisons: From Hemlock to Botox to the Killer Bean of Calabar*. New York: Arcade Pub., 2005. Print.

Weed, Susun S. *Wise Woman Herbal for the Childbearing Year*. Woodstock, NY: Ash Tree Pub., 1986. Print.

Part II: Body Traditions

Chapter 6: Ayurveda

1 "Facts: Cow Urine Cure," National Geographic Channel
Anne McIntyre FNIMH, Women's Herbal Conference 2008
Patnaik, Naveen. *The Garden of Life*. New York; Doubleday, 1993.

"India" sidebar:

1 "Facts: Cow Urine Cure." *National Geographic Channel* (n.d.): n. pag. *National Geographic - Inspiring People to Care About the Planet Since 1888*. From the Witch Doctor Will See You Now: India. Web.

2 Gogtay, N.J., et al. "The use and safety of non-allopathic Indian medicines." Department of Clinical Pharmacology, Seth GS Medical College and KEM Hospital, Mumbai, India. Drug Saf. 2002; 25(14):1005-19. Accessed on PubMed.gov November 2013.

3 Ibid

4 Griffith, Ralph T. H. "Rig Veda, 1895: Book 10, Hymn XCVII, "Praise of Herbs" *Sacred-Texts.com* November (2013): n. pag. Web.

"Ginger" sidebar:

Katzer, Gernot. "Spice Pages." *Institut Für Chemie, University of Graz, Austria* (2013): n. pg. Web.

The Holy Qur'an. Translated by M.H. Shakir and published by Tahrike Tarsile Qur'an, Inc., 1983. (accessed online at http://quod.lib.umich.edu/k/koran/, January 15, 2009)

Lunde, Paul. "The Explorer Marco Polo." *Saudi Aramco World* July/August 56.4 (2005): n. pag. Web.

Patnaik, Naveen. *The Garden of Life: An Introduction to the Healing Plants of India.* New York: Doubleday, 1993. Print.

Chapter 7: Eastern Oriental Medicine

Avedon, John. "Exploring the Mysteries of Tibetan Medicine." *The New York Times* 11 Jan. 1981: n. pag. Web.

Personal interview, The Shang Shung Institute, Conway, MA, USA.

"Leaves" sidebar:

"Online Etymology Dictionary." *Online Etymology Dictionary.* Douglas Harper, 2001-2013. Web. <http://www.etymonline.com/>.

"China" sidebar:

Macleod, Calum. *Eyewitness Travel Guide China.* London: Dorling Kindersley, 2005. Print.

"Hibiscus" sidebar:

Patnaik, Naveen. *The Garden of Life: An Introduction to the Healing Plants of India.* New York: Doubleday, 1993. Print.

Stearn, William T. *Stearn's Dictionary of Plant Names for Gardeners: A Handbook on the Origin and Meaning of the Botanical Names of Some Cultivated Plants.* Portland, Or.: Timber, 2002. Print.

Tierra, Michael. *The Way of Herbs: Fully Updated --with the Latest Developments in Herbal Science.* New York: Pocket, 1990. Print.

Whistler, W. Arthur. *Polynesian Herbal Medicine.* Lawai, Kauai, Hawaii: National Tropical Botanical Garden, 1992. Print.

"Compassion" sidebar:

"Online Etymology Dictionary." *Online Etymology Dictionary.* Douglas Harper, 2001-2013. Web. <http://www.etymonline.com/>.

Withington, Edward T. "Medical History from the Earliest Times: A Popular History of the Healing Art." *The Scientific Press* 27th ser. January (2006): n. pag. Harvard University. Web.

"Tibet" sidebar:

"Central Tibetan Administration." *Central Tibetan Administration.* N.p., n.d. Web. 30 Dec. 2013. <http://tibet.net/>.

Avedon, John. "Exploring the Mysteries of Tibetan Medicine." *The New York Times* 11 Jan. 1981: n. pag. Web.

"Tea" sidebar:

Dillman, Erika. *The Little Book of Healthy Teas.* New York: Warner, 2002. Print.

Heiss, Mary Lou, and Robert J. Heiss. *The Story of Tea: A Cultural History and Drinking Guide.* Berkeley, CA: Ten Speed, 2007. Print.

Claus, Edward P., and Varro E. Tyler. *Pharmacognosy.* Philadelphia: Lea & Febiger, 1965. Print.

Chapter 8: Midwifery

"Childbirth: Nature v. Drugs." Leupp, Constance and Tracy, Marguerite. *Time* magazine, Monday May 25, 1936. Accessed online May 20, 2009.

"Websites that Address Epidural Anesthesia for Chilbirth." Cubera, Sabrina and Montgomery, Kristen. *Journal of Perinatal Education.* 2004 Fall; 13(4): 53–56.

Adrian Feldhusen is a New Hampshire Certified Midwife and CPM, as reported in "The History of Midwifery and Childbirth in America: A Time Line," *Midwifery Today,* 2000.

"Outcomes of planned home births with certified professional midwives: large prospective study in North America." By epidemiologist Kenneth Johnson and project manager Betty-Anne Daviss. *British Medical Journal* 2005; 330:1416 (18 June).

Personal interview, Caroline Weaver, 2000.

Marie-Henriette LeJeune Ross

"Canadian Women in Science." *Library and Archives Canada.* N.p., n.d. Web. 23 Apr. 2010.

"Dictionary of Canadian Biography. Volume III. 2000. Toronto: University of Toronto Press." *Marie-Henriette LeJeune Ross* (2000): 489-99. Web.

"Tincture" sidebar:

"Online Etymology Dictionary." *Online Etymology Dictionary.* Douglas Harper, 2001-2013. Web. <http://www.etymonline.com/>.

"Nova Scotia" sidebar:

Landry, Peter. *The Lion and the Lily: Nova Scotia between 1600-1760.* [Victoria, B.C.]: Trafford, 2007. Print.

"Conceive" sidebar:

"Online Etymology Dictionary." *Online Etymology Dictionary.* Douglas Harper, 2001-2013. Web. <http://www.etymonline.com/>.

Chapter 9: Allopathic (Modern) Medicine

"To Err Is Human: Building a Safer Health System." The Institute of Medicine Committee on the Quality of Health Care in America, a Private Non-profit Organization under the National Academy of Sciences, 1999-2000. Web.

Van Der Zee, Barbara. *Green Pharmacy: The History and Evolution of Western Herbal Medicine.* Rochester, VT: Healing Arts, 1997. Print.

Trotula of Salerno:

1 Green, Monica Helen. *The Trotula: A Medieval Compendium of Women's Medicine.* Philadelphia: University of Pennsylvania, 2001. Print. p. 47.

2 Ibid , p. 49

3 Ibid , p. 94

4 Ibid , p. 49

5 Ibid , p. 50

6 Ibid , p. 48

7 Hamilton, George L. "Trotula." *Modern Philology* October 4.2 (1906): 377-80. Web.

8 Green, Monica Helen. *The Trotula: A Medieval Compendium of Women's Medicine.* Philadelphia: University of Pennsylvania, 2001. Print. p. 48.

9 Chaucer, Geoffrey, and Robert A. Pratt. *The Tales of Canterbury: Complete.* Boston: Houghton Mifflin, 1974. Print.; p. 268.

10 Green, Monica Helen. *The Trotula: A Medieval Compendium of Women's Medicine.* Philadelphia: University of Pennsylvania, 2001. Print. p. 93-109.

11 Ibid , p.114

12 Ibid , introduction

13 Ibid , p. 41

14 Ibid , p. 41

15 Ibid , p. 41

16 Ibid , p. 91

17 Ibid , p. 104

Additional references:

Green, Monica H. "In Search of an Authentic Women's Medicine: The Strange Fates of Trota of Salerno and Hildegard of Bingen." *DYNAMIS.* Acta Hisp. Med. Sci. Hist. Illus., 1999. Web.pp: 25-54.

Bifulco, M. "The First Cosmetic Treatise of History. A Female Point of View." *International Journal of Cosmetic Science* 30 (2008): 79-86. Web.

Ferraris, Zoe, and Victor Ferraris. "The Women of Salerno: Contribution to the Origins of Surgery from Medieval Italy." *The Society of Thoracic Surgeons* 1855-7 64 (1997): n. pag. Web.

Brooke, Elisabeth. *Women Healers: Portraits of Herbalists, Physicians, and Midwives.* Rochester, VT: Healing Arts, 1996. Print.

"Salerno, Italy" sidebar:

1 "University History." *Universita Degli Studi Di Salerno.* N.p., n.d. Web. 4 Nov. 2013.

"Stinging Nettle" sidebar:

Harris, Ben Charles. *The Compleat Herbal: Being a Description of the Origins, the Lore, the Characteristics, the Types, and the Prescribed Uses of Medicinal Herbs, including an Alphabetical Guide to All Common Medicinal Plants.* Barre, MA: Barre, 1972. Print.

Gibbons, Euell. *Stalking the Healthful Herbs.* New York: D. McKay, 1966. Print.

"Remedy" sidebar:

"Online Etymology Dictionary." *Online Etymology Dictionary.* Douglas Harper, 2001-2013. Web. <http://www.etymonline.com/>.

"Tucson, Arizona" sidebar:

DesertUSA.com, 2008; Web.

Nabokov, Peter, and Robert Easton. *Native American Architecture.* New York: Oxford UP, 1989. Print.

Stearn, William T. *Stearn's Dictionary of Plant Names for Gardeners: A Handbook on the Origin and Meaning of the Botanical Names of Some Cultivated Plants.* Portland, Or.: Timber, 2002. Print.

"Chaste-tree Berry" sidebar:

Stearn, William T. *Stearn's Dictionary of Plant Names for Gardeners: A Handbook on the Origin and Meaning of the Botanical Names of Some Cultivated Plants.* Portland, Or.: Timber, 2002. Print.

Gladstar, Rosemary. *Herbal Healing for Women: Simple Home Remedies for Women of All Ages.* New York: Simon & Schuster, 1993. Print.

"Online Etymology Dictionary." *Online Etymology Dictionary*. Douglas Harper, 2001-2013. Web. <http://www.etymonline.com/>.

Chapter 10: Pharmacology

Tierra, Michael. *The Way of Herbs: Fully Updated–with the Latest Developments in Herbal Science*. New York: Pocket, 1990. Print.

Claus, Edward P., and Varro E. Tyler. *Pharmacognosy*. Philadelphia: Lea & Febiger, 1965. Print.

Locusta of Gaul

Macinnis, Peter. *Poisons: From Hemlock to Botox to the Killer Bean of Calabar*. New York: Arcade Pub., 2005. Print.

León, Vicki. *Outrageous Women of Ancient Times*. New York: Wiley, 1998. Print.

Baldwin, James. "Nero" *Fifty Famous Stories Retold*. [United States]: Filiquarian, 2007. Print.

Barrett, Anthony. *Agrippina: Sex, Power, and Politics in the Early Empire*. New Haven: Yale UP, 1996. Print.

Barrett, Anthony. *Nero*. Boston: Belknap of Harvard UP, 2005. Print.

"Poison" sidebar:

"Online Etymology Dictionary." *Online Etymology Dictionary*. Douglas Harper, 2001-2013. Web. <http://www.etymonline.com/>.

"Apothecary" sidebar:

1 "Online Etymology Dictionary." *Online Etymology Dictionary*. Douglas Harper, 2001-2013. Web. <http://www.etymonline.com/>.

"Rome, Italy" sidebar:

1 Hayes, A. Wallace, and Claire L. Kruger. *Principles and Methods of Toxicology*. Sept. ed.: CRC, 2007. Print. p. 14.

2 Von Stackelberg, Katharine T. *The Roman Garden: Space, Sense and Society*. Routledge Monographs in Classical Studies. London: Routledge, 2009. Web.

3 Ibid

"Foxglove" sidebar:

Grieve, Mrs. Maude. *A Modern Herbal: The Medicinal, Culinary, Cosmetic and Economic Properties, Cultivation and Folk-Lore of Herbs, Grasses, Fungi, Shrubs & Trees with Their Modern Scientific Uses*. Dover, New York: 1971.

Jordan, Michael. *The Green Mantle: An Investigation into Our Lost Knowledge of Plants*. London: Cassell, 2001. Print.

Claus, Edward P., and Varro E. Tyler. *Pharmacognosy*. Philadelphia: Lea & Febiger, 1965. Print.

"Cooperate" sidebar:

"Online Etymology Dictionary." *Online Etymology Dictionary*. Douglas Harper, 2001-2013. Web. <http://www.etymonline.com/>.

"Morocco" sidebar:

Morocco. London: Dorling Kindersley, 2002. Print.

"Argan tree" sidebar:

1 Wall, Tim. "Tree-Going Goats Threaten Oil Supply." *Beta News* 22nd ser. Sept. (2011): n. pag. Web.

"Hyssop" sidebar:

Musselman, Lytton J. "Bible Plants." *Old Dominion University* (n.d.): n. pag. 19 Feb. 2013. Web. <http://ww2.odu.edu/~lmusselm/plant/bible/bible.php>.

Part III: Spirit Traditions

Chapter 11: Flower Essence Therapy

"Salve" sidebar:

"Online Etymology Dictionary." *Online Etymology Dictionary*. Douglas Harper, 2001-2013. Web. <http://www.etymonline.com/>.

Starbird, Margaret. *The Woman with the Alabaster Jar: Mary Magdalen and the Holy Grail*. Santa Fe, NM: Bear & Pub., 1993. Print.

Baring, Anne, and Jules Cashford. *The Myth of the Goddess: Evolution of an Image*. New York: Penguin, 1991. Print. p. 589.

Harper, Robert Francis. *Assyrian and Babylonian Literature: Selected Translations*. New York: Appleton, 1904. Print.

"Adirondacks, New York" sidebar:

"GoAdirondack.com-Home Page." *GoAdirondack.com-Home Page.* Adirondack Coast Visitors and Convention Bureau, n.d. Web. 30 Dec. 2013. <http://goadirondack.com/>.

"Adirondack History Network." *The Adirondack Museum.* Blue Mountain Lake, 2000. Web.

Smith, Greg. "The Adirondacks: More than Just Mountains." *Greg Smith.* N.p., 2000. Web. <www.adirondackpark.net>.

"Hawthorn" sidebar:

Frazer, James George. *The Golden Bough; a Study in Magic and Religion.* New York: Macmillan, 1951. Print.

Gibbons, Euell. *Stalking the Healthful Herbs.* New York: D. McKay, 1966. Print.

Van Der Zee, Barbara. *Green Pharmacy: The History and Evolution of Western Herbal Medicine.* Rochester, VT: Healing Arts, 1997. Print.

Winston, David. *Herbal Therapeutics: Specific Indications for Herbs & Herbal Formulas.* Broadway, NJ: Herbal Therapeutics Research Library, 2003. Print.

Chapter 12: Homeopathy

Van Der Zee, Barbara. *Green Pharmacy: The History and Evolution of Western Herbal Medicine.* Rochester, VT: Healing Arts, 1997. Print.

Mary Baker Eddy

"The Mary Baker Eddy Library." *The Mary Baker Eddy Library.* The Mary Baker Eddy Library for the Betterment of Humanity, Inc., 2013. Web. <http://www.marybakereddylibrary.org/>.

"Grateful" sidebar:

"Online Etymology Dictionary." *Online Etymology Dictionary.* Douglas Harper, 2001-2013. Web. <http://www.etymonline.com/>.

"Garlic and Onion" sidebar:

Lockie, Andrew. *Homeopathy Handbook.* New York: Dorling Kindersley Pub., 2001. Print.

Rose, Barry. *The Family Health Guide to Homeopathy.* Berkeley, CA: Celestial Arts, 1993. Print.

Mabey, Richard, and Michael McIntyre. *The New Age Herbalist: How to Use Herbs for Healing, Nutrition, Body Care, and Relaxation.* New York: Collier, 1988. Print.

Howard, Lois Jean. "Herbs in Mythology." *The South Texas Unit of the American Herb Society* (n.d.): n. pag. Web. <http://www.herbsociety-stu.org/Mythology.htm>.

"Arnica" sidebar:

1 Mars, Brigitte. "Arnica." Gladstar, Rosemary, and Pamela Hirsch. *Planting the Future: Saving Our Medicinal Herbs.* Healing Arts: Rochester, VT. 2000. Print.

Chapter 13: Gaelic Pharmacy

Ross, Anne. *The Folklore of the Scottish Highlands.* Totowa, NJ: Rowman and Littlefield, 1976. Print.

"Inspire" sidebar:

"Online Etymology Dictionary." *Online Etymology Dictionary.* Douglas Harper, 2001-2013. Web. <http://www.etymonline.com/>.

"Scotland" sidebar:

1 *Fodor's Exploring Scotland.* New York: Fodor's Travel Publications, 1995. Print.

Humphreys, Rob, Donald Reid, and Helena Smith. *The Rough Guide to Scotland.* London: Rough Guides, 2011. Print.

"Bogbean" sidebar:

Harris, Ben Charles. *The Compleat Herbal: Being a Description of the Origins, the Lore, the Characteristics, the Types, and the Prescribed Uses of Medicinal Herbs, including an Alphabetical Guide to All Common Medicinal Plants.* Barre, MA: Barre, 1972. Print.

Hoffmann, David. *The Herbal Handbook: A User's Guide to Medical Herbalism.* Rochester, VT: Healing Arts, 1988. Print.

"Gorse" sidebar:

Grieve, Mrs. Maude. *A Modern Herbal: The Medicinal, Culinary, Cosmetic and Economic Properties, Cultivation and Folk-Lore of Herbs, Grasses, Fungi, Shrubs & Trees with Their Modern Scientific Uses.* Dover, New York: 1971.

Chapter 14: Shamanism and Spirit Medicine

Personal interview, Dona Enriqueta Contreras, 2009.

Balick, Michael J., and Paul Alan Cox. *Plants, People, and Culture: The Science of Ethnobotany.* New York: Scientific American Library, 1996. Print.

Van Der Zee, Barbara. *Green Pharmacy: The History and Evolution of Western Herbal Medicine*. Rochester, VT: Healing Arts, 1997. Print.

Minnis, Paul E. *Ethnobotany: A Reader*. Norman: University of Oklahoma, 2000. Print.

"Witch" sidebar:

"Online Etymology Dictionary." *Online Etymology Dictionary*. Douglas Harper, 2001-2013. Web. <http://www.etymonline.com/>.

Susun Weed, Baba Yaga lecture, 2007 International Herb Symposium

"Mullein" sidebar:

Moerman, Daniel. "Mullein." *Native American Ethnobotany Database*. University of Michigan–Dearborn, n.d. Web.

"Chicory and Succor" sidebar:

Silverman, Maida. *A City Herbal: A Guide to the Lore, Legend & Usefulness of 34 Plants That Grow Wild in Cities, Suburbs and Country Places*. Boston: David R. Godine, 1990. Print.

"Online Etymology Dictionary." *Online Etymology Dictionary*. Douglas Harper, 2001-2013. Web. <http://www.etymonline.com/>.

"Gabon, Africa" sidebar:

The World Book Encyclopedia. Chicago, IL: World Book, 2009. Print.

"Iboga" sidebar:

Fernandez, James W. *Bwiti: An Ethnography of the Religious Imagination in Africa*. Princeton, NJ: Princeton UP, 1982. Print.

Samorini, Giorgio. "Adam, Eve and Iboga." *Integration* 4 (2009): 4-10. Web.

Part IV: Land Traditions

Chapter 15: Conservation and Gardening

1 Short, P. S. *In Pursuit of Plants: Experiences of Nineteenth & Early Twentieth Century Plant Collectors*. Portland: Timber, 2004. Print.

2 Ibid

3 Gladstar, Rosemary, and Pamela Hirsch. *Planting the Future: Saving Our Medicinal Herbs*. Rochester, VT: Healing Arts, 2000. Print. p. ix.

Pharaoh Hatshepsut

Brown, Chip. "The King Herself." *National Geographic Channel* April (2009): 88-111. Print.

Bancroft-Hunt, Norman. *Living in Ancient Egypt*. New York: Chelsea House, 2009. Print.

"Vegetable" sidebar:

"Online Etymology Dictionary." *Online Etymology Dictionary*. Douglas Harper, 2001-2013. Web. <http://www.etymonline.com/>.

"Myrrh" sidebar:

"Online Etymology Dictionary." *Online Etymology Dictionary*. Douglas Harper, 2001-2013. Web. <http://www.etymonline.com/>.

Raver, Miki. *Listen to Her Voice: Women of the Hebrew Bible*. San Francisco, CA: Chronicle, 1998. Print.

Anne McIntyre, Lecture at Women's Herbal Conference 2008.

"Lettuce" sidebar:

Culpeper, Nicholas. *Culpeper's Complete Herbal and English Physician: Wherin Several Hundred Herbs with a Display of Their Medicinal and Occult Properties, Are Physically Applied to the Cure of All Disorders Incident to Mankind : To Which Are Added, Rules for Compounding Medicines ...* Leicester, UK: Magna, 1992. Print.

Gibbons, Euell. *Stalking the Healthful Herbs*. New York: D. McKay, 1966. Print.

Lorenzi, Rossella. "Egyptians Ate Lettuce to Boost Sex Drive." *Sydney, NSW: ABC Science, News in Science* 29th ser. June (2005): n. pag. Web.

Empress Josephine

HRH Princess Michael of Kent. "Josephine's Garden." *Orient Express Magazine* 19.1 (2002): n. pag. Web.

Brittain, Julia. *The Plant Lover's Companion: Plants, People & Places*. Boston: Horticulture, 2006. Print.

Erickson, Carolly. *Josephine: A Life of the Empress*. New York: St. Martin's, 1999. Print.

Grieve, M. *A Modern Herbal; the Medicinal, Culinary, Cosmetic and Economic Properties, Cultivation and Folk-lore of Herbs, Grasses,*

Fungi, Shrubs, & Trees with All Their Modern Scientific Uses,. New York: Dover Publications, 1971. Print.

Mundt, Klara Muller. *The Empress Josephine: An Historical Sketch of the Days of Napoleon.* McClure, 1867. University of California, 2007. Web.

"Museum" sidebar:

"Online Etymology Dictionary." *Online Etymology Dictionary.* Douglas Harper, 2001-2013. Web. <http://www.etymonline. com/>.

"France" sidebar:

A Guide to the European Market for Medicinal Plants and Extracts. London: Commonwealth Secretariat, 2001. Print.

"Conservation" sidebar:

"Online Etymology Dictionary." *Online Etymology Dictionary.* Douglas Harper, 2001-2013. Web. <http://www.etymonline. com/>.

"Jordan" sidebar:

National Geographic Atlas of the Middle East. Washington D.C.: National Geographic, 2003. Print.

The World: Afghanistan to Zimbabwe. Chicago, IL: Rand McNally, 1998. Print.

"Black Cumin" sidebar:

Hajhashemi, Valiollah, Alireza Ghannadi, and Hadi Jafarabadi. "Black Cumin Seed Essential Oil, as a Potent Analgesic and Antiinflammatory Drug." *Phytotherapy Research* 18.3 (2004): 195-99. Print.

Chapter 16: Ethnobotany

Moerman, Daniel. "Mullein." *Native American Ethnobotany Database.* University of Michigan–Dearborn, n.d. Web.

Schultes, Richard Evans. and Reis Siri Von. "The Urgent Need for the Study of Medicinal Plants." *Ethnobotany: Evolution of a Discipline.* Portland, Or.: Dioscorides, 1995. N. pag. Print.

Rocio Alarcon

Joyce, Christopher. *Earthly Goods: Medicine-hunting in the Rainforest.* Boston: Little, Brown, 1994. Print.

"Earth" sidebar:

"Online Etymology Dictionary." *Online Etymology Dictionary.* Douglas Harper, 2001-2013. Web. <http://www.etymonline. com/>.

"Ecuador" sidebar:

Adès, Harry, Mellisa Graham, and Carlos Villafuerte. *The Rough Guide to Ecuador.* London: Rough Guides, 2010. Print.

The World: Afghanistan to Zimbabwe. Chicago, IL: Rand McNally, 1998. Print.

"Walnut" sidebar:

Collingwood, G. H., W. D. Brush, and D. Butcher. *Knowing Your Trees: With More than 900 Illustrations Showing Typical Trees and Their Leaves, Bark, Flowers and Fruits.* Washington: American Forestry Association, 1974. Print.

Johnson, Hugh. *The International Book of Trees ; a Guide and Tribute to the Trees of Our Forests and Gardens.* New York: Simon and Schuster, 1973. Print.

Stearn, William T. *Stearn's Dictionary of Plant Names for Gardeners: A Handbook on the Origin and Meaning of the Botanical Names of Some Cultivated Plants.* Portland, Or.: Timber, 2002. Print.

Howard, Lois Jean. "Herbs in Mythology." *The South Texas Unit of the American Herb Society* (n.d.): n. pag. Web. <http://www. herbsociety-stu.org/Mythology.htm>.

Photo Credits

The author expresses sincere gratitude to the following people and organizations for graciously providing their images and photographs for inclusion in this book:

Chapter 1   Vik Martin, Kia Ingenlath, Rick Marquart, Rosemary Gladstar, Tom Iraci, Isla Burgess, Harry Beach
Chapter 2   Jody Noé, Angelina Bellebuono, Ada-Belinda DancingLion
Chapter 4   HRH Princess Basma bint Ali, James Prineas, Patricia and Cindy Flanders, Ann McIntyre, Katie Bowers

Part II   Leslie Roberts
Chapter 6   Anne McIntyre, Priya and Uma Datta
Chapter 7   Dr. Ysiang Chang, Harry Beach, Phuntsog Wangmo
Chapter 8   Sara Figlow, Doña Enriqueta Contreras, Mary Margaret Navar,
Chapter 9   Dr. Tieraona Low Dog, Arizona Center for Integrative Medicine, Karin Stanley, Phyllis Savides
Chapter 10 Dr. Zoubida Charrouf, Jib Ellis
Chapter 11 Ian White, Australian Bush Flower Essences, Kate Gilday
Chapter 13 Mary Beith, Leslie H. Roberts
Chapter 14 Susun Weed, Marisol Villanueva, Ann Rosencranz, Center for Sacred Studies and the Grandmother's Council, Gina Boltz, Native Village Publications

Part IV   Harry Beach
Chapter 15 Harry Beach, Gia Rae Winsryg-Ulmer, Dia Saleh, HRH Princess Basma bint Ali
Chapter 16 Roçio Alarcon

For individual photo credits, please refer to the photos within.

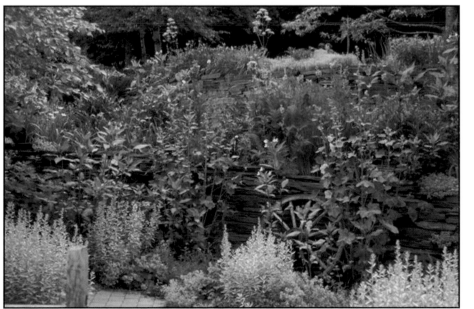

Photo credit: Rosemary Gladstar

GENERAL BIBLIOGRAPHY

"About The Faculty of Herb College Providing Herbal Studies." *About The Faculty of Herb College Providing Herbal Studies*. Burgess, Isla. Web. 20 Aug. 2009. <http://www.herbcollege. com/aboutfaculty.asp?id=1>.

Achterberg, Jeanne. *Woman as Healer*. Boston: Shambhala, 1990. Print.

"Agriculture." *FLORA and FAUNA of MIDDLE AMERICA.* Web. 01 Jan. 2010. <http://www.utexas.edu/courses/stross/ant322m_ files/florafaun.htm>.

Amt, Emilie. *Women's Lives in Medieval Europe: A Sourcebook*. New York: Routledge, 1993. Print.

Baker, Jeannine Parvati. *Hygieia: A Woman's Herbal*. [Albion, Calif.]: Freestone, 1978. Print.

Baldwin, James. "Nero" *Fifty Famous Stories Retold*. [United States]: Filiquarian, 2007. Print.

Balick, Michael J., and Paul Alan Cox. *Plants, People, and Culture: The Science of Ethnobotany*. New York: Scientific American Library, 1996. Print.

Bairacli-Levy, Juliette De. *Common Herbs for Natural Health*. Woodstock, NY: Ash Tree Pub., 1997. Print.

Bairacli-Levy, Juliette De. *Herbal Handbook for Everyone*. London: Faber and Faber Limited, 1966. Print.

Bairacli-Levy, Juliette De. *Nature's Children*. Woodstock, NY: Ash Tree Pub., 1997. Print.

Baring, Anne, and Jules Cashford. *The Myth of the Goddess: Evolution of an Image*. New York: Penguin, 1991. Print.

Barrett, Anthony A. *Nero*. Cambridge: Belknap of Harvard UP, 2005. Print.

Barrett, Anthony. *Agrippina: Sex, Power, and Politics in the Early Empire*. New Haven: Yale UP, 1996. Print.

Bellebuono, Holly. *The Essential Herbal for Natural Health: How to Transform Easy-to-find Herbs into Healing Remedies for the Whole Family*. Boston: Roost, 2012. Print.

Bellebuono, Holly H. *The Authentic Herbal Healer: The Complete Guide to Herbal Formulary & Plant-inspired Medicine for Every Body System*. Bloomington, IN: Balboa, 2012. Print.

Brittain, Julia. *Plants, People & Places: The Plant Lover's Companion*. Newton Abbot: David & Charles, 2006. Print.

Brooke, Elisabeth. *Women Healers: Portraits of Herbalists, Physicians, and Midwives*. Rochester, VT: Healing Arts, 1996. Print.

Cameron, Elizabeth. *A Floral ABC*. New York: Morrow, 1983. Print.

Castleman, Michael, and Michael Castleman. *The New Healing Herbs: The Classic Guide to Nature's Best Medicines Featuring the Top 100 Time-tested Herbs*. Emmaus, PA: Rodale, 2001. Print.

Claus, Edward P., and Varro E. Tyler. *Pharmacognosy*. Philadelphia: Lea & Febiger, 1965. Print.

Collingwood, G. H., W. D. Brush, and D. Butcher. *Knowing Your Trees: With More than 900 Illustrations Showing Typical Trees and Their Leaves, Bark, Flowers and Fruits*. Washington: American Forestry Association, 1974. Print.

Crawford, Amanda McQuade. *Herbal Remedies for Women: Discover Nature's Wonderful Secrets Just for Women*. Rocklin, CA: Prima Pub., 1997. Print.

Crowell, Robert L. *The Lore & Legends of Flowers*. New York: Thomas Y. Crowell, 1992. Print.

Culpeper, Nicholas. *Culpeper's Complete Herbal and English Physician: Wherin Several Hundred Herbs with a Display of Their Medicinal and Occult Properties, Are Physically Applied to the Cure of All Disorders Incident to Mankind : To Which Are Added, Rules for Compounding Medicines ...* Leicester, UK: Magna, 1992. Print.

Dante, Alighieri, Lawrence Grant White, and Gustave Doré. *The Divine Comedy: The Inferno, Purgatorio, and Paradiso*. New York: Pantheon, 1948. Print.

"Discover Biography." *Bio.com*. A&E Networks Television. Web. 20 Mar. 2011. <http://www.biography.com/people>.

DuBois, W.E.B. *The Negro*. Ed. Robert Gregg. Philadelphia: University of Pennsylvania, 2001. Print.

Edwards, Amelia Ann Blanford. *Pharaohs, Fellahs and Explorers*. New York: Harper & Brothers, 1891. Print.

Edwards, Carolyn McVickar. *The Storyteller's Goddess: Tales of the Goddess and Her Wisdom from around the World*. New York, NY: HarperSanFrancisco, 1991. Print.

Elliot, Doug. *Wild Roots: A Forager's Guide to the Edible and Medicinal Roots, Tubers, Corms, and Rhizomes of North America*. Rochester, VT: Healing Arts, 1995. Print.

Erickson, Carolly. *Josephine: A Life of the Empress*. New York: St. Martin's, 1999. Print.

Feierman, Steven, and John M. Janzen. *The Social Basis of Health and Healing in Africa*. Berkeley: University of California, 1992. Print.

Fernauld, Merritt L., and Alfred C. Kinsey. *Herbs for Use and for Delight: An Anthology from the Herbarist, A Publication of the Herb Society of America*. New York, NY: Dover Publications, 1974. Print.

"First National Botanic Garden Founded in Jordan." *First National Botanic Garden Founded in Jordan*. Web. 01 Jan. 2009. <http://www.bgci.org/resources/news/0022/>.

Foster, Steven, James A. Duke, and Steven Foster. *A Field Guide to Medicinal Plants and Herbs of Eastern and Central North America*. Boston: Houghton Mifflin, 2000. Print.

"Franck Goddio: Homepage." *Franck Goddio: Homepage*. Web. 22 Sept. 2009. <http://www.franckgoddio.org/>.

Frazer, James George. *The Golden Bough; a Study in Magic and Religion*. New York: Macmillan, 1951. Print.

Gibbons, Euell. *Stalking the Healthful Herbs*. New York: D. McKay, 1966. Print.

Gladstar, Rosemary, and Pamela Hirsch. *Planting the Future: Saving Our Medicinal Herbs*. Rochester, VT: Healing Arts, 2000. Print.

Gladstar, Rosemary. *Herbal Healing for Women: Simple Home Remedies for Women of All Ages*. New York: Simon & Schuster, 1993. Print.

Graves, Robert. *The White Goddess: A Historical Grammar of Poetic Myth*. New York: Vintage, 1960. Print.

Green, James. *The Herbal Medicine-makers' Handbook: A Home Manual*. Freedom, CA: Crossing, 2000. Print.

Green, Monica Helen. *The Trotula: A Medieval Compendium of Women's Medicine*. Philadelphia: University of Pennsylvania, 2001. Print.

Grieve, M. *A Modern Herbal; the Medicinal, Culinary, Cosmetic and Economic Properties, Cultivation and Folk-lore of Herbs, Grasses, Fungi, Shrubs, & Trees with All Their Modern Scientific Uses*. New York: Dover Publications, 1971. Print.

A Guide to the European Market for Medicinal Plants and Extracts. London: Commonwealth Secretariat, 2001. Print.

Guthrie, W. K. C. *The Greeks and Their Gods*. Boston: Beacon, 1962. Print.

Gwinne, Matthew, and Heinz-Dieter Leidig. *Nero: (print. 1603); Prepared with an Introd*. Hildesheim U.a.: Olms, 1983. Web.

Halpenny, Frances G., and Andre Vachon. "Marie-Henriette LeJeune Ross." *Dictionary of Canadian Biography*. 1741-1770 ed. Vol. III. Toronto: University of Toronto, 1974. Print.

Harper, Robert Francis. *Assyrian and Babylonian Literature: Selected Translations*. New York: Appleton, 1904. Print.

Harris, Ben Charles. *The Compleat Herbal: Being a Description of the Origins, the Lore, the Characteristics, the Types, and the Prescribed Uses of Medicinal Herbs, including an Alphabetical Guide to All Common Medicinal Plants*. Barre, MA: Barre, 1972. Print.

"The Hashemites: Jordan's Royal Family." *The Hashemites: Jordan's Royal Family*. Web. 01 Jan. 2009. <http://www.kinghussein.gov.jo/hash_intro.html>.

"Herodotus Wept." *Herodotus Wept*. Web. 01 Jan. 2013. <http://herodotuswept.wordpress.com/>.

"Hinduism." *Sacred-Texts:*. Web. 01 Jan. 2010. <http://www.sacred-texts.com/hin/index.htm>.

"HistoryWorld History and Timelines." *HistoryWorld - History and Timelines*. Web. 22 Dec. 2009. <http://www.historyworld.net/>.

Hoffmann, David. *The Herbal Handbook: A User's Guide to Medical Herbalism*. Rochester, VT: Healing Arts, 1988. Print.

Hoffmann, David. *The New Holistic Herbal*. Rockport: Element, 1990. Print.

Hoffmann, David. *The Complete Illustrated Holistic Herbal: A Safe and Practical Guide to Making and Using Herbal Remedies*. Boston: Element, 1996. Print.

"Home | Center for Sacred Studies." *Home | Center for Sacred Studies*. Web. 08 June 2008. <http://centerforsacredstudies.org/>.

Hozeski, Bruce W. *Hildegard's Healing Plants: From Her Medieval Classic Physical*. Boston: Beacon, 2001. Print.

"HRH Princess Michael of Kent." *Josephine's Garden*. Web. 22 May 2013. <http://www.princessmichael.org.uk/articles/josephines-garden/>.

"Hurd-Mead, Kate Campbell, 1867-1941. Papers, 1939: A Finding Aid." *Hurd-Mead, Kate Campbell, 1867-1941. Papers, 1939: A Finding Aid*. Web. 01 Jan. 2010. <http://oasis.lib.harvard.edu/oasis/deliver/~sch00733>.

Huxley, Anthony Julian. *Green Inheritance: The World Wildlife Fund Book of Plants*. Garden City, NY: Anchor/Doubleday, 1985. Print.

Jarvis, D. C. *Folk Medicine; a Vermont Doctor's Guide to Good Health.* New York: Holt, 1958. Print.

Johnson, Hugh. *The International Book of Trees ; a Guide and Tribute to the Trees of Our Forests and Gardens.* New York: Simon and Schuster, 1973. Print.

"JORDAN." *Jordan2.* Web. 01 Jan. 2009. <http://www.royalark. net/Jordan/jordan2.htm>.

Jordan, Michael. *The Green Mantle: An Investigation into Our Lost Knowledge of Plants.* London: Cassell, 2001. Print.

"Journey Through Jordan: The Royal Botanic Garden." *Journey Through Jordan: The Royal Botanic Garden.* Web. 01 Jan. 2009. <http://www.projectexplorer.org/hs/jo/garden.php>.

Joyce, Christopher. *Earthly Goods: Medicine-hunting in the Rainforest.* Boston: Little, Brown, 1994. Print.

Kavasch, E. Barrie. *Native Harvests: Recipes and Botanicals of the American Indian.* New York: Vintage, 1979. Print.

Kennell, Frances. *Folk Medicine: Fact and Fiction.* London: Marshall Cavendish, 1976. Print.

Klara, Virginia, and Diane Relf. *Roses: A Colorful History.* Virginia Cooperative Extension, 1997. Print.

Kloss, Jethro. *Back to Eden: A Human Interest Story of Health and Restoration to Be Found in Herb, Root, and Bark.* Loma Linda, CA: Back to Eden, 1982. Print.

Krochmal, Arnold, and Connie Krochmal. *A Field Guide to Medicinal Plants.* New York, NY: Times, 1984. Print.

León, Vicki. *Outrageous Women of Ancient Times.* New York: Wiley, 1998. Print.

León, Vicki. *Uppity Women of Ancient Times.* Berkeley, CA: Conari, 1995. Print.

Lindsay, Jack. *The Origins of Alchemy in Graeco-Roman Egypt.* New York: Barnes & Noble, 1970. Print.

Loewenfeld, Claire, and Philippa Back. *The Complete Book of Herbs and Spices.* New York: Putnam, 1974. Print.

Mabey, Richard, and Michael McIntyre. *The New Age Herbalist: How to Use Herbs for Healing, Nutrition, Body Care, and Relaxation.* New York: Collier, 1988. Print.

Macinnis, Peter. *Poisons: From Hemlock to Botox to the Killer Bean of Calabar.* New York: Arcade Pub., 2005. Print.

"Marie-Henriette LeJeune Ross, Midwife and Healer." *Collections Canada, Library and Archives.* Web. 01 Jan. 2012. <http://www. collectionscanada.gc.ca/women/030001-1413-e.html>.

McCleod, Dawn. *Herb Handbook: A Practical Guide to Herbs and Their Uses.* N. Hollywood: Wilshire Book, 1968. Print.

"The Meanings and Origins of Sayings and Phrases." *RSS.* Web. 01 Jan. 2010. <http://phrases.org.uk/>.

Meyer, Joseph Ernest. *The Herbalist and Herb Doctor.* Hammond, IN: Indiana Herb Gardens, 1918. Print.

Minnis, Paul E. *Ethnobotany: A Reader.* Norman: University of Oklahoma, 2000. Print.

Miyano, Leland, and Douglas Peebles. *Hawai'i's Beautiful Trees.* Honolulu: Mutual Pub., 1997. Print.

Moerman, Daniel. "Mullein." *Native American Ethnobotany Database.* University of Michigan–Dearborn, n.d. Web.

Mundt, Klara Muller. *The Empress Josephine: An Historical Sketch of the Days of Napoleon.* McClure, 1867. University of California, 2007. Web.

National Audubon Society. *Field Guide to Wildflowers, Eastern Region.* New York: A. Knopf, 2001. Print.

"National Geographic - Inspiring People to Care About the Planet Since 1888." *National Geographic - Inspiring People to Care About the Planet Since 1888.* Web. 09 Nov. 2010. <http://www. nationalgeographic.com/>.

"Native Village Publications." *Native Village Publications.* Web. 03 June 2008. <http://www.nativevillage.org/>.

Navar, Mary M. *Zapotec Woman of the Clouds: The Life of the Midwife-Healer Enriqueta Contreras Contreras.* Austin: Zapotec, 2001. Print.

Neumann, Erich. *The Great Mother.* Princeton: Princeton UP, 1963. Print.

Ody, Penelope. *Essential Guide to Natural Home Remedies.* London: Kyle Cathie, 2003. Print.

Patnaik, Naveen. *The Garden of Life: An Introduction to the Healing Plants of India.* New York: Doubleday, 1993. Print.

Peterson, Lee, and Roger Tory Peterson. *A Field Guide to Edible Wild Plants of Eastern and Central North America.* Boston: Houghton Mifflin, 1977. Print.

Phillips, Nancy, and Michael Phillips. *The Village Herbalist: Sharing Plant Medicines with Your Family and Community.* White River Junction, VT: Chelsea Green Pub., 2001. Print.

Philpot, J. H. *The Sacred Tree in Religion and Myth.* Mineola, NY: Dover Publications, 2004. Print.

"PJ Online." *PJ Online.* Web. 01 Jan. 2012. <http://www.pjonline. com/>.

Plant Names Explained: Botanical Terms and Their Meaning. Boston, MA: Horticulture, 2005. Print.

Pratt, H. Douglas. *A Pocket Guide to Hawai'i's Trees and Shrubs.* Honolulu, HI: Mutual Pub., 1998. Print.

Ramos-e-Silva, Marcia, M.D. "St. Hildegard Von Bingham: The Light of Her People and of Her Time." Lecture. Women in Dermatology Symposium, History of Dermatology Society Meeting. Florida, Orlando. Sector of Dermatology and the Post Graduation Course in Dermatology, HUCFF_UFRJ, School of Medicine, Federal University of Rio De Janeiro, Brazil, 26 Feb. 1998. Web. 01 Jan. 2012.

Raver, Miki. *Listen to Her Voice: Women of the Hebrew Bible.* San Francisco, CA: Chronicle, 1998. Print.

"Readings In Ancient History Illustrative Extracts From The Sources." *Readings In Ancient History Illustrative Extracts From The Sources.* Web. 01 Jan. 2013. <http://archive.org/stream/readingsinancien011109mbp>.

Robinson, James M., and Richard Smith. *The Nag Hammadi Library in English.* San Francisco: Harper & Row, 1990. Print.

"Roses for Sale - East Sussex, Kent, Tenterden, Rye, Hastings, Ashford, Tunbridge Wells." Web. 01 Jan. 2010. <http://theoldrosenursery.co.uk/>.

Ross, Anne. *The Folklore of the Scottish Highlands.* Totowa, NJ: Rowman and Littlefield, 1976. Print.

Sanders, Jack. *The Secrets of Wildflowers: A Delightful Feast of Little-known Facts, Folklore, and History.* Guilford, CT: Lyons, 2003. Print.

Saville, Carole. *Exotic Herbs: A Compendium of Exceptional Culinary Herbs.* New York: H. Holt, 1997. Print.

Schiff, Paul L., PhD. "Ergot and Its Alkaloids." *American Journal of Pharmaceutical Education* 70.5 (2006): 98. Print.

Schultes, Richard Evans, and Reis Siri Von. *Ethnobotany: Evolution of a Discipline.* Portland, Or.: Dioscorides, 1995. Print.

"The Search for Cleopatra." *National Geographic Magazine - NGM.com.* Web. 01 Jan. 2012. <http://ngm.nationalgeographic.com/print/2011/07/cleopatra/brown-text>.

Silverman, Maida. *A City Herbal: A Guide to the Lore, Legend & Usefulness of 34 Plants That Grow Wild in Cities, Suburbs and Country Places.* Boston: David R. Godine, 1990. Print.

Soule, Deb. *The Roots of Healing: A Woman's Book of Herbs.* Secaucus, NJ: Carol Pub. Group, 1995. Print.

"St. Anthony's Fire." *Time Magazine* 10 Sept. 1951. Print.

Starbird, Margaret. *Mary Magdalen: Bride in Exile.* Rochester, VT: Bear & Pub., 2005. Print.

Starbird, Margaret. *The Woman with the Alabaster Jar: Mary Magdalen and the Holy Grail.* Santa Fe, NM: Bear & Pub., 1993. Print.

Stearn, William T. *Stearn's Dictionary of Plant Names for Gardeners: A Handbook on the Origin and Meaning of the Botanical Names of Some Cultivated Plants.* Portland, Or.: Timber, 2002. Print.

Stearn, William Thomas. *Botanical Latin.* Portland, Or.: Timber, 2004. Print.

Stone, Julie, and Joan Matthews. *Complementary Medicine and the Law.* Oxford: Oxford UP, 1996. Print.

Stone, Merlin. *Ancient Mirrors of Womanhood: A Treasury of Goddess and Heroine Lore from around the World.* Boston: Beacon, 1984. Print.

Tierra, Michael. *The Way of Herbs: Fully Updated—with the Latest Developments in Herbal Science.* New York: Pocket, 1990. Print.

"Travel Guide." *Marvelous Egypt Travel Egypt Travel PackagesEgypt Tours Egypt Tours for Christmas.* Web. 22 July 2011. <http://www.marvelousegypttravel.com/>.

"28th April 2008 NEWS, National Botanic Gardens, Glasnevin." Web. 01 Dec. 2010. <http://www.botanicgardens.ie/news/20080416.htm>.

Van Der Zee, Barbara. *Green Pharmacy: The History and Evolution of Western Herbal Medicine.* Rochester, VT: Healing Arts, 1997. Print.

Weed, Susun S. *Wise Woman Herbal for the Childbearing Year.* Woodstock, NY: Ash Tree Pub., 1986. Print.

Weed, Susun S. *Wise Woman Herbal Healing Wise.* Woodstock, NY: Ash Tree Pub., 1989. Print.

Whistler, W. Arthur. *Polynesian Herbal Medicine.* Lawai, Kauai, Hawaii: National Tropical Botanical Garden, 1992. Print.

Whitman, Walt, and Francis Murphy. *The Complete Poems.* Harmondsworth, Middlesex: Penguin, 1986. Print.

Whitmont, Edward C. *The Alchemy of Healing: Psyche and Soma.* Berkeley, CA: Homeopathic Educational Services, 1993. Print.

Winston, David. *Herbal Therapeutics: Specific Indications for Herbs & Herbal Formulas.* Broadway, NJ: Herbal Therapeutics Research Library, 2003. Print.

Wood, Matthew. *The Earthwise Herbal: A Complete Guide to Old World Medicinal Plants.* North Atlantic Books, Berkeley, CA: 2008. p. 11.

Acknowledgments

Over the course of the seven years of researching, curating, and writing this book, I've been blessed to have met so many wonderful people, those who are included within the pages and also those who helped me "behind the scenes" with information, housing, travel, guidance, encouragement, and support.

First, many heartfelt thanks go to my husband, Rocco, who has supported this project from its inception and who has championed my herbal business, my books, and all my endeavors. He is certainly the "better half"!

Warm thanks go to Leslie Roberts, Tom Owens, Angelina Bellebuono, Mary Ambulos, Laurisa Rich, and Nancy Leport for their ongoing friendship and encouragement; thanks to Margie Navar for her good advice and counsel; to Susan Larsen for her translation services; to Noli Hoye, Lorrin Pang, his parents Mr. and Mrs. Pang, and to Lisa Salkever for their gracious hospitality and support in Oahu; to Rosemary Gladstar for her kindness and guidance; to Raylene Kawaiae'a for her hugs and her listening ear; to Harry Beach for the generous use of so many of his world-class photos; to Tracy Thorpe for agreeing to paint these gorgeous watercolors because she believed in this project; and to Leslie Roberts, Kristina West, Kim Klaren, Gia Winsryg-Ulmer, Blaire Edwards, Laura Coit, and Gail Tipton for being the beautiful photo models for the ancient women portrayed and celebrated here.

Much grateful appreciation to Nicole Frail, my editor, and a warm thank-you to my agent, Jody Klein, whose enthusiasm for this project has grown over the years and whom I greatly admire for her perseverance and compassion.

And especially to all the women I've profiled within these pages; I am excited, honored, and humbled to share your stories with the world.

ABOUT THE AUTHOR

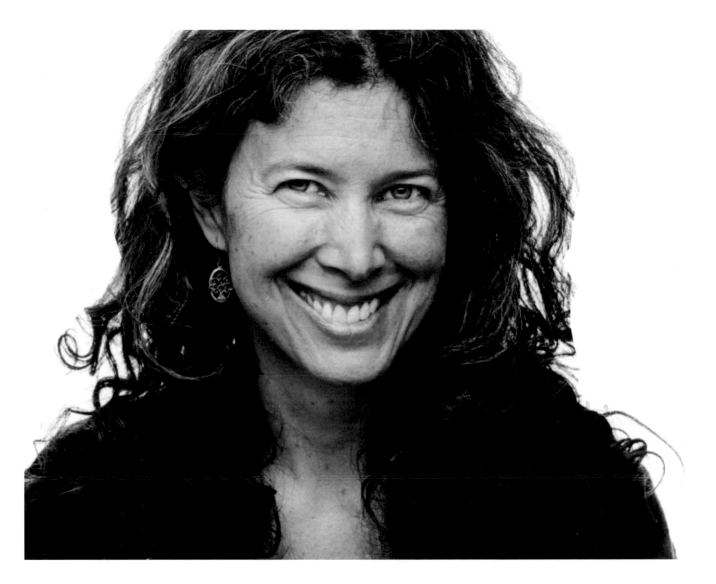

Award-winning herbalist, speaker and author Holly Bellebuono inspires audiences with motivational lectures and down-to-earth workshops that empower women and share the experience of medical herbalism. Both entrepreneur and educator, Holly trains and certifies students through the Bellebuono School of Herbal Medicine, teaches pharmacology and formulary, and is a leading presenter at regional and national workshops and retreats. Holly founded and directs the artisan retailer Vineyard Herbs Teas & Apothecary, producing Martha's Vineyard Teas. Her books include *The Essential Herbal for Natural Health* (Roost Books), *The Authentic Herbal Healer* (Balboa Press), the audio CD collection *How to Use Herbs for Natural Health*, and several e-books. Holly, her husband, and their two children live on Martha's Vineyard.

Index